Eye Diseases: Diagnosis and Treatment, 2nd Edition

Eye Diseases: Diagnosis and Treatment, 2nd Edition

Guest Editors

Alba Martín-Gil
Laura De Diego-García

MDPI

Basel • Beijing • Wuhan • Barcelona • Belgrade • Novi Sad • Cluj • Manchester

Guest Editors
Alba Martín-Gil
Department of Optometry
And Vision
Complutense University
of Madrid
Madrid
Spain

Laura De Diego-García
Department of Biochemistry
And Molecular Biology
Complutense University
Of Madrid
Madrid
Spain

Editorial Office
MDPI AG
Grosspeteranlage 5
4052 Basel, Switzerland

This is a reprint of the Special Issue, published open access by the journal *Life* (ISSN 2075-1729), freely accessible at: https://www.mdpi.com/journal/life/special_issues/2CSICDW893.

For citation purposes, cite each article independently as indicated on the article page online and as indicated below:

Lastname, A.A.; Lastname, B.B. Article Title. *Journal Name* **Year**, *Volume Number*, Page Range.

ISBN 978-3-7258-8407-0 (Hbk)
ISBN 978-3-7258-8408-7 (PDF)
https://doi.org/10.3390/books978-3-7258-8408-7

Contents

About the Editors

Alba Martín-Gil

Alba Martín-Gil is a Lecturer at the Department of Optometry and Vision, Faculty of Optics and Optometry at the Complutense University of Madrid (UCM). She obtained her PhD with the doctoral thesis titled "Cellular Mechanisms Activated by P2Y2 Receptors in the Ciliary Processes: Implication in Ocular Hypertension and Glaucoma", for which she received the Extraordinary Doctorate Award. Her academic and research activity is focused on ocular physiology and the molecular mechanisms involved in ocular hypertension and glaucoma. She is the author of more than 30 scientific publications, and she has participated in more than 75 international conferences, including three invited lectures, and serves as reviewer for several international scientific journals.

Laura De Diego-García

Laura De Diego-García is an Assistant Professor at the Department of Biochemistry and Molecular Biology, Faculty of Optics and Optometry, Complutense University of Madrid (UCM), Spain. She obtained her PhD in Biochemistry, Molecular Biology and Biomedicine from UCM after completing her MSc in Optometry and Vision and her degree in Optics and Optometry at the same institution. She carried out postdoctoral research stays at the Royal College of Surgeons in Ireland (Dublin, Ireland), and at Ludwig Maximilian University (Munich, Germany). Her research focuses on the molecular mechanisms involved in central nervous system disorders and on the identification of novel therapeutic strategies for epilepsy and glaucoma, combining molecular biology, neurobiology, and translational approaches. She has published more than 25 articles and participated in more than 50 national and international conferences.

Preface

The second edition of Eye Diseases: Diagnosis and Treatment continues the objective of bringing together current research focused on the mechanisms, diagnosis, and therapeutic management of ocular diseases. Vision disorders remain one of the leading causes of disability and reduced quality of life worldwide, representing an important clinical and public health challenge. Diseases affecting the retina, optic nerve, and ocular surface, including glaucoma, diabetic retinopathy, dry eye disease, keratoconus, and cataract, involve complex molecular and cellular alterations that require multidisciplinary approaches for their study and treatment.

The contributions included in this Reprint provide complementary perspectives ranging from molecular and experimental studies to clinical and translational research. Several articles address oxidative stress, inflammation, neurodegeneration, retinal injury, and ocular surface dysfunction, while others explore novel biomarkers, diagnostic methodologies, and emerging therapeutic strategies with potential clinical relevance. Together, these studies reflect the growing integration of basic science and clinical ophthalmology in the development of more precise and personalized approaches to eye care.

This Reprint is intended for researchers, clinicians, healthcare professionals, and students working in ophthalmology, vision science, molecular biology, and related biomedical disciplines. By compiling recent advances from different areas of ocular research, this collection aims to contribute to the understanding of eye diseases and to encourage future developments in diagnosis and treatment.

Alba Martín-Gil and Laura De Diego-García
Guest Editors

life

MDPI

Article

Evaluation of Ocular and Systemic Oxidative Stress Markers in Patients with Diabetic Retinopathy

Ana Karen López-Contreras [1], Diana Esperanza Arévalo-Simental [2], Fermín Paúl Pacheco-Moisés [3], María Guadalupe Martínez-Ruíz [1], Cecilia Olvera-Montaño [1], Ricardo Raúl Robles-Rivera [1], Sonia Sifuentes-Franco [4], Tannia Isabel Campos-Bayardo [1], Selene Guadalupe Huerta-Olvera [5] and Adolfo Daniel Rodríguez-Carrizalez [1,*]

[1] Institute of Clinical and Experimental Therapeutics, Department of Physiology, Health Sciences University Center, University of Guadalajara, Guadalajara 44340, Jalisco, Mexico; ana.lopez3430@alumnos.udg.mx (A.K.L.-C.); maria.mruiz@alumnos.udg.mx (M.G.M.-R.); cecilia.olvera3372@alumnos.udg.mx (C.O.-M.); ricardo.robles3334@alumnos.udg.mx (R.R.R.-R.); tannia.campos@academicos.udg.mx (T.I.C.-B.)
[2] Department of Ophthalmology, Hospital Civil de Guadalajara "Fray Antonio Alcalde", Guadalajara 44280, Jalisco, Mexico; diana.arevalo1673@alumnos.udg.mx
[3] Department of Chemistry, University Centre of Exact and Engineering Sciences, University of Guadalajara, Guadalajara 44430, Jalisco, Mexico; fermin.pacheco@academicos.udg.mx
[4] Department of Health Sciences—Disease as an Individual Process, Tonalá Campus, University of Guadalajara, Tonala 45425, Jalisco, Mexico; sonia.sifuentes@academicos.udg.mx
[5] Medical and Life Sciences Department, La Ciénega University Center, University of Guadalajara, Ocotlan 47810, Jalisco, Mexico; selene.huerta@academicos.udg.mx
* Correspondence: adolfo.rodriguez@academicos.udg.mx

Abstract: Proliferative diabetic retinopathy (PDR) is the most severe complication of chronic hyperglycaemi stimulates oxidative stress that changes the retinal basement membrane function and provokes neovascularization, macular edema and retinal detachment. But an oxidative–antioxidant biomarker assessment in ocular matrices, such as aqueous humor (AH) and vitreous, might show the oxidative stress (OS) status in the posterior segment. Here, we show a cross-sectional analytical study of 39 patients who had a vitrectomy and assess the levels of different oxidative–antioxidant biomarkers in blood, aqueous and vitreous humor in three groups: diabetes mellitus 2 (DM2) with PDR [DM(+)PDR(+)] (n =13), DM2 without PDR [DM(+)PDR(−)] (n = 13) and non-DM2 non-PDR [DM(−)PDR(−)] as the control group (n = 13). Our finding suggests the presence of oxidative stress in diabetic retinopathy, as evidenced by increased levels of 8-isoprostanes and decreased levels of total antioxidant capacity from stages before the development of diabetic retinopathy. Our results reveal a notable increment in catalase levels in the DM(+)PDR(+) group in blood and vitreous humor. Likewise, we identified that the DM(+)PDR(−) group presents significant levels in 8-IP and SOD in vitreous humor and blood versus aqueous humor. These finding suggest the role of antioxidant enzymes in compensating oxidative stress mechanisms in PDR development.

Keywords: oxidative stress; diabetic retinopathy; aqueous; vitreous

1. Introduction

Diabetic retinopathy (DR) is a serious sight-threatening complication that is closely associated with diabetes mellitus. It is characterized by incessant damage to the blood capillaries of the retina, which is attributed to various alterations caused by high levels of glucose [1]. In diabetic retinopathy due to chronic hyperglycemia, the microvascular damage in the basement membrane of the retina and capillarity thickening increases vascular permeability, tissue ischemia and the release of several angiogenic factors that results in neovascularization, macular edema and retinal detachment [2]. These events are indicators of the progression in proliferative diabetic retinopathy (PDR), which represents one of the most severe complications of diabetes [1–3]. Oxidative stress (OS) occurs when the production of reactive oxygen species (ROS) and reactive nitrogen species (RNS) is higher than the antioxidant defenses present in organisms like superoxide dismutase, glutathione peroxidase, catalase and non-enzymatic antioxidants; therefore, the balance between them disappears [4–6]. Thus, OS is increased by the activation of secondary signaling pathways mediated by protein kinase C (PKC) and the overactivity of the hexosamine and polyol pathways, being considered one of the factors in the development of DR [6,7].

There are also different microenvironments in the body, where each organ and tissue may have its own environment, including blood and cells. A given biomarker may be present at multiple sites, and its relationship to retinopathy status may vary depending on the site where it is measured [8]. The variety of ocular matrices that can be collected and analyzed to measure biomarkers is wide, but the application of a biomarker at a clinic depends on the type of ocular matrix to be sampled [9]. In humans, aqueous humor (AH) and vitreous humor are the most suitable matrices for assessing biomarkers relevant to posterior segment disorders, such as DR [9,10]. AH is composed mainly of water (99.9%), plus small amounts of sugars, vitamins, proteins along with other nutrients, as well as growth factors and cytokines. It is primarily responsible for maintaining ocular pressure and oxygenating structures such as the cornea and lens [11,12]. The vitreous is located between the lens and the retina, and due to its close contact with the retina, which has high levels of polyunsaturated fatty acids in addition to greater oxygen absorption and glucose oxidation compared to other tissues, it is susceptible to oxidative stress [13], making the passage of radicals possible towards the vitreous body, which, together with its anatomical position, makes it ideal for sampling to reflect biochemical and pathophysiological changes in retinal disease states, including PDR. The vitreous body is mainly composed of water and a meshwork of fine collagen fibrils embedded with dissolved hyaluronan molecules, inorganic salts, lipids, proteins such as albumin, globulins, coagulation proteins and complement factors that have accumulated from blood filtration [14,15]. The aim of this study was to evaluate the ocular and systemic oxidative stress markers in patients with diabetic retinopathy.

2. Patients and Methods

This cross-sectional study was approved by the ethics committee of Hospital Civil de Guadalajara "Fray Antonio Alcalde" Guadalajara, Jalisco, Mexico (folio 058/19), and conducted in accordance with the principles of the Declaration of Helsinki. Written informed consent was obtained from all the participants.

2.1. Subjects

All participants were recruited from the Department of Ophthalmology, Hospital Civil de Guadalajara Fray Antonio Alcalde in Guadalajara from 1 February 2019 to 31 January 2021.

Inclusion criteria were as follows:

(a) Aged $\geq$ 18 years

2.1.1. First Group:

(b) Type 2 diabetic patients with proliferative diabetic retinopathy [DM(+)PDR(+)] undergoing vitrectomy for vitreous hemorrhage (VH) or tractional retinal detachment (TRD) or epiretinal membrane and vitreomacular traction (ERM), (c) HbA1c $\leq$ 9%, (d) systolic blood pressure $\leq$ 160 mmHg, (e) diastolic blood pressure $\leq$ 100 mmHg, (f) serum total cholesterol $\leq$ 250 mg/dL, and (g) blood Triglycerides $\leq$ 300 mg/dL.

2.1.2. Second Group:

(h) Type 2 diabetic patients without proliferative diabetic retinopathy [DM(+)PDR(−)] undergoing vitrectomy for vitreous hemorrhage (VH) or tractional retinal detachment (TRD) or epiretinal membrane and vitreomacular traction (ERM), (i) HbA1c $\leq$ 9%, (j) systolic blood pressure ≤ 160 mmHg, (k) diastolic blood pressure ≤ 100 mmHg, (l) serum total cholesterol ≤ 250 mg/dL, and (m) blood triglycerides ≤ 300 mg/dL.

2.1.3. Third Group:

(n) Non-diabetic controls patients without diabetic retinopathy [DM(−)PDR(−)] undergoing vitrectomy for vitreous hemorrhage (VH) or tractional retinal detachment (TRD) or epiretinal membrane and vitreomacular traction (ERM) due to accident and/or ocular trauma, (o) HbA1c ≤ 5.7%, (p) systolic blood pressure < 130 mmHg, (q) diastolic blood pressure < 85 mmHg, (r) serum total cholesterol ≤ 200 mg/dL, and (s) blood triglycerides ≤ 150 mg/dL.

2.1.4. Healthy Volunteer Group:

Healthy age- and sex-matched volunteers were included as a systemic reference for improving the understanding of the biochemical markers.

Non-inclusion criteria were as follows: (a) subjects who had undergone vitreoretinal surgery or laser surgery in the last six months, (b) subjects who received an intravitreal application of antiangiogenics in the last two months, (c) subjects who had taken oral antioxidants above the recommended intake in the last six months, systemic corticosteroid therapy or cytostatic, and all those without controlled cardiovascular status, (d) those who had prior ophthalmic surgeries, intravitreal corticosteroid, or ocular infections, (e) diabetic complications other than diabetic retinopathy, (f) pregnancy or breast-feeding, and (g) acute or chronic kidney disease.

2.2. *Examination Procedures*

The diagnosis of Diabetes mellitus type 2 was based on criteria outlined by the American Diabetes Association in 1997 and clinical history. The evaluation of DR was according to the diagnostic criteria of the American Academy of Ophthalmology 2001 Annual Meeting by retinal examination using an ophthalmoscope by Retina Specialist.

Laboratory tests were performed to determine 8-isoprostanes (8-IP) and nitric oxide (NO) levels as markers of OS, as well as total antioxidant capacity (TAC), catalase, superoxide dismutase and glutathione peroxidase (GPx) activity. All of these were measured in blood, aqueous humor and vitreous humor.

2.3. *Sample Collection*

Blood, AH and vitreous samples were collected from all participants on the day of surgery. Blood samples for serum and plasma analysis (5 mL) were simultaneously collected from the cubital vein, in vials containing EDTA and without it, and were centrifuged at 1200× *g* at room temperature for 15 min. Serum and plasma samples were stored at −80 °C. AH samples (50–100 µL) were collected at the beginning of cataract surgery with a 27-gauge needle on an insulin syringe. Special care was taken to avoid blood contamination. Samples were immediately cooled and stored at −80 °C. Vitreous humor samples (300–400 µL) were taken immediately after setting the trocars and before turning on the infusion system to avoid dilution. Samples were placed in individual Eppendorf tubes, stored at −80 °C. At the time of analysis, all samples were dissolved at room temperature.

2.4. *8-Isoprostanes ELISA Assay*

The quantification of 8-isoprostanes was performed according to the methodology described by the kit's manufacturer (8-isoprostanes ELISA kit, Item No. 516351, Cayman chemicals, Ann Arbor, MI, USA). This assay is based on the competition between 8-isoprostanes and an 8-isoprostane-acetylcholinesterase (AChE) conjugate for a limited number of specific rabbit antiserum binding sites. Since the concentration of the 8-isoprostane conjugate was constant while the concentration of 8-isoprostanes in the samples was variable, the amount of the 8-isoprostane conjugate capable of binding to the rabbit antiserum was inversely proportional to the concentration of 8-isoprostanes per sample, and the absorbance measurement was performed at 405–420 nm.

2.5. Nitric Oxide (NO) Assay

Before starting the assay, the samples were deproteinized by the addition of zinc sulfate [16]. A colorimetric test was performed according to the instructions of the kit (Nitric Oxide Assay Kit, User Protocol 482650, Calbiochem®, San Diego, CA, USA). Eighty five microliters of the standard or sample was placed in wells and 10 μL of nitrate reductase and 10 μL of 2 mM NADH were added. The plate was agitated for 20 min at room temperature, 50 μL of colorant 1 was added and agitated, and 50 μL of colorant 2 was added, agitated at room temperature, and read at 540 nm.

2.6. Total Antioxidant Capacity (TAC) Assay

TAC was measured according to the kit's instructions (Total Antioxidant Power Kit, No. TA02.120530, Oxford Biomedical Research®, Rochester Hills, MI, USA) to obtain a concentration in μM Trolox equivalents. Standards and samples were diluted 1:40, and 200 μL aliquots were placed in each well. The plate was read at 450 nm as a reference value, 50 μL of copper solution was added and incubated for 3 min at room temperature, then 50 μL of stop solution was added, and finally, the microplate was read at 450 nm.

2.7. Catalase Assay

Catalase was determined according to the kit manufacturer's instructions (Bioxytech Catalase-520®, cat. 21042, OXIS Int, Tampa, FL, USA), where 30 μL of the diluted standard or sample and 500 μL of substrate (10 mM of H_2O_2) were added into tubes, samples were incubated for 1 min at room temperature, and 500 μL of the stop reagent was added. The sample/standard was covered and mixed by immersion, and 20 μL of each reagent was added to a microplate. Two milliliters of HRP/reactive chromogen were deposited, mixed in a water bath, and incubated for 10 min at room temperature. The absorbance was read at 520 nm.

2.8. Superoxide Dismutase (SOD) Assay

Measure SOD activity according to the kit manufacturer's instructions (Superoxide dismutase Assay Kit, Item No. 706002, Cayman Chemicals). Start by adding 200 μL of the diluted radical detector and 10 μL of the standard and sample per well. Start the reaction by adding 20 μL of xanthine oxidase to all previously loaded wells. Record the precise time of the start and addition of xanthine oxidase. Mix the microplate for a few seconds and cover with the lid. Incubate in a mixer for 30 min at room temperature and then read the absorbance at 440–460 nm.

2.9. Glutathione Peroxidase (GPx) Assay

The measurement of the GPx activity was performed according to the manufacturer's instructions (Bioxytech GPx-340®, cat. 21017, Richmond, CA, USA). The reagent was based on the oxidation of reduced glutathione in the presence of tert-butyl hydroperoxide, glutathione reductase, and NADPH. The decrease in absorbance at 340 nm following substrate addition was recorded; the rate of decrease in absorbance was directly proportional to GPx activity.

2.10. Statistical Analysis

Sample size was calculated using a formula to compare means, where n of 13 subjects per group was calculated using a 95% confidence interval, to achieve a power of 80% and a level of significance of $p < 0.05$ to detect a difference in means between the test and reference group (117.13 U/Min/Mg severe Non-proliferative diabetic retinopathy group vs. 100.32 U/Min/Mg mild non-proliferative diabetic retinopathy group, respectively) and 14.84 U/Min/Mg of the standard deviation [17].

The distribution of variables was assessed with the Shapiro–Wilk test, where the measured values were mainly non-normally distributed. For a better understanding, the results are expressed as the mean ± standard error of the mean (SEM). The significance of the difference between groups was evaluated using the Mann–Whitney test, and the Kruskal–Wallis test were used to compare values among study groups. Frequencies were determined per category, as well as percentages and the $\chi 2$ (or Fisher's exact) test. All data were computed using an Excel database and SPSS PC for Windows version 26 (Chicago, IL, USA) for the statistical analysis.

3. Results

A total of 53 patients were evaluated in the study, and only 39 patients were included, with 13 patients in each study group. As shown in Table 1, there were no significant differences between the ages of the patients in each group, nor in clinical parameters such as heart rate, respiratory rate, weight and height, or in analytes such as glucose, creatinine and cholesterol. However, there were significant differences between patients in the DM2(+)RDP(+) and DM2(+)RDP(−) groups with respect to years with the diagnosis of diabetes, and HbA1c levels were also significantly higher in the DM2(+)RDP(+) and DM2(+)RDP(−) groups compared to the group without diabetes. A fourth group with 13 healthy volunteers was included as a systemic reference for improving the understanding of the biochemical markers: 8-isoprostanes, nitrites/nitrates, total antioxidant capacity, catalase, and superoxide dismutase. See the dotted line in the graphics.

Table 1. Demographic data and results of laboratory tests.

	DM2(+)PDR(+)	DM2(+)PDR(−)	DM2(−)PDR(−)	*p*-Value
n	13	13	13	*K-W*
Age (years)	55.81 ± 2.64	61.77 ± 2.09	50.92 ± 4.73	NS
Duration of DM (years)	16.18 ± 1.37 †	9.31 ± 1.92 *	N/A	<0.001
SBP (mmHg)	140.59 ± 2.96 ‡	143.00 ± 5.44 ‡	120.23 ± 3.42 *,†	0.001
DBP (mmHg)	85.41 ± 2.06 †	75.31 ± 1.73 *	78.15 ± 2.99	0.004
Heart frequency (b/min)	78.48 ± 2.27	76.85 ± 1.73	77.31 ± 2.86	NS
Respiratory rate (r/min)	17.00 ± 0.44	18.85 ± 1.02	18.54 ± 0.53	NS
Weight (kg)	73.53 ± 3.08	68.19 ± 2.57	79.45 ± 5.13	NS
Height (cm)	160.67 ± 1.86	165.31 ± 3.24	166.69 ± 2.52	NS
BMI (kg/m^2)	28.41 ± 1.07	24.92 ± 0.69	28.49 ± 1.68	NS
RIOP (mmHg)	14.89 ± 0.86 †,‡	12.61 ± 1.04 *	11.08 ± 0.58 *	0.004
LIOP (mmHg)	16.15 ± 1.50 †	11.00 ± 1.35 *	13.00 ± 0.94	0.009
RVA (LogMar)	1.41 ± 0.20	1.29 ± 0.30	1.47 ± 0.28	NS
LVA (LogMar)	1.62 ± 0.21	1.41 ± 0.29	1.31 ± 0.32	NS
HbA1c (%)	7.39 ± 0.22 ‡	6.54 ± 0.51 ‡	5.20 ± 0.12 *,†	<0.001
Glucose (mg/dL)	112.93 ± 6.35	111.69 ± 4.24	93.81 ± 3.11	NS
Urea (mg/dL)	44.76 ± 3.30 †,‡	27.16 ± 2.95 *	28.25 ± 2.48 *	0.003
Creatinine (mg/dL)	1.48 ± 0.29	0.96 ± 0.17	0.85 ± 0.06	NS
TC (mg/dL)	190.33 ± 9.13	220.41 ± 14.64	181.54 ± 4.49	NS
TG (mg/dL)	193.23 ± 14.88 ‡	214.07 ± 12.62 ‡	106.69 ± 8.34 *,†	0.001

Unless indicated otherwise, data are the mean ± SEM (standard error of the mean). DM, diabetes mellitus; SBP, systolic blood pressure; DBP, diastolic blood pressure; BMI, body mass index; RIOP, right intraocular pressure; LIOP, left intraocular pressure; RVA, right visual acuity; LVA, left visual acuity; TC, total cholesterol; TG, triglycerides. K-W, Kruskal–Wallis test; NS, not significant. $p < 0.05$ between groups: *, [DM2(+)RDP(+)]; †, [DM2(+)RDP(−)]; ‡, [DM2(−)RDP(−)].

3.1. 8-Isoprostanes

Blood levels of 8-IP in the controls were 14.62 ± 1.73 pg/mL. Blood levels increased with the presence of diabetes and retinopathy in all three study groups from 14.88 ± 1.94 to 24.68 ± 3.79 and 21.68 ± 2.77 pg/mL ([DM(−)PDR(−)], [DM(+)PDR(−)] and [DM(+)PDR(+)], respectively). In AH, 8.41 ± 1.27, 4.04 ± 0.37 and 2.63 ± 0.27 pg/mL, and in vitreous humor, 3.59 ± 0.76, 38.90 ± 5.83 and 4.29 ± 0.59 pg/mL were also obtained, respectively, indicating their presence in these matrices. Since 8-IPs are metabolic degradation products of lipoperoxides, these findings suggest cellular and systemic OS.

3.2. Nitric Oxide

Levels of the NO catabolites nitrites/nitrates (NOx) in the controls were 11.97 ± 1.22 μM/mL. The NOx levels found in the different biological matrices in the study groups were, in serum, 8.02 ± 1.70, 6.55 ± 0.73 and 5.50 ± 0.60 μM/mL; in AH, 2.72 ± 0.13, 3.01 ± 0.13 and 3.04 ± 0.11 μM/mL; and finally, in vitreous, 3.16 ± 0.29, 2.77 ± 0.12 and 3.62 ± 0.46 μM/mL [DM(−)PDR(−)], [DM(+)PDR(−)] and [DM(+)PDR(+)], respectively (as seen in Table 2). These results suggest nitrosative stress at the ocular and circulatory levels.

Table 2. Oxidants and antioxidants.

	DM2(+)PDR(+)	DM2(+)PDR(−)	DM2(−)PDR(−)	*p*-Value
n	13	13	13	*K-W*
8-IP (S) (pg/mL)	21.68 ± 2.77	24.68 ± 3.79	14.88 ± 1.94	NS
8-IP (A) (pg/mL)	2.63 ± 0.27 †,‡	4.04 ± 0.37 *,‡	8.41 ± 1.27 *,†	<0.001
8-IP (V) (pg/mL)	4.29 ± 0.59 †	38.90 ± 5.83 *,‡	3.59 ± 0.76 †	<0.001
NO (S) (μM/mL)	5.50 ± 0.60	6.55 ± 0.73	8.02 ± 1.70	NS
NO (A) (μM/mL)	3.04 ± 0.11	3.01 ± 0.13	2.72 ± 0.13	NS
NO (V) (μM/mL)	3.62 ± 0.46	2.77 ± 0.12	3.16 ± 0.29	NS
TAC (S) (mMEq)	4.39 ± 0.23 †	2.86 ± 0.60 *,‡	5.22 ± 0.57 †	<0.001
TAC (A) (mMEq)	4.40 ± 0.35	4.30 ± 0.31	4.94 ± 0.46	NS
TAC (V) (mMEq)	4.31 ± 0.45	3.36 ± 0.19	3.55 ± 0.47	NS
SOD (S) (U/mL)	5.43 ± 0.40	4.65 ± 0.18	5.59 ± 0.51	NS
SOD (A) (U/mL)	4.41 ± 0.37 ‡	3.59 ± 0.24 ‡	9.02 ± 0.55 *,†	<0.001
SOD (V) (U/mL)	8.54 ± 0.81 †	16.94 ± 0.39 *,‡	9.46 ± 0.53 †	<0.001
Catalase (S) (U/mL)	285.64 ± 5.40 †,‡	132.72 ± 5.23 *,‡	198.73 ± 2.77 *,†	<0.001
Catalase (A) (U/mL)	148.72 ± 2.82 †,‡	131.67 ± 1.55 *	122.89 ± 2.65 *	<0.001
Catalase (V) (U/mL)	253.96 ± 4.73 †,‡	109.64 ± 1.23 *	129.79 ± 4.57 *	<0.001
GPx (S) (U/min/mg)	106.20 ± 4.97 †	147.36 ± 3.94 *,‡	153.03 ± 6.83 †	<0.001
GPx (A) (U/min/mg)	28.88 ± 1.31 †	110.13 ± 2.46 *,‡	32.95 ± 3.72 †	<0.001
GPx (V) (U/min/mg)	6.37 ± 0.28	5.46 ± 0.14	5.74 ± 0.49	NS

Values expressed as arithmetic mean ± SEM. S, systemic; A, aqueous; V, vitreous; 8-IP, 8-isoprostane; ON, nitric oxide; TAC, total antioxidant capacity; SOD, superoxide dismutase; GPx, glutathione peroxidase; K–W, Kruskal–Wallis test; NS, not significant. $p < 0.05$ between groups: *, [DM2(+)RDP(+)]; †, [DM2(+)RDP(−)]; ‡, [DM2(−)RDP(−)].

3.3. Total Antioxidant Capacity

The TAC represents a set of physiological responses to OS composed of enzymes and different molecules. In the controls, the values found in serum were 2.62 ± 0.17 mM, in the study groups at the systemic level, they were 5.22 ± 0.57, 2.86 ± 0.60 and 4.39 ± 0.23 mM, in vitreous humor, they were 3.55 ± 0.47, 3.36 ± 0.19 and 4.31 ± 0.45 mM, and in AH, they were 4.94 ± 0.46, 4.30 ± 0.31 and 4.40 ± 0.35 mM from [DM(−)PDR(−)], [DM(+)PDR(−)] and [DM(+)PDR(+)], respectively.

3.4. Catalase

Catalase activity in blood samples was 198.73 ± 2.77, 132.72 ± 5.23 and 285.64 ± 5.40 U/mL, in AH, it was 122.89 ± 2.65, 131.67 ± 1.55 and 148.72 ± 2.82 U/mL, and in the vitreous body, 129. 79 ± 4.57, 109.64 ± 1.23 and 253.96 ± 4.73 U/mL in each study group [DM(−)PDR(−)], [DM(+)PDR(−)] and [DM(+)PDR(+)], respectively, in contrast to the controls (92.39 ± 2.08 U/mL).

3.5. Superoxide Dismutase

Superoxide dismutase is a metalloenzyme that catalyzes the dismutation of superoxide anion by decomposing it into hydrogen peroxide and oxygen molecules for catalase and GPx to act. Levels of 5.59 ± 0.51, 4.65 ± 0.18 and 5.43 ± 0.40 U/mL were found in blood samples, in AH, they were 9.02 ± 0.55, 3.59 ± 0.24 and 4.41 ± 0.37 U/mL, and in vitreous humor, they were 9.46 ± 0.53, 16.94 ± 0.39 and 8.54 ± 0.81 U/mL ([DM(−)PDR(−)], [DM(+)PDR(−)] and [DM(+)PDR(+)], respectively) (Table 2). This contrasts with the controls, who exhibited 10.67 ± 1.95 U/mL.

3.6. Glutathione Peroxidase

In the controls, GPx activity was 32.83 ± 3.24 U/min/mg protein. GPx activity decreased in vitreous humor in all groups (5.74 ± 0.49, 5.46 ± 0.14 and 6.37 ± 0.28 U/min/mg), in AH, it oscillated between each group with 32.95 ± 3.72, 110.13 ± 2.46 and 28.88 ± 1.31 U/min/mg, and at the systemic level, there was an increase with 153.03 ± 6.83, 147.36 ± 3.94 and 106.20 ± 4.97 U/min/mg in the [DM(−)PDR(−)], [DM(+)PDR(−)] and [DM(+)PDR(+)] study groups, respectively (Figure 1).

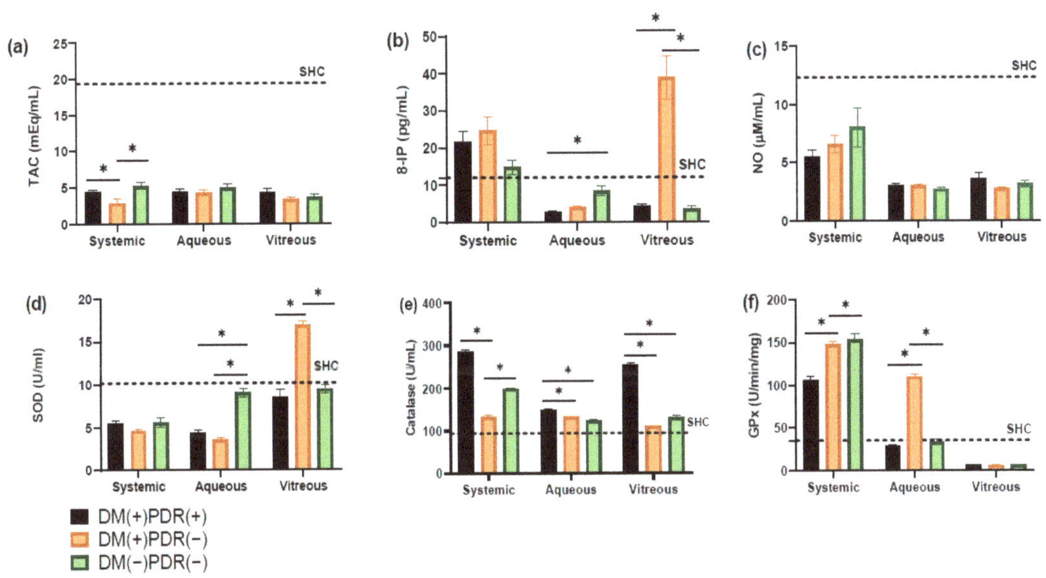

Figure 1. Comparative oxidative stress (OS) biomarkers levels on three study groups, diabetes mellitus 2 (DM2) with PDR [DM(+)PDR(+)], DM2 without PDR [DM(+)PDR(−)] and non-DM2 non-PDR [DM(−)PDR(−)]. OS biomarkers: (**a**) TAC, total antioxidant capacity, (**b**) 8-IP, 8-isoprostane; (**c**) NO, nitric oxide; (**d**) SOD, superoxide dismutase; (**e**) catalase; (**f**) GPx, glutathione peroxidase; SHC, systemic healthy controls. Data are the mean ± SE. * $p < 0.05$.

4. Discussion

Due to its location, the retina is directly exposed to light and also has a high fatty acid content and high oxygen consumption, which makes it susceptible to OS [18]. There is increasing evidence of the contribution of OS in the pathogenesis of RD [1]. We determined the levels of different markers of oxidant–antioxidant status in blood and aqueous and vitreous humor of patients with PDR and made comparisons between them and with healthy controls. It has been described that the composition of the AH is altered according to the pathophysiology and severity of DR [19]. Also, low-molecular-weight scavengers such as α-tocopherol, glutathione and ascorbic acid are present in the retina, and their mechanisms help minimize OS [20]. 8-IPs are potent vasoconstrictors and act as a mitogen for fibroblasts and vascular smooth muscle cells; these biological actions help explain the reason for the microvascular abnormalities reported in the retinal vasculature in both diabetic and RDP patients, which may contribute to hypoxia and hypoperfusion in the anterior segment of these patients [21,22]. Furthermore, we found increased levels of this biomarker in the three study groups; this also coincides with that reported in other pathologies of ocular origin such as cataracts and exfoliative syndrome [23,24]. Our results reaffirm the findings reported by Lahaie et al. as they propose that 8-IPs contribute to the pathogenesis of retinal ischemia–reperfusion injury, as in the retinopathy of prematurity and diabetes. However, there were no significant differences between the groups. On the contrary, both in aqueous and vitreous humor, we found their levels decreased [25].

The overproduction of NO has been implicated in several pathological processes, from tissue damage together with inflammation and ischemia, followed by cell apoptosis, to something more serious such as acute and chronic neurodegenerative diseases mainly [26]. Kulaksizoglu and Karalezli, in a prospective study with 35 diabetic patients compared with healthy controls who were underwent cataract surgery, found that patients with DM had significantly higher NO levels in the AH, and healthy subjects had significantly higher serum TAC levels. The authors then concluded that the development of PDR is associated with elevated levels of NO in the AH coupled with reduced serum antioxidant defenses [27,28]. The results that we obtained differ from this study because the levels of NO in both aqueous and vitreous humor were lower, and in serum, when compared with healthy controls, there was also a decrement in their concentrations (Table 2), so in the determination of this biomarker, we did not find significant differences between the study groups. More studies are needed to properly understand the effect of NO in the pathogenesis of retinopathy since it is not as simple as saying that the increase or decrease in NO levels is directly related to the severity of the pathology. This is because, according to the findings of different studies, NO concentrations vary according to the area of the retina affected or the severity of diabetes, including the intensity of hypoxia present at the time [26,28].

Each antioxidant system can carry out its activity with a variety of mechanisms and efficacy, according to the chemical structure and stage of the disease. For this reason, TAC is considered an excellent biomarker of the endogenous antioxidant defense system and is widely used since its determination could be much more important than the concentration of individual antioxidants [18]. The levels of TAC in blood, AH and vitreous humor were lower in the group with diabetes but without retinopathy (DM(+)PDR(−)) in comparison to the other two groups; additionally, in blood, there were also lower values compared to healthy controls, which coincides with the behavior of biomarkers reported by Mancino et al. Our results reaffirm that endogenous antioxidant defenses are reduced in patients with diabetes and PDR because their capacity to neutralize oxygen radicals is lower.

Regarding enzymatic antioxidants, SOD activity is very variable in some ocular compartments, even low, as is the case of tears, the aqueous humor and the vitreous body as they are acellular, so the importance of other oxygen radical scavengers must also be considered. Therefore, the eye is almost free of inflammatory reactions, which can be explained by the low levels of SOD isoenzymes [29,30]. This supports the results obtained in our study since the SOD activity found in blood was lower in the three study groups with respect to the healthy controls, Kernell et al. reported that, in non-diabetic patients, total SOD activity was much lower in the anterior chamber, with 9.9 U/mL, than in the vitreous humor, with 106.3 U/mL. We obtained similar results in aqueous humor (9.02 U/mL) but not in the vitreous body (9.46 U/mL). However, the group without diabetes [DM(−)PDR(−)] in the AH had a significant increase in SOD activity compared to the other two groups ($p < 0.001$). In the vitreous body, the group with diabetes but without retinopathy [DM(+)PDR(−)] also had a significant increase in SOD activity relative to the other study groups ($p < 0.001$) [31,32]. Catalase concentrations were higher in the group with retinopathy [DM(+)PDR(+)] compared to the other groups studied in all matrices analyzed; this increase was significant in the aqueous and vitreous humors compared to the other two groups ($p < 0.001$). Information on the determination of catalase at the ocular level is limited; however, currently, antioxidant enzyme activities can be reliably assessed, and the method we used allowed us to effectively detect low concentrations of the enzyme in all matrices [33,34]. On the other hand, in the case of GPx, Huang et al. reported serum concentrations of 3.81(0.84) mg/L (mean(S.D.)) and, in AH, of 0.66(0.18) mg/L in cataract patients. However, there was no significant association between AH and serum levels [35]. Our GPx results obtained in blood were elevated in all study groups with respect to the healthy control, but its detection in AH and vitreous humor was reduced. These values coincide with the results of Pavlovschi et al., who established that a progressive increase in the activity of the GSH system is manifested by an increase in GPx activities [36]. Another important point to take into consideration in the groups without diabetes and without retinopathy that were vitrectomized due to ocular trauma is that this event by itself is proven to generate an increase in oxidative stress, which could explain the behavior of the different biomarkers in this group, where levels were expected to be closer to the healthy groups, but on the contrary, they were comparable to the groups with diabetes [37,38]. The findings so far for all antioxidant enzymes suggest that any imbalance between oxidative and antioxidant defense mechanisms contribute to the development of the proliferative process in diabetic retinopathy [39].

5. Conclusions

Our finding suggests the presence of oxidative stress in diabetic retinopathy, as evidenced by increased levels of 8-isoprostanes and decreased levels of total antioxidant capacity from stages before the development of diabetic retinopathy. This indicates that metabolic dysregulation significantly contributes to the depletion of ocular and systemic antioxidant defenses. Consequently, the persistence of this disorder favors the progression of diabetic retinopathy. Determining biomarkers in the vitreous, aqueous humor, and serum enhances our understanding of their behavior, aiming to design a therapeutic strategy that could aid in managing complications associated with diabetic retinopathy. The evaluation of OS biomarkers in matrices such as HA and the vitreous has been standardized, but further studies are still needed to achieve a comparison and to elucidate the role of the antioxidant defense system in PDR.

In terms of the limitations of this study, we accept that it was a cross-sectional study; thus, only one sample was used to decide about the inflammation and OS markers. The levels of the markers do not have static behavior and a follow-up throughout the study with multiple determinations in time is required to corroborate these findings. The study design provides a snapshot of oxidative stress status but does not establish causal relationships or allow for an assessment of disease progression over time.

A cross-sectional study cannot determine the causality between alterations in retina function, OS, and the severity of the disease.

Author Contributions: Conceptualization, A.K.L.-C. and A.D.R.-C.; methodology, A.K.L.-C. and A.D.R.-C.; formal analysis, A.K.L.-C.; investigation, C.O.-M. and S.S.-F.; sampling, D.E.A.-S.; data curation, M.G.M.-R.; writing—original draft preparation, A.K.L.-C., F.P.P.-M. and A.D.R.-C.; writing—review and editing, R.R.R.-R., T.I.C.-B., C.O.-M. and S.G.H.-O.; project administration, A.D.R.-C. All authors have read and agreed to the published version of the manuscript.

Funding: This research received no external funding.

Institutional Review Board Statement: The study was approved by the Ethics and Research Committee of Hospital Civil de Guadalajara Fray Antonio Alcalde (No. 051/19) and was conducted at the Department of Ophthalmology in accordance with the updated Declaration of Helsinki and Good Clinical Practice.

Informed Consent Statement: Coded numbers were assigned to ensure patient confidentiality and written informed consent has been obtained from the patients to publish this paper.

Data Availability Statement: The data contained in this article are part of the research project registered in Clinical Trials with the identifier NCT04071977.

Acknowledgments: We offer our thanks to the Department of Ophthalmology, Hospital Civil de Guadalajara "Fray Antonio Alcalde", Guadalajara, Jalisco, Mexico.

Conflicts of Interest: The authors have no conflicts of interest to report. This research did not receive any specific grant from funding agencies in the public, commercial, or not-for-profit sectors.

References

1. Behl, T.; Kaur, I.; Kotwani, A. Implication of oxidative stress in progression of diabetic retinopathy. *Surv. Ophthalmol.* **2016**, *61*, 187–196. [CrossRef]
2. Safi, H.; Safi, S.; Hafezi-Moghadam, A.; Ahmadieh, H. Early detection of diabetic retinopathy. *Surv. Ophthalmol.* **2018**, *63*, 601–608. [CrossRef] [PubMed]
3. Zhang, X.; Saaddine, J.B.; Chou, C.F.; Cotch, M.F.; Cheng, Y.J.; Geiss, L.S.; Gregg, E.W.; Albright, A.L.; Klein, B.E.K.; Klein, R. Prevalence of diabetic retinopathy in the United States, 2005–2008. *JAMA—J. Am. Med. Assoc.* **2010**, *304*, 649–656. [CrossRef] [PubMed]
4. Miyamoto, N.; de Kozak, Y.; Jeanny, J.C.; Glotin, A.; Mascarelli, F.; Massin, P.; BenEzra, D.; Behar-Cohen, F. Placental growth factor-1 and epithelial haemato-retinal barrier breakdown: Potential implication in the pathogenesis of diabetic retinopathy. *Diabetologia* **2007**, *50*, 461–470. [CrossRef]
5. Géhl, Z.; Bakondi, E.; Resch, M.D.; Hegedus, C.; Kovács, K.; Lakatos, P.; Szabó, A.; Nagy, Z.; Virág, L. Diabetes-induced oxidative stress in the vitreous humor. *Redox Biol.* **2016**, *9*, 100–103. [CrossRef] [PubMed]
6. Darenskaya, M.A.; Kolesnikova, L.I.; Kolesnikov, S.I. Oxidative Stress: Pathogenetic Role in Diabetes Mellitus and Its Complications and Therapeutic Approaches to Correction. *Bull. Exp. Biol. Med.* **2021**, *171*, 179–189. [CrossRef]
7. Giacco, F.; Brownlee, M. Oxidative stress and diabetic complications. *Circ. Res.* **2010**, *107*, 1058–1070. [CrossRef]
8. Li, S.; Fu, X.A.; Zhou, X.F.; Chen, Y.Y.; Chen, W.Q. Angiogenesis-related cytokines in serum of proliferative diabetic retinopathy patients before and after vitrectomy. *Int. J. Ophthalmol.* **2012**, *5*, 726–730. [CrossRef]
9. López-Contreras, A.K.; Martínez-Ruiz, M.G.; Olvera-Montaño, C.; Robles-Rivera, R.R.; Arévalo-Simental, D.E.; Castellanos-González, J.A.; Hernández-Chávez, A.; Huerta-Olvera, S.G.; Cardona-Muñoz, E.G.; Rodríguez-Carrizalez, A.D. Importance of the use of oxidative stress biomarkers and inflammatory profile in aqueous and vitreous humor in diabetic retinopathy. *Antioxidants* **2020**, *9*, 891. [CrossRef]
10. Tamhane, M.; Cabrera-Ghayouri, S.; Abelian, G.; Viswanath, V. Review of Biomarkers in Ocular Matrices: Challenges and Opportunities. *Pharm. Res.* **2019**, *36*, 40. [CrossRef]
11. Chowdhury, U.R.; Madden, B.J.; Charlesworth, M.C.; Fautsch, M.P. Proteome analysis of human aqueous humor. *Investig. Ophthalmol. Vis. Sci.* **2010**, *51*, 4921–4931. [CrossRef] [PubMed]
12. Johnson, M.; McLaren, J.W.; Overby, D.R. Unconventional aqueous humor outflow: A review. *Exp. Eye Res.* **2017**, *158*, 94–111. [CrossRef] [PubMed]
13. Oguntibeju, O.O. Type 2 diabetes mellitus, oxidative stress and inflammation: Examining the links. *Int. J. Physiol. Pathophysiol. Pharmacol.* **2019**, *11*, 45–63.
14. Mishra, D.; Gade, S.; Glover, K.; Sheshala, R.; Singh, T.R.R. Vitreous Humor: Composition, Characteristics and Implication on Intravitreal Drug Delivery. *Curr. Eye Res.* **2023**, *48*, 208–218. [CrossRef]
15. Ulrich, J.N.; Spannagl, M.; Kampik, A.; Gandorfer, A. Components of the fibrinolytic system in the vitreous body in patients with vitreoretinal disorders. *Clin. Experiment. Ophthalmol.* **2008**, *36*, 431–436. [CrossRef]
16. Rodríguez-Carrizalez, A.D.; Castellanos-González, J.A.; Martínez-Romero, E.C.; Miller-Arrevillaga, G.; Pacheco-Moisés, F.P.; Román-Pintos, L.M.; Miranda-Díaz, A.G. The effect of ubiquinone and combined antioxidant therapy on oxidative stress markers in non-proliferative diabetic retinopathy: A phase IIa, randomized, double-blind, and placebo-controlled study. *Redox Rep.* **2016**, *21*, 155–163. [CrossRef]
17. Rodríguez-Carrizalez, A.D.; Castellanos-González, J.A.; Martínez-Romero, E.C.; Miller-Arrevillaga, G.; Villa-Hernández, D.; Hernández-Godínez, P.P.; Ortiz, G.G.; Pacheco-Moisés, F.P.; Cardona-Muñoz, E.G.; Miranda-Díaz, A.G. Oxidants, antioxidants and mitochondrial function in non-proliferative diabetic retinopathy. *J. Diabetes* **2014**, *6*, 167–175. [CrossRef]
18. Martínez-Fernández de la Cámara, C.; Salom, D.; Sequedo, M.D.; Hervás, D.; Marín-Lambíes, C.; Aller, E.; Jaijo, T.; Díaz-LLopis, M.; Millán, J.M.; Rodrigo, R. Altered Antioxidant-Oxidant Status in the Aqueous Humor and Peripheral Blood of Patients with Retinitis Pigmentosa. *PLoS ONE* **2013**, *8*, e74223. [CrossRef]
19. Mancino, R.; Di Pierro, D.; Varesi, C.; Cerulli, A.; Feraco, A.; Cedrone, C.; Pinazo-Duran, M.D.; Coletta, M.; Nucci, C. Lipid peroxidation and total antioxidant capacity in vitreous, aqueous humor, and blood samples from patients with diabetic retinopathy. *Mol. Vis.* **2011**, *17*, 1298–1304.
20. Tokarz, P.; Kaarniranta, K.; Blasiak, J. Role of antioxidant enzymes and small molecular weight antioxidants in the pathogenesis of age-related macular degeneration (AMD). *Biogerontology* **2013**, *14*, 461–482. [CrossRef]
21. Praticò, D.; Lawson, J.A.; Rokach, J.; FitzGerald, G.A. The isoprostanes in biology and medicine. *Trends Endocrinol. Metab.* **2001**, *12*, 243–247. [CrossRef] [PubMed]

22. Kähler, J.; Ewert, A.; Weckmüller, J.; Stobbe, S.; Mittmann, C.; Köster, R.; Paul, M.; Meinertz, T.; Münzel, T. Oxidative Stress Increases Endothelin-1 Synthesis in Human Coronary Artery Smooth Muscle Cells. *J. Cardiovasc. Pharmacol.* **2001**, *38*, 49–57. [CrossRef] [PubMed]
23. Koliakos, G.G. 8-Isoprostaglandin F2a and ascorbic acid concentration in the aqueous humour of patients with exfoliation syndrome. *Br. J. Ophthalmol.* **2003**, *87*, 353–356. [CrossRef] [PubMed]
24. Rahim, A. 8-Isoprostaglandin F2a Levels in Aqueous Humor of Senile and Diabetic Cataract Patients. *IOSR J. Dent. Med. Sci.* **2012**, *2*, 40–42. [CrossRef]
25. Lahaie, I.; Hardy, P.; Hou, X.; Hasséssian, H.; Asselin, P.; Lachapelle, P.; Almazan, G.; Varma, D.; Morrow, J.; Roberts, L.; et al. A novel mechanism for vasoconstrictor action of 8-isoprostaglandin F2 alpha on retinal vessels. *Am. J. Physiol.* **1998**, *274*, R1406. [CrossRef]
26. Toda, N.; Nakanishitoda, M. Nitric oxide: Ocular blood flow, glaucoma, and diabetic retinopathy. *Prog. Retin. Eye Res.* **2007**, *26*, 205–238. [CrossRef]
27. Kulaksızoglu, S.; Karalezli, A. Aqueous Humour and Serum Levels of Nitric Oxide, Malondialdehyde and Total Antioxidant Status in Patients with Type 2 Diabetes with Proliferative Diabetic Retinopathy and Nondiabetic Senile Cataracts. *Can. J. Diabetes* **2016**, *40*, 115–119. [CrossRef]
28. Opatrilova, R.; Kubatka, P.; Caprnda, M.; Büsselberg, D.; Krasnik, V.; Vesely, P.; Saxena, S.; Ruia, S.; Mozos, I.; Rodrigo, L.; et al. Nitric oxide in the pathophysiology of retinopathy: Evidences from preclinical and clinical researches. *Acta Ophthalmol.* **2018**, *96*, 222–231. [CrossRef]
29. Kost, O.A.; Beznos, O.V.; Davydova, N.G.; Manickam, D.S.; Nikolskaya, I.I.; Guller, A.E.; Binevski, P.V.; Chesnokova, N.B.; Shekhter, A.B.; Klyachko, N.L.; et al. Superoxide dismutase 1 nanozyme for treatment of eye inflammation. *Oxid. Med. Cell. Longev.* **2016**, *2016*, 5194239. [CrossRef]
30. Zhang, W.; Zhao, M.; Chu, D.; Chen, H.; Cui, B.; Ning, Q.; Wang, X.; Li, Z.; Cao, S.; Li, J. Dual-ROS-scavenging and dual-lingering nanozyme-based eye drops alleviate dry eye disease. *J. Nanobiotechnol.* **2024**, *22*, 229. [CrossRef]
31. Izuta, H.; Chikaraishi, Y.; Adachi, T.; Shimazawa, M.; Sugiyama, T.; Ikeda, T.; Hara, H. Extracellular SOD and VEGF are increased in vitreous bodies from proliferative diabetic retinopathy patients. *Mol. Vis.* **2009**, *15*, 2663–2672.
32. Kernell, A.; Lundh, B.L.; Marklund, S.L.; Skoog, K.O.; Björkstén, B. Superoxide dismutase in the anterior chamber and the vitreous of diabetic patients. *Investig. Ophthalmol. Vis. Sci.* **1992**, *33*, 3131–3135.
33. Sawada, H.; Fukuchi, T.; Abe, H. Oxidative Stress Markers in Aqueous Humor of Patients with Senile Cataracts. *Curr. Eye Res.* **2009**, *34*, 36–41. [CrossRef]
34. Giordano, C.R.; Roberts, R.; Krentz, K.A.; Bissig, D.; Talreja, D.; Kumar, A.; Terlecky, S.R.; Berkowitz, B.A. Catalase Therapy Corrects Oxidative Stress-Induced Pathophysiology in Incipient Diabetic Retinopathy. *Investig. Ophthalmol. Vis. Sci.* **2015**, *56*, 3095. [CrossRef] [PubMed]
35. Huang, W.; Koralewska-Makár, A.; Bauer, B.; Åkesson, B. Extracellular glutathione peroxidase and ascorbic acid in aqueous humor and serum of patients operated on for cataract. *Clin. Chim. Acta* **1997**, *261*, 117–130. [CrossRef] [PubMed]
36. Pavlovschi, E.; Pantea, V.; Borovic, D.; Tagadiuc, O. Glutathione-related antioxidant defense system in patients with hypertensive retinopathy. *Rom. J. Ophthalmol.* **2021**, *65*, 46–53. [CrossRef] [PubMed]
37. Kotzampassi, K.; Kolios, G.; Manousou, P.; Kazamias, P.; Paramythiotis, D.; Papavramidis, T.S.; Heliadis, S.; Kouroumalis, E.; Eleftheriadis, E. Oxidative stress due to anesthesia and surgical trauma: Importance of early enteral nutrition. *Mol. Nutr. Food Res.* **2009**, *53*, 770–779. [CrossRef]
38. Rosenfeldt, F.; Wilson, M.; Lee, G.; Kure, C.; Ou, R.; Braun, L.; de Haan, J. Oxidative stress in surgery in an ageing population: Pathophysiology and therapy. *Exp. Gerontol.* **2013**, *48*, 45–54. [CrossRef] [PubMed]
39. Cicik, E.; Tekin, H.; Akar, S.; Ekmekçi, Ö.B.; Donma, O.; Koldaş, L.; Özkan, Ş. Interleukin-8, Nitric Oxide and Glutathione Status in Proliferative Vitreoretinopathy and Proliferative Diabetic Retinopathy. *Ophthalmic Res.* **2003**, *35*, 251–255. [CrossRef]

life

MDPI

Article

Erosive Tarsal Conjunctival Lesions Following Immunogenic Events in Early Development of Ocular Graft-vs-Host Disease

Marcus G. Kohnstam [1], Pier Luigi Surico [1,2,3] and Zhonghui K. Luo [1,*]

1 Massachusetts Eye and Ear, Department of Ophthalmology, Harvard Medical School, Boston, MA 02114, USA
2 Department of Ophthalmology, Campus Bio-Medico University Hospital, 00128 Rome, Italy
3 Department of Organs of Sense, La Sapienza University of Rome, 00185 Rome, Italy
* Correspondence: zhonghui_luo@meei.harvard.edu

Abstract: Purpose: Ocular graft-versus-host disease (oGVHD) affects more than half of the patients following allogeneic hematopoietic stem cell transplantation (HSCT). The disease onset and the pathogenesis of oGVHD are not well understood. We hope to identify the triggers and explore the clinical signs and symptoms of oGVHD development at the early stages. Methods: The records of post-HSCT patients seen consecutively in a 1-year span in a single provider's clinic were reviewed. The history, symptoms, and clinical findings of the patients with erosive tarsal conjunctival lesions (ETCLs) were analyzed. Results: Out of the 228 patients screened, 19 had clinically witnessed ETCL in at least one eye during the period. Twelve (63%) patients had a never-before-described nodular erosion on the subtarsal conjunctiva; seven (37%) had previously described pseudomembranous erosions. The ocular symptom onset was within 1 month after immunosuppression (IS) taper, vaccination, or donor lymphocyte infusion (DLI) in 16 of the 19 patients. While 16 (84%) patients reported painless mucous discharge, only 9 (47%) reported dryness as the initial symptom. Within 6 months, only 4 (21%) had discharge but 15 (82%) patients endorsed dryness. Subepithelial conjunctival fibrosis followed ETCL immediately in situ. Corneal punctate staining increased with time, while aqueous tear production decreased. Conclusions: The ETCL described is likely one of the earliest detectable findings of oGVHD and triggered by certain immunogenic events. The ocular symptoms of wet mucous discharge should be considered a warning sign for oGVHD onset, particularly when it occurs shortly after prominently immunogenic events.

Keywords: stem cell transplantation; ocular graft-versus-host disease; inflammation; conjunctival fibrosis; pseudomembrane

1. Introduction

Allogeneic hematopoietic stem cell transplantation (allo-HSCT) is an increasingly common treatment for many otherwise-fatal hematologic malignancies and disorders [1]. Chronic graft-versus-host disease (cGVHD) is the leading cause of morbidity and mortality following stem cell transplantation, affecting 30–70% of all the HSCT recipients [1–3].

Ocular graft-versus-host disease (oGVHD) is one of the most common presentations of cGVHD, found in about half of the patients with other types of cGVHD [4,5]. It has been shown that a donor T-cell-mediated inflammatory cascade leads to lacrimal gland fibrosis, meibomian gland dysfunction, and ocular surface inflammation, which severely affects all the components of the tear film and causes the most recognized feature of oGVHD, keratoconjunctivitis sicca (KCS) [1,6–11]. Detrimental outcomes can range widely from ocular discomfort to cicatricial deformation to corneal perforation [12,13]. Currently, treatment is mostly supportive; oGVHD can still result in debilitating pain and blindness in many patients [14].

Despite the well-recognized impact on quality of life from oGVHD [15,16], the early stages of oGVHD are not well understood. Due to the limitation of resources and the burden of diseases on patients undergoing allo-HSCT, most of them do not undergo baseline evaluation by an ophthalmologist prior to HSCT [16]. Patients often do not receive ophthalmologic care until they are severely symptomatic; therefore, mild to moderate early symptoms could go unnoticed, and the preliminary manifestations of oGVHD go undocumented and untreated. Without early recognition, early intervention is not possible, which can lead to more serious complications. It has long been recognized that early diagnosis and treatment are crucial for reducing the morbidity of oGVHD [17].

In our practice, we repeatedly found that two types of erosive tarsal conjunctival lesions (ETCLs) preceded conjunctival subepithelial fibrosis (CSEF) in situ, often before the development of keratoconjunctivitis sicca (KCS), the most recognized oGVHD clinical presentation. Although both CSEF and serosanguinous conjunctivitis have been reported before [18], there is no literature that has described a direct connection between the two. We are the first to describe the nodular type of erosive lesions on the tarsal conjunctiva, and to report the proximity in time to certain systemic immunogenic events. Our retrospective series describes what we suspect to be a critical event in the early development of oGVHD.

2. Materials and Methods

We conducted a retrospective observational series at Massachusetts Eye and Ear. Approval for this study (2021P003700) was obtained from the Mass General Brigham Human Research Committee of Mass General Brigham, Boston, MA, USA. All research adhered to the tenets of the Declaration of Helsinki. The electronic medical records of all the patients with a history of allo-HSCT and a diagnosis of oGVHD seen in the clinic of a single cornea specialist between 10 May 2021 and 9 May 2022 were reviewed. Among them, the patients with active erosive conjunctival lesions including nodular and/or pseudomembranous lesions involving at least one tarsus (ETCL) during at least one of the encounters were identified, and the electronic medical records of these patients were reviewed. The allo-HSCT history, immunosuppression (IS) regimen, vaccination record, and previous ocular history were summarized. The ophthalmological findings including the slit lamp examinations of the eyelids; bulbar and palpebral conjunctiva with lid eversion, cornea, and other ocular surface structures; and intraocular pressure were reviewed and analyzed. The patients underwent various treatments such as systemic immunosuppression, topical steroids (preservative-free 1% prednisolone acetate, 0.5% loteprednol etabonate suspension/ointment, or 0.05% difluprednate), punctal plugs, preservative-free artificial tears, and/or 40% autologous serum tears. Some patients required intraocular pressure control with topical agents during this period. Slit lamp photographs were obtained using Streit Haag Imaging Module 900. Anterior segment optical coherence tomography (OCT) was performed using Heidelberg Spectralis HRA + OCT. Schirmer 1 test was performed without topical anesthesia for 5 min.

3. Results

The electronic medical records of 228 patients with a history of allo-HSCT and a diagnosis of oGVHD were reviewed. A total of 19 patients, with a mean age of 60 years (range 29 to 72), were seen in the clinic with active ETCL involving at least one tarsus in a total of 35 eyes during the one-year period. The patients' characteristics are shown in Table 1.

Seventeen patients presented with their ETCL at the first visit to our clinic, with or without previous ophthalmologic evaluation at other institutions following their HSCT; the other two patients presented with a new onset of ETCL with established care at our clinic following their HSCT. The 19 patients were seen in our clinic from a few days to several weeks after their symptom onset. The patients were followed in the clinic at various frequencies, and the course of ETCL was documented. In most patients, the ETCL episode was only observed once, lasting several weeks to months; in 3 eyes of 2 patients, the ETCL was witnessed to have resolved and then recurred at a later date. The diagnosis of oGVHD was either pre-existing or established after the observation of ETCL later in the course according to the NIH 2014 criteria [3].

Table 1. Patients' characteristics.

	Male (n = 12)	Female (n = 7)	Total (n = 19)
Age-year (SD)	58.9 (11.7)	62.6 (7.8)	60.3 (10.6)
	Ethnicity		
Non-Hispanic Caucasian	10	7	17
Hispanic Caucasian	1	0	1
Hispanic African American	1	0	1
Conditioning Regimen			
Myeloablative	4	2	6
Reduced Intensity	8	5	13
	Donor		
Matched Related Donor (Sister)	3	0	3
Matched Related Donor (Brother)	2	0	2
Matched Unrelated Donor	7	7	14
Stem Cell Source			
Peripheral Blood	11	7	18
Bone Marrow	1	0	1

Fifteen patients (79%) had distinctive nodular erosions (Figures 1 and 2) in a total of 27 eyes; eight patients (42%) had pseudomembranous erosions (Figure 3) in a total of 14 eyes; and four patients (21%) had co-existing nodular and pseudomembranous erosions on the same tarsal conjunctiva in 6 eyes. Three eyes of 3 patients (16%) did not have any observed ETCL while the fellow eyes were actively involved.

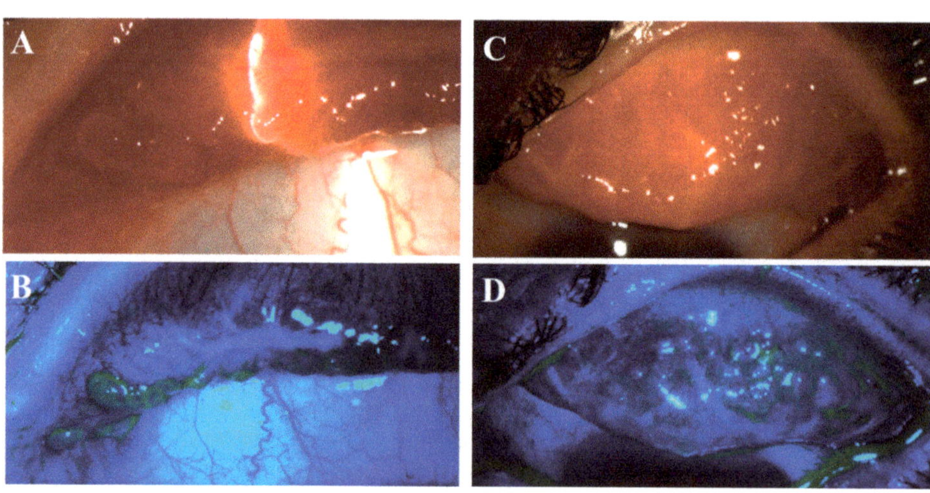

Figure 1. Nodular erosive tarsal conjunctival lesions (ETCLs). The slit lamp color images of everted superior palpebral conjunctiva with nodular ETCL in two representative patients following fluorescein staining without (**A**,**C**) or with (**B**,**D**) cobalt blue filter. The epithelium over the nodules displays different degrees of erosion.

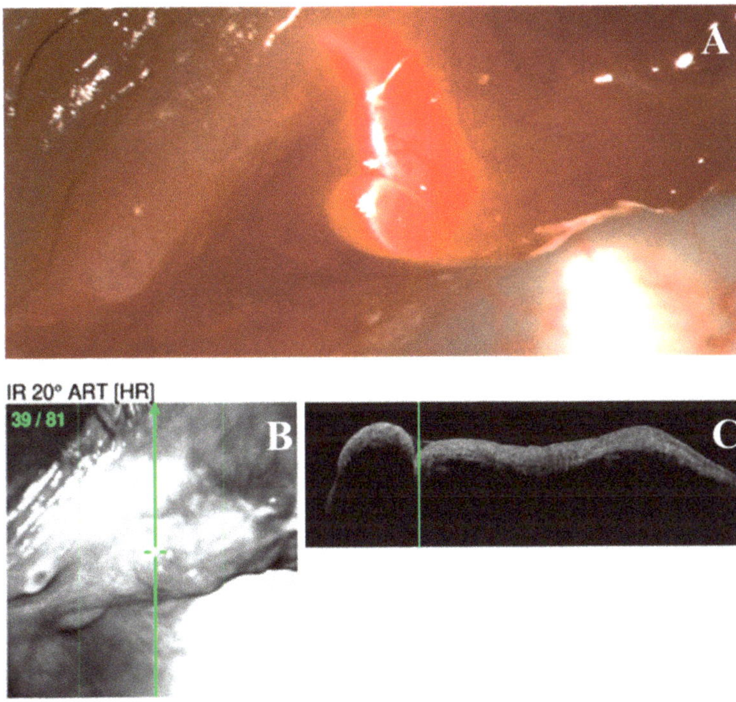

Figure 2. Optical coherence tomography (OCT) scan of a nodular erosive tarsal conjunctival lesion (ETCL). (**A**). The slit lamp color image of the nodule. (**B**,**C**). OCT image showing a uniformly hypo-reflective nodule without any fibrous internal structure.

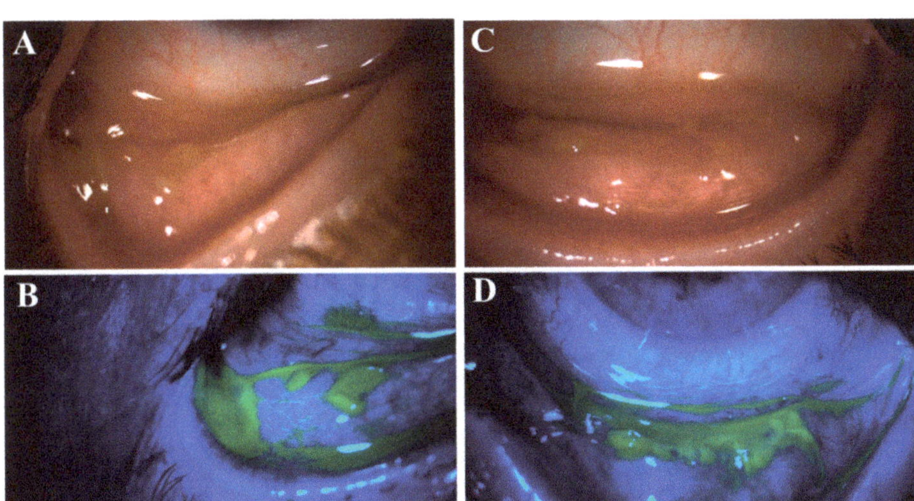

Figure 3. Pseudomembranous erosive tarsal conjunctival lesions (ETCLs). Slit lamp color images of inferior palpebral conjunctivae with pseudomembranous ETCL in one representative patient following fluorescein staining without (**A**,**C**) or with (**B**,**D**) cobalt blue filter.

Of the 35 eyes with ETCL, 15 eyes had lesions (nodular and/or pseudomembranous erosions) on both superior and inferior tarsal conjunctivae (Figure 4); in the other 20 eyes, the lesions were only found on one tarsal conjunctiva, with 17 superiorly and 3 inferiorly. The superior tarsal conjunctival lesions were only visible when the upper lids were everted.

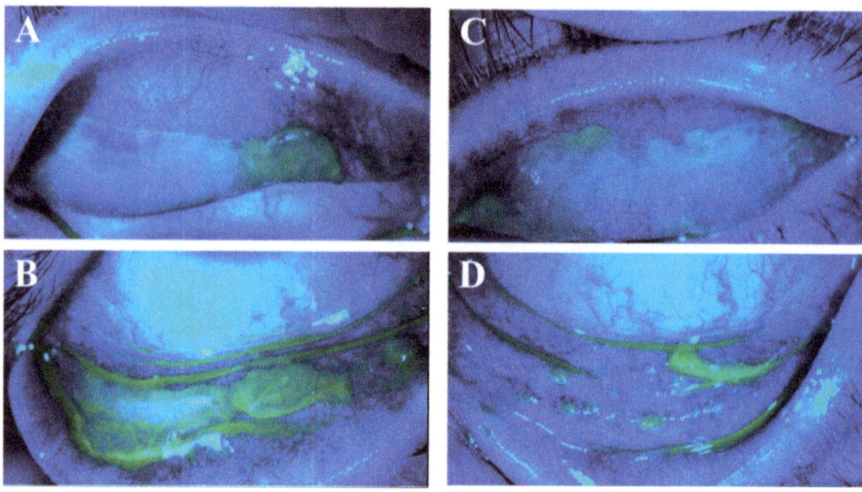

Figure 4. Co-existing nodular and pseudomembranous erosive tarsal conjunctival lesions (ETCLs). Slit lamp color images of all four palpebral conjunctivae with co-existing nodular and pseudomembranous ETCL in one representative patient following fluorescein staining with cobalt blue filter. (**A**). Right superior palpebral conjunctiva. (**B**). Left superior palpebral conjunctiva. (**C**). Right inferior palpebral conjunctiva. (**D**). Left inferior palpebral conjunctiva.

All tarsal conjunctivae of the 35 eyes following ETCL resolved and re-epithelialized with new fibrosis formation. The ETCL in 20 eyes (57%) also resulted in inferior fornix foreshortening, including inferior symblepharon formation in 3 eyes. In 16 eyes of 9 patients, both tarsal conjunctivae were free of fibrosis at the initial encounter of ETCL. In the other 19 eyes, CSEF was found adjacent to the active ETCL, and new fibrosis developed at the sites of erosions during re-epithelialization (Figures 5 and 6). In the aforementioned 13 patients (23 eyes) with frequent follow-up visits, the observed ETCL completely resolved into CSEF by a mean of 2.7 months (0.5 to 6.2).

The most common initial symptoms of the 19 patients were mucous discharge or "thick tears" or "goop" (84%), morning crusting (79%), dryness (47%), and irritation/foreign body sensation (42%). Thirteen patients followed up regularly within the first 6 months after the initial presentation with ETCL. They returned to the clinic 4.6 times on average (median 4.0, range 2–9 times) within a period of 5.3 to 7.8 months after the initial encounter. The most common symptoms of these 13 patients at 6 months were irritation or foreign body sensation (69%) and dryness (77%). Concurrently, mucous discharge was only reported in 31% and crusting in 23% of the followed-up patients (Table 2).

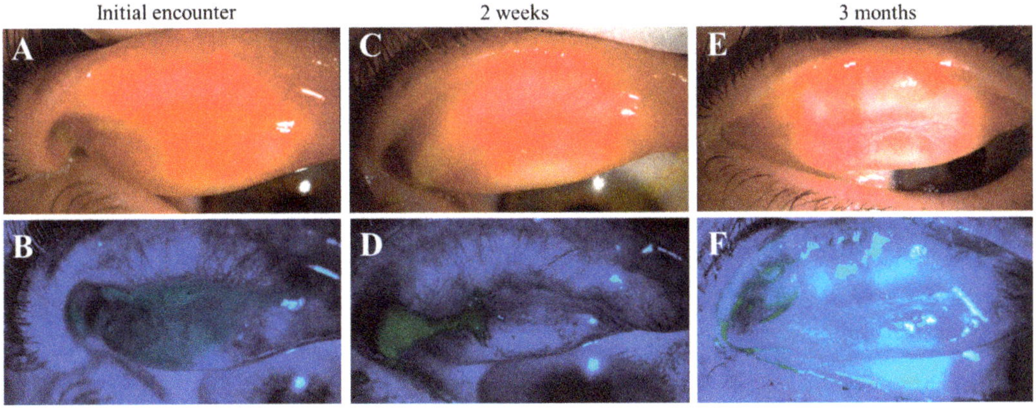

Figure 5. Progression of pseudomembranous erosive tarsal conjunctival lesions (ETCLs) into fibrosis. Slit lamp color images of superior palpebral conjunctivae with pseudomembranous ETCL in one representative patient following fluorescein staining without (**A**,**C**,**E**) or with (**B**,**D**,**F**) cobalt blue filter, showing progressive fibrotic changes. (**A**,**B**). At initial encounter. (**C**,**D**). Two weeks after the initial encounter. (**E**,**F**). Three months after the initial encounter.

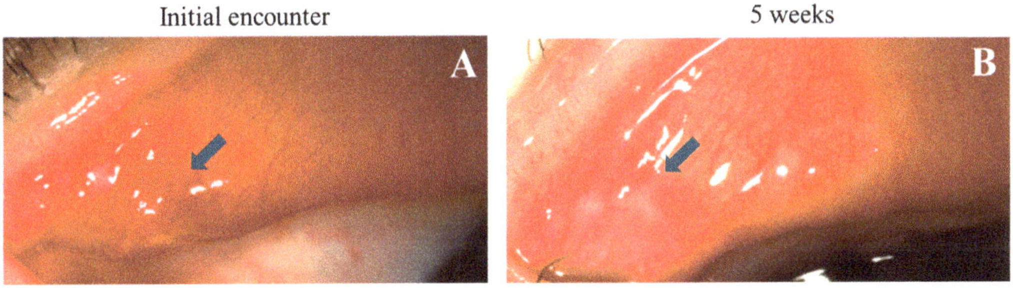

Figure 6. Progression of nodular erosive tarsal conjunctival lesions (ETCLs) into fibrosis. Slit lamp color images of the same superior palpebral conjunctiva (**A**). At initial encounter, a single nodular lesion (blue arrow) with adjacent pre-existing fibrosis. (**B**). Five weeks after the initial encounter, fibrosis seen at the exact location of the resolved nodule (blue arrow).

Table 2. Patients' symptom records at erosive tarsal conjunctival lesions (ETCLs) onset and at 6 ± 1 month follow-up.

Symptom	At ETCL Onset (19 Patients)	At 6 ± 1 Month (13 Patients) *
Mucous discharge	16 (84%)	4 (31%)
Heavy morning Crusting	15 (79%)	3 (23%)
Dryness	9 (47%)	10 (77%)
Irritation/FBS	8 (42%)	9 (69%)

* Thirteen patients had follow-up regularly and had visits at 6 +/− 1 month. Among them, 7 had increased corneal fluorescein staining (CFS), 3 had decreased and 1 had unchanged CFS, and 2 had therapeutic scleral lens. ETCL = erosive tarsal conjunctival lesions; FBS = foreign body sensation. Significant percentages are bolded.

Five patients (9 eyes) had aqueous tear production measured during the active ETCL, with the average Schirmer 1 score of 15 mm/5′ (range 0–35). Repeated tests were performed 3 to 5 months later when the conjunctiva had re-epithelialized, with the average Schirmer 1 score decreased to 4 mm/5′ (range 0–13).

The mean onset of the symptoms associated with the ETCL was 9.6 months after HSCT (range 4.2 to 21.5 months). However, the mean time between the reported symptom onset and most recent immunosuppressive drug (IS) tapering (12 patients), COVID vaccination (5 patients), post-HSCT 9-month immunization bundle (4 patients), or donor lymphocyte infusion (DLI) (1 patient) was 0.7 months (range 0.1 to 1.2). In 16 out of the 19 patients, the symptoms started within 1 month after one or more of these immunogenic events (Table 3).

Table 3. Mean time from hematopoietic stem cell transplantation (HSCT), systemic immune-suppressive (IS) drug taper, vaccination, or donor lymphocyte infusion (DLI) to erosive tarsal conjunctival lesions (ETCL)-related symptom onset.

Patient	Symptom Onset (Months after HSCT)	IS Taper (Months before Symptom Onset)	Vaccination (Months before Symptom Onset)	DLI (Months Before Symptom Onset)
1	5.6	0.5	-	-
2	12.6	4.3	-	0.6
3	5.6	0.6	0.9 (COVID)	-
4	Unclear	Unclear	-	-
5	21.4	4	0.8 (COVID)	-
6	10.5	0.6	0.7 (COVID)	-
7	9	1.2	-	-
8	6.3	0.3	-	-
9	10.5	1	-	-
10	9	0.9	-	-
11	9.6	-	0.8 (Bundle)	-
12	4.4	1.1	-	-
13	9.7	0.5	0.5 (Bundle)	-
14	8	0.2	-	-
15	9.6	4	1 (COVID)	-
16	8.8	1	2	-
17	9.1	2.9	0.1 (Bundle)	-
18	8	2.3	0.3 (COVID)	-
19	9.6	0.6	0.9 (Bundle)	-

HSCT—allogeneic hematopoietic stem cell transplantation; DLI—donor lymphocyte infusion; IS taper—most recent systemic immunosuppressive drug taper; Vaccination—any vaccination received within 3 months prior to ocular symptom onset; Bundle—post-HSCT 9-month vaccination bundle (DTap, 5 Pertussis antigens, Hib, PRP-T, Pneumococcal conjugate PCV20, Polio—IPV, Zoster recombinant); Unclear—patient's ocular symptom onset timing was not documented.

A qualitative description of corneal fluorescein staining (CFS) at 5–7 months was available in these 13 patients. In seven patients, there was increased CFS in one or both eyes. Two other patients started wearing therapeutic scleral lenses after the ETCL episode; therefore, the corneal staining was non-descriptive. Three patients had decreased CFS in both eyes on an exam, and one patient never had any CFS in either eye.

All the patients had intraocular pressure (IOP) within the normal range at their initial encounters; however, three patients (16% of 19) developed an IOP greater than 21 mm Hg (mean Tmax 30.5, range 25 to 34), which required topical therapy for IOP control.

4. Discussion

Allo-HSCT serves as an effective cure for various hematological disorders, encompassing both malignant and non-malignant conditions. Despite significant progress in the field over the recent decades, graft-versus-host disease (GVHD) still affects more than half of the recipients and causes significant mortality and morbidity [2,19,20]. The focus of care of this population is now shifting from simple survival to quality of life of the transplantation survivors, which is significantly dependent on their ocular health. It is our hope that this retrospective series brings attention to the earlier stage of oGVHD, occurring prior to the commonly recognized, established stages when aqueous deficiency and eyelid deconfiguration have already developed from the fibrotic processes involving the ocular adnexa [18,21].

Structural changes such as conjunctival fibrosis, fornix foreshortening, and symblepharon can lead to lid retraction, entropion, ectropion, trichiasis, lagophthalmos, ankyloblepharon, and other distortions that threaten ocular surface health [22–25]. The corneal epithelium is vulnerable to exposure, particularly in the context of aqueous tear deficiency and meibomian gland disease which are both common manifestations of oGVHD [26]. Any corneal epithelial defect is more likely to lead to stromal melting, ulcer, and perforation [10]. In addition to infection, pain, and scarring, irreversible vision loss can be a very unfortunate result [25]. Furthermore, lacrimal gland fibrosis and meibomian gland damage likely happen simultaneously as the conjunctival inflammation is taking place [2,6,27,28]. Therefore, the prevention of such changes is very meaningful and only possible when the conjunctival inflammation is recognized early.

One of the most enlightening findings from our retrospective series is that during the early stage of ETCL, the most common ocular symptoms are mucous discharge and crusting, not dryness or irritation. Within 6 months, dryness becomes predominant compared to other symptoms. As oGVHD has long been recognized for and often incorrectly equated to the dry eye disease/keratoconjunctivitis sicca (KCS), the early symptoms rarely catch the attention of HSCT providers or even eyecare providers. Therefore, we should modify the expectation: the most common late manifestation of oGVHD is dryness; however, the early stage can be rather "wet", with excessive tearing or mucous discharge. One should not rule out oGVHD simply because of a lack of dry eye complaints or findings. In addition, the onset of ETCL seems to be more associated with certain immunogenic events than the number of months after allo-HSCT, which should encourage us to arrange ophthalmic examinations in accordance with patients' IS taper, DLI, or vaccination schedules rather than every 3 or 6 months. Certainly, whenever patients complain about painless mucous discharge, tearing, and crusting, they should be seen immediately.

Another finding is that ETCL is more likely to involve the superior tarsal conjunctivae (32 of 35 eyes) than the inferior ones (18 of 35 eyes). Therefore, the careful inspection of all ocular surfaces including the everted upper tarsal conjunctivae should be adopted in routine practice.

According to the 2014 National Institutes of Health Consensus, there are two principal categories of graft-versus-host disease: chronic (cGVHD) and acute (aGVHD), differentiated according to clinical presentations and features [1,29]. aGVHD occurs when the donor stem cells successfully populate into a functional immune system and start to attack the host. The typical target organs of aGVHD include the skin, the gastrointestinal tract, and the liver. The ocular involvement in aGVHD is probably under-recognized in the context of other, more life-threatening conditions. Ocular aGVHD has been reported to be associated with dry eye sensation (often without epitheliopathy), foreign body sensation, (bulbar) conjunctival hyperemia, and, in severe cases, pseudomembranous conjunctivitis [3,18,30,31]. Chronic oGVHD is often diagnosed at a late stage when the ocular irritation has exceeded the patient's high tolerance threshold. It has been reported to be associated with prominent fibrosis of the conjunctiva, and with ocular surface epitheliopathy, KCS, and a greater risk of corneal perforation in extreme cases [32]. A subset of cGVHD—overlap syndrome—is described as a combination of traditional cGVHD symptoms and one or more aGVHD symptoms [17,32]. Such categorization of GVHD is still dominant in the HSCT and ophthalmology communities. What we have observed in this series supports the more unifying theory: regardless of the length of time following allo-HSCT, oGVHD activity can lead to an erosive conjunctival process. It is a similar process in both early and later stages, triggered by the donor immune system activation, the intensity of which determines the severity of ETCL. IS taper or immunizations typically trigger a milder form of ETCL than that from the immune reconstitution in acute GVHD, and therefore, is much less noticeable. Even when noticed, it is often misdiagnosed as "infectious conjunctivitis" and treated with topical antibiotics. Further understanding of the ETCL process will significantly increase our understanding of oGVHD pathogenesis.

This is the first ever report of such nodular erosion lesions in the literature. The nodules (Figure 1) were different from the fine papillae seen in allergic conjunctivitis, or the clear, fluid-filled follicles seen in viral conjunctivitis. The nodules can appear individually or in clusters with variable sizes from 1 mm to over 5 mm in diameter. In previous studies, a serosanguineous exudate was reported to progress into pseudomembrane [5], but such nodular lesions were never described. Several studies examining pseudomembrane in the setting of oGVHD have demonstrated that donor-derived immune cells, particularly Natural Killer T-cells, are active in infiltrating the host epithelium [6,33,34]. We hypothesize that nodular ETCL may represent the initial sites of donor immune cell infiltration, with the potential to progress into a larger area of deeper involvement—the pseudomembranous erosion.

To avoid iatrogenic trauma, we did not biopsy any lesions because trauma can lead to non-healing defects in such populations and detrimental outcomes [35]. Instead, we performed an anterior segment OCT and found the lesion to be uniform and hypo-reflective without any fibrous internal structure. Future investigation into the histopathology of the nodular lesions is needed to elucidate the pathogenesis.

We have repeatedly observed the formation of CSEF as the nodular or pseudomembranous ETCL resolves (Figure 3). All the tarsal conjunctivae of the 16 eyes were free of fibrosis prior to developing fibrosis at the exact location of ETCL. Therefore, our observation indicates an origin of the CSEF reported previously [18]. We treated the ETCL in all the eyes empirically with topical steroids. Although this is not a controlled study and no comparisons were made between fibrosis formation in other treatment regimens, we hope the early treatment decreased the level of inflammation and helped preserve the conjunctival epithelium and normal eyelid anatomy, therefore decreasing the risk of severe ocular surface complications in the future [16].

5. Limitations

Our series is limited by its retrospective nature, as well as the dependence on patients' recollection, who have all undergone extensive chemotherapy, conditioning, and treatment for other forms of GVHD. Despite an extensive chart review of the patients' medical records from their clinic encounters with the HSCT providers, not all ocular complaints were documented prior to our encounters. The self-reported timeline of symptoms and events was limited by their memory. Only 13 out of the 19 patients had rigorous follow-ups in the first 6 months. The others were not seen regularly due to various reasons such as hospitalization and long travel distances. It reflects the difficulty of studying this group of patients whose systemic conditions are very challenging to manage.

This study is a retrospective case series with purely observational findings and is reliant on active processes at the time of examination. It is possible that other unobserved aspects of the disease may have been present at times when the patients were not in the clinic, and/or not apparent due to the lack of physical presentation while in the clinic. Additionally, as most patients did not have documented eye exams prior to their allo-HSCT, there were few documented baseline findings to compare to. Future longitudinal observational studies including a pre-HSCT eye exam are warranted to further elucidate the natural history of oGVHD as strongly recommended by the NIH consensus group [16].

Future controlled studies should also be carried out to explore early treatment options and effects.

6. Conclusions

We have observed that ETCL can occur shortly after certain immunogenic events in patients with an established diagnosis of oGVHD and those who developed oGVHD soon after, and that ETCL precedes CSEF in situ. Patients at this stage mostly experience thick mucous discharge and morning crusting with less dryness or other ocular discomfort. Our findings present an opportunity to diagnose and investigate oGVHD much earlier in the disease course.

Author Contributions: Conceptualization, Z.K.L.; methodology, Z.K.L., M.G.K. and P.L.S.; software, Z.K.L. and M.G.K.; validation, Z.K.L.; formal analysis, Z.K.L., M.G.K. and P.L.S.; investigation, Z.K.L.; resources, Z.K.L.; data curation, Z.K.L., M.G.K. and P.L.S.; writing—original draft preparation, Z.K.L., M.G.K. and P.L.S.; writing—review and editing, Z.K.L. and M.G.K.; visualization, Z.K.L. and P.L.S.; supervision, Z.K.L.; project administration, Z.K.L. All authors have read and agreed to the published version of the manuscript.

Funding: This research received no external funding.

Institutional Review Board Statement: The study was conducted at Massachusetts Eye and Ear. Approval for this study (2021P003700) was obtained from the Mass General Brigham Human Research Committee of Mass General Brigham, Boston, MA. All research adhered to the tenets of the Declaration of Helsinki.

Informed Consent Statement: Patient consent was waived due to the retrospective nature of the study.

Data Availability Statement: The data that support the findings of this study are available upon request from the corresponding author, Z.K.L.

Conflicts of Interest: The authors declare no conflicts of interest.

References

1. Qiu, Y.; Hong, J.; Peng, R. Manifestation of Clinical Categories of Ocular Graft-versus-Host Disease. *J. Ophthalmol.* **2018**, *2018*, 6430953. [CrossRef]
2. Jagasia, M.H.; Greinix, H.T.; Arora, M.; Williams, K.M.; Wolff, D.; Cowen, E.W.; Palmer, J.; Weisdorf, D.; Treister, N.S.; Cheng, G.S.; et al. National Institutes of Health Consensus Development Project on Criteria for Clinical Trials in Chronic Graft-versus-Host Disease: I. The 2014 Diagnosis and Staging Working Group Report. *Biol. Blood Marrow Transplant.* **2015**, *21*, 389–401. [CrossRef]
3. Ogawa, Y.; Kim, S.K.; Dana, R.; Clayton, J.; Jain, S.; Rosenblatt, M.I.; Perez, V.L.; Shikari, H.; Riemens, A.; Tsubota, K. International Chronic Ocular Graft-vs-Host-Disease (GVHD) Consensus Group: Proposed Diagnostic Criteria for Chronic GVHD (Part I). *Sci. Rep.* **2013**, *3*, 3419. [CrossRef]
4. Jeppesen, H.; Gjærde, L.K.; Lindegaard, J.; Julian, H.O.; Heegaard, S.; Sengeløv, H. Ocular Chronic Graft-versus-Host Disease and Its Relation to Other Organ Manifestations and Outcomes after Allogeneic Hematopoietic Cell Transplantation. *Transplant. Cell. Ther.* **2022**, *28*, 833.e1–833.e7. [CrossRef]
5. Rojas, B.; Cuhna, R.; Zafirakis, P.; Ramirez, J.M.; Lizan-Garciía, M.; Zhao, T.; Foster, C.S. Cell Populations and Adhesion Molecules Expression in Conjunctiva before and after Bone Marrow Transplantation. *Exp. Eye Res.* **2005**, *81*, 313–325. [CrossRef]
6. Ogawa, Y.; Kawakami, Y.; Tsubota, K. Cascade of Inflammatory, Fibrotic Processes, and Stress-Induced Senescence in Chronic GVHD-Related Dry Eye Disease. *Int. J. Mol. Sci.* **2021**, *22*, 6114. [CrossRef]
7. Janin, A.; Facon, T.; Castier, P.; Mancel, E.; Jouet, J.P.; Gosselin, B. Pseudomembranous Conjunctivitis Following Bone Marrow Transplantation: Immunopathological and Ultrastructural Study of One Case. *Hum. Pathol.* **1996**, *27*, 307–309. [CrossRef]
8. Perez, V.L.; Mousa, H.M.; Soifer, M.; Beatty, C.; Sarantopoulos, S.; Saban, D.R.; Levy, R.B. Meibomian Gland Dysfunction: A Route of Ocular Graft-Versus-Host Disease Progression That Drives a Vicious Cycle of Ocular Surface Inflammatory Damage. *Am. J. Ophthalmol.* **2023**, *247*, 42–60. [CrossRef]
9. Tatematsu, Y.; Ogawa, Y.; Shimmura, S.; Dogru, M.; Yaguchi, S.; Nagai, T.; Yamazaki, K.; Kameyama, K.; Okamoto, S.; Kawakami, Y.; et al. Mucosal Microvilli in Dry Eye Patients with Chronic GVHD. *Bone Marrow Transplant.* **2012**, *47*, 416–425. [CrossRef]
10. Shimizu, E.; Aketa, N.; Yazu, H.; Uchino, M.; Kamoi, M.; Sato, Y.; Tsubota, K.; Ogawa, Y. Corneal Higher-Order Aberrations in Eyes with Chronic Ocular Graft-versus-Host Disease. *Ocul. Surf.* **2020**, *18*, 98–107. [CrossRef]

11. Singh, R.B.; Cho, W.; Liu, C.; Naderi, A.; Surico, P.L.; Kahale, F.; Dohlman, T.H.; Chauhan, S.K.; Dana, R. Immunopathological Mechanisms and Clinical Manifestations of Ocular Graft-versus-Host Disease Following Hematopoietic Stem Cell Transplantation. *Bone Marrow Transplant.* **2024**, *59*, 1049–1056. [CrossRef]
12. Inamoto, Y.; Valdés-Sanz, N.; Ogawa, Y.; Alves, M.; Berchicci, L.; Galvin, J.; Greinix, H.; Hale, G.A.; Horn, B.; Kelly, D.; et al. Ocular Graft-versus-Host Disease after Hematopoietic Cell Transplantation: Expert Review from the Late Effects and Quality of Life Working Committee of the CIBMTR and Transplant Complications Working Party of the EBMT. *Bone Marrow Transplant.* **2019**, *54*, 662–673. [CrossRef]
13. Suzuki, M.; Usui, T.; Kinoshita, N.; Yamagami, S.; Amano, S. A Case of Sterile Corneal Perforation after Bone Marrow Transplantation. *Eye* **2007**, *21*, 114–116. [CrossRef]
14. Sun, Y.C.; Chai, X.; Inamoto, Y.; Pidala, J.; Martin, P.J.; Flowers, M.E.D.; Shen, T.T.; Lee, S.J.; Jagasia, M. Impact of Ocular Chronic Graft-versus-Host Disease on Quality of Life. *Biol. Blood Marrow Transplant.* **2015**, *21*, 1687–1691. [CrossRef]
15. Saboo, U.S.; Amparo, F.; Abud, T.B.; Schaumberg, D.A.; Dana, R. Vision-Related Quality of Life in Patients with Ocular Graft-versus-Host Disease. *Ophthalmology* **2015**, *122*, 1669–1674. [CrossRef]
16. Kitko, C.L.; Pidala, J.; Schoemans, H.M.; Lawitschka, A.; Flowers, M.E.; Cowen, E.W.; Tkaczyk, E.; Farhadfar, N.; Jain, S.; Steven, P.; et al. National Institutes of Health Consensus Development Project on Criteria for Clinical Trials in Chronic Graft-versus-Host Disease: IIa. The 2020 Clinical Implementation and Early Diagnosis Working Group Report. *Transplant. Cell. Ther.* **2021**, *27*, 545–557. [CrossRef]
17. Jabs, D.A.; Wingard, J.; Green, W.R.; Farmer, E.R.; Vogelsang, G.; Saral, R. The Eye in Bone Marrow Transplantation. III. Conjunctival Graft-vs-Host Disease. *Arch. Ophthalmol.* **1989**, *107*, 1343–1348. [CrossRef]
18. Kheirkhah, A.; Coco, G.; Satitpitakul, V.; Dana, R. Subtarsal Fibrosis Is Associated with Ocular Surface Epitheliopathy in Graft-Versus-Host Disease. *Am. J. Ophthalmol.* **2018**, *189*, 102–110. [CrossRef]
19. Copelan, E.A.; Chojecki, A.; Lazarus, H.M.; Avalos, B.R. Allogeneic Hematopoietic Cell Transplantation; the Current Renaissance. *Blood Rev.* **2019**, *34*, 34–44. [CrossRef]
20. Wolff, D.; Radojcic, V.; Lafyatis, R.; Cinar, R.; Rosenstein, R.K.; Cowen, E.W.; Cheng, G.S.; Sheshadri, A.; Bergeron, A.; Williams, K.M.; et al. National Institutes of Health Consensus Development Project on Criteria for Clinical Trials in Chronic Graft-versus-Host Disease: IV. The 2020 Highly Morbid Forms Report. *Transplant. Cell. Ther.* **2021**, *27*, 817–835. [CrossRef]
21. Ogawa, Y.; Shimmura, S.; Dogru, M.; Tsubota, K. Immune Processes and Pathogenic Fibrosis in Ocular Chronic Graft-versus-Host Disease and Clinical Manifestations after Allogeneic Hematopoietic Stem Cell Transplantation. *Cornea* **2010**, *29*, S68–S77. [CrossRef]
22. Dulz, S.; Wagenfeld, L.; Richard, G.; Schrum, J.; Muschol, N.; Keserü, M. A Case of a Bilateral Cicatricial Upper Eyelid Entropion After Hematopoietic Stem Cell Transplantation in Mucopolysaccharidosis Type I. *Ophthalmic Plast. Reconstr. Surg.* **2017**, *33*, S75–S77. [CrossRef]
23. Giannaccare, G.; Bernabei, F.; Pellegrini, M.; Arpinati, M.; Bonifazi, F.; Sessa, M.; Versura, P.; Campos, E. Eyelid Metrics Assessment in Patients with Chronic Ocular Graft Versus-Host Disease. *Ocul. Surf.* **2019**, *17*, 98–103. [CrossRef]
24. Riemens, A.; Te Boome, L.; Imhof, S.; Kuball, J.; Rothova, A. Current Insights into Ocular Graft-versus-Host Disease. *Curr. Opin. Ophthalmol.* **2010**, *21*, 485–494. [CrossRef]
25. Ogawa, Y.; Okamoto, S.; Wakui, M.; Watanabe, R.; Yamada, M.; Yoshino, M.; Ono, M.; Yang, H.Y.; Mashima, Y.; Oguchi, Y.; et al. Dry Eye after Haematopoietic Stem Cell Transplantation. *Br. J. Ophthalmol.* **1999**, *83*, 1125–1130. [CrossRef]
26. Sinha, S.; Singh, R.B.; Dohlman, T.H.; Taketani, Y.; Yin, J.; Dana, R. Prevalence and Risk Factors Associated with Corneal Perforation in Chronic Ocular Graft-Versus-Host-Disease. *Cornea* **2021**, *40*, 877–882. [CrossRef]
27. Wang, Y.; Ogawa, Y.; Dogru, M.; Tatematsu, Y.; Uchino, M.; Kamoi, M.; Okada, N.; Okamoto, S.; Tsubota, K. Baseline Profiles of Ocular Surface and Tear Dynamics after Allogeneic Hematopoietic Stem Cell Transplantation in Patients with or without Chronic GVHD-Related Dry Eye. *Bone Marrow Transplant.* **2010**, *45*, 1077–1083. [CrossRef]
28. Ban, Y.; Ogawa, Y.; Ibrahim, O.M.A.; Tatematsu, Y.; Kamoi, M.; Uchino, M.; Yaguchi, S.; Dogru, M.; Tsubota, K. Morphologic Evaluation of Meibomian Glands in Chronic Graft-versus-Host Disease Using in Vivo Laser Confocal Microscopy. *Mol. Vis.* **2011**, *17*, 2533.
29. Franklin, R.M.; Kenyon, K.R.; Tutschka, P.J.; Saral, R.; Richard Green, W.; Santos, G.W. Ocular Manifestations of Graft-vs-Host Disease. *Ophthalmology* **1983**, *90*, 4–13. [CrossRef]
30. Johnson, D.A.; Jabs, D.A. The Ocular Manifestations of Graft-versus-Host Disease. *Int. Ophthalmol. Clin.* **1997**, *37*, 119–133. [CrossRef]
31. Hayashi, S.; Shimizu, E.; Uchino, M.; Yazu, H.; Aketa, N.; Tsubota, K.; Ogawa, Y. The Overlap Syndrome: A Case Report of Chronic Graft-Versus-Host Disease After the Development of a Pseudomembrane. *Cornea* **2021**, *40*, 1188–1192. [CrossRef]
32. Filipovich, A.H.; Weisdorf, D.; Pavletic, S.; Socie, G.; Wingard, J.R.; Lee, S.J.; Martin, P.; Chien, J.; Przepiorka, D.; Couriel, D.; et al. National Institutes of Health Consensus Development Project on Criteria for Clinical Trials in Chronic Graft-versus-Host Disease: I. Diagnosis and Staging Working Group Report. *Biol. Blood Marrow Transplant.* **2005**, *11*, 945–956. [CrossRef]
33. Shamloo, K.; Weng, J.; Ross, C.; Lee, J.; Alfuraih, S.; Totonchy, J.; Sharma, A. Local Renin-Angiotensin System Activation and Myofibroblast Formation in Graft Versus Host Disease-Associated Conjunctival Fibrosis. *Investig. Ophthalmol. Vis. Sci.* **2021**, *62*, 10. [CrossRef]

34. Gehlsen, U.; Faust, C.; Blecha, C.; Dietrich-Ntoukas, T.; Eberwein, P.; Issleib, S.; Meyer-ter-Vehn, T.; Braun, R.; Westekemper, H.; Steven, P. Outcomes and Complications of Cataract Surgery in Patients with Chronic Ocular Graft-versus-Host-Disease-a Multicenter, Retrospective Analysis. *Graefes Arch. Clin. Exp. Ophthalmol.* **2022**, *260*, 2613–2622. [CrossRef]
35. Mudhar, H. Update on Conjunctival Pathology. *Indian J. Ophthalmol.* **2017**, *65*, 797–807. [CrossRef]

life

MDPI

Article

Corneal Biomechanics and Other Factors Associated with Postoperative Astigmatism after Cataract Surgery

Kata Čulina [1], Martina Tomić [2], Tomislav Bulum [2,3,*], Aleksej Medić [1], Ivan Šoša [4], Kristina Ivanišević [5] and Tomislav Jukić [1,3,6]

1 Eye Clinic "Medić, Jukić", 21000 Split, Croatia
2 Vuk Vrhovac University Clinic for Diabetes, Endocrinology and Metabolic Diseases, Merkur University Hospital, 10000 Zagreb, Croatia
3 School of Medicine, University of Zagreb, 10000 Zagreb, Croatia
4 School of Medicine, University of Rijeka, 51000 Rijeka, Croatia
5 Ophthalmological Office "Ante Vuković", 21300 Makarska, Croatia
6 Department of Ophthalmology, Zagreb University Hospital Center, 10000 Zagreb, Croatia
* Correspondence: tomobulum@gmail.com; Tel.: +385-12353887; Fax: +385-12331515

Abstract: This study aimed to investigate the impact of the cornea's biomechanical properties, corneal hysteresis (CH), and corneal resistance factor (CRF) on postoperative astigmatism after cataract surgery and determine the other factors that influence it. Forty eyes of 40 patients (13M/27F; the median age of 74) were included in this prospective study, underwent 2.75 mm incision cataract surgery, and were followed for 30 days. Visits were scheduled at baseline before surgery (V0), the 1st (V1), the 7th (V2), and the 30th (V3) postoperative days. The main parameters estimated and analyzed with Statistica® 14.0.1 were CH, CRF, astigmatism diopter, and axis. Following the cataract surgery, the CH did not significantly change during the study visits ($p = 0.109$). However, there was a significant change in the CRF from baseline during the study visits (per protocol set) ($p = 0.002$). After a slight but insignificant increase from V0 to V1, post hoc analysis found a significant decrease in the mean CRF from V1 to V2 ($p = 0.049$) with no substantial change from V2 to V3. According to the post hoc analysis, the median astigmatism diopter increased significantly only from V0 to V1 ($p = 0.001$) and slightly but not significantly decreased to the end of the study with the achievement of a near-baseline value. The main predictors for the final astigmatism diopter ($R^2 = 0.898$) obtained by stepwise regression analysis were its values at V0, V1, and V2 ($p < 0.001$). The CRF at V1 was marginally significant, with a negative parameter estimate of -0.098303 ($p = 0.0623$). In conclusion, there was no correlation between preoperative CH and CRF and postoperative astigmatism using 2.75 mm incision cataract surgery. However, the final astigmatism diopter's main predictors were its baseline values before cataract surgery, the first, and the seventh postoperative days.

Keywords: corneal hysteresis; corneal resistance factor; cataract surgery; preoperative and postoperative astigmatism

1. Introduction

Cataract surgery today is no longer just removing a clouded eye lens but also a refractive procedure aiming to achieve emmetropia. Choosing the appropriate intraocular lens (IOL) is one of the essential factors in achieving the best possible refractive results. Another equally important factor is the size of the surgical incision, since it can affect postoperative astigmatism, a significant cause of poor uncorrected visual acuity after cataract surgery. Today's microincision cataract surgery minimizes the prevalence of postoperative surgically induced astigmatism (SIA) [1,2].

Except for the incision size, SIA also depends on other factors. The factors that have been mainly studied so far are the position and architecture of the incision. Regarding the position of the incision, there are corneal, limbal, scleral, and corneoscleral incisions.

The most frequently used approach in modern cataract surgery is a corneal incision, and the postoperative astigmatism is smaller with increasing distance from the cornea [3,4]. Most studies suggest that the temporal position of the incision results in smaller surgically induced astigmatism if there is mild preoperative astigmatism and against-the-rule astigmatism [5–7]. In contrast, the superior position is more adequate for more significant preoperative astigmatism and with-the-rule astigmatism [8,9]. Regarding the architecture of the incision, there are several incision forms: uniplanar, biplanar, triplanar, and hinged corneal incision [10]. The incision architecture is essential for wound stability, which implies proper adhesion of incision edges, protection from infection, adequate wound healing, and reduction in surgically induced astigmatism [11,12].

However, the cornea's biological influence is still insufficiently understood, but it may play a role in postoperative astigmatism. The cornea's biological factors are its biomechanical properties: corneal hysteresis (CH) and corneal resistance factor (CRF) [13–15]. The CH refers to the cornea's elastic properties, that is, its ability to return to its original position after temporary deformation, and the CRF indicates the cornea's resistance to stress. The correlation between CH, CRF, and SIA is still unclear and dependent on other factors.

The biomechanical properties of the cornea may relate to SIA because cataract surgery causes a kind of stress in the cornea. In a clinical setting, it would be important to better understand the cornea's reaction to cataract surgery and to detect whether and how much cataract surgery affects the cornea's biomechanical properties and the cornea's postoperative return to its original state. This study aimed to investigate the impact of the cornea's biomechanical properties, CH and CRF, and other factors on postoperative astigmatism after cataract surgery.

2. Patients and Methods

2.1. Study Design and Patients

This prospective, observational cohort study was conducted at the Eye Clinic "Medic, Jukic" in Split, Croatia, following the Declaration of Helsinki, and was approved by the Eye Clinical Ethics Committee. The study's patients received written and oral information about the study and signed written informed consent.

Forty patients (13 males and 27 females) referred to the Eye Clinic because of low visual acuity were included in this study, underwent cataract surgery, and were followed for 30 days. All included patients had best-corrected visual acuity (BCVA) ≤ 0.5 and immature cataracts graded as C2N3P2 to C4N4P4 according to the Lens Opacities Classification System (LOCS) [16]. Exclusion criteria were ocular surface disease, i.e., dry eye disease (Schirmer test < 10 mm, tear break-up time (TBUT) < 5 s, fluorescein positive test), pathology of the cornea, glaucoma, ocular hypertension, high refractive errors (myopia > −6 Dsph, hypermetropia > +5 Dsph), pseudoexfoliative syndrome, and intraoperative and postoperative complications.

2.2. Scheduled Visits and Ophthalmological Examinations

The first baseline visit (V0) was the inclusion visit in the study, performed before the cataract surgery, while the three further follow-up visits were scheduled on the first (V1), seventh (V2), and thirtieth postoperative days (V3).

At the first baseline visit, all patients underwent standard ophthalmological examinations and special diagnostics. Standard examinations included Snellen visual acuity and refraction testing, Goldman applanation tonometry, slit-lamp examination of the anterior eye segment in the physiological state and after mydriasis with eye drops containing 0.5% tropicamide, and indirect slit-lamp fundoscopy, both performed using the Zeiss Slit-lamp (Carl Zeiss Meditec AG, Jena, Germany).

After standard examinations, special diagnostics included corneal topography using the WaveLight Oculyzer™ II diagnostic system (Alcon, Freiburg im Breisgau, Germany) for the determination of corneal astigmatism diopter and axis, measurement of CH and CRF by the Ocular Response Analyzer G3 (ORA G3) (Reichert Inc., Buffalo, NY, USA), and examination at the Zeiss IOL Master 700 (Carl Zeiss Meditec AG, Jena, Germany), the first swept-source OCT-based biometer that enables OCT imaging and visualization of the entire length of the eyeball to determine the appropriate intraocular lens. Surgically induced astigmatism (SIA) diopter and axis were calculated using the corneal SIA tool available online on the American Society of Cataract and Refractive Surgery website (https://ascrs.org/tools/corneal-sia-tool (accessed on 1 March 2024)) [17].

At the further three follow-up visits (per protocol set), all patients underwent the following clinical and diagnostic examinations: Snellen visual acuity and refraction testing, corneal topography, corneal biomechanics (CH and CRF) measurements, and SIA diopter and axis calculation. All examinations and measurements at the first baseline and further follow-up visits were performed by the first author of this manuscript.

2.3. Measurement of Corneal Hysteresis and Corneal Resistance Factor

With its electro-optical system, the Ocular Response Analyzer (ORA) allows cornea-compensated intraocular pressure (IOP) measurements and can estimate CH and CRF [18,19]. It is designed to improve the accuracy of the IOP measurement by using corneal biomechanical data to calculate a biomechanically adjusted estimate of IOP. ORA measures the IOP at the moment when the deformation (i.e., applanation) of the cornea begins (P1) and the IOP at the moment when the deformation (i.e., applanation) ends (P2). During applanation, the cornea absorbs part of the energy; because of this, there is a difference in the initial and final applanation pressures, respectively. The pressure at which the applanation ends is lower than when the applanation begins. This pressure difference, P1–P2, represents the cornea's elastic property or CH and is measured in mmHg. A higher CH indicates a greater ability of the cornea to return to its initial state after applying stress. The CRF represents the cornea's resistance to stress and is calculated using the formula $CRF = P1 - kP2$, where k denotes a constant obtained by empirical evaluation of the relationship between the initial applanation intraocular pressure (P1), final applanation intraocular pressure (P2), and central corneal thickness. The CRF is also measured in mmHg. A higher CRF indicates a higher cornea's resistance to permanent deformation after applied stress.

2.4. Cataract Surgery

Cataract surgery was performed by a single operator, the last author of this manuscript, using the ophthalmic microscope OPMI Lumera 700 (Carl Zeiss Meditec AG, Jena, Germany) and phacoemulsification device Centurion Vision System (Alcon Laboratories, Inc., Fort Worth, TX, USA). The operation was performed through a 2.75 mm corneal incision positioned at 12 o'clock in the superior position using the phacoemulsification method with IOL implantation in the capsular bag. Postoperatively, all patients received the same therapy: Maxitrol Eye Drops four times a day and Maxitrol Eye Ointment once a day for the first seven days, and then Maxitrol Eye Drops three times a day for the next two weeks.

2.5. Statistical Analysis

Statistical analysis was performed, and the graphs were created using the statistical package Statistica™ 14.0.1. In all analyses, a p-value < 0.05 was considered statistically significant. After testing the normality of the data distribution with the Shapiro–Wilk test, normally distributed continuous variables were expressed as mean $\pm$ SD and non-normally distributed variables as median (min, max). The categorical variable (gender) was presented as a number. Differences in the distributions of dependent continuous data were evaluated by parametric (repeated measures ANOVA) and nonparametric (Friedman ANOVA) tests. A nonparametric test was used when the assumption of homogeneity of variance for the tested variables was not met. The Scheffe and Wilcoxon tests were used for post hoc analyses. The Spearman rank correlation test was used to evaluate the relationship between the studied variables, and stepwise regression was used to detect the main predictors of the final astigmatism diopter.

3. Results

Forty eyes of 40 patients, with a median age of 74 (min 48, max 83) years, were included in this study. Their baseline characteristics at the inclusion visit before cataract surgery (V0) are presented in Table 1.

Table 1. Baseline characteristics of 40 patients (eyes) included in the study.

Characteristics	Patients/Eyes (n = 40)
CH (mmHg) *	8.86 ± 2.44
CRF (mmHg) *	10.04 ± 2.32
BCVA (decimal) *	0.29 ± 0.18
Refraction (SE) **	−0.75 (−6.0, 3.5)
Astigmatism (D) **	0.4 (−4.5, 2.4)
Axis (°) **	78.2 (1.6, 177.3)

* mean ± SD. ** median (min, max). Abbreviations: CH—corneal hysteresis, CRF—corneal resistance factor, BCVA—best-corrected visual acuity, SE—spherical equivalent, D—diopter of corneal astigmatism determined by corneal topography, °—degrees of corneal astigmatism axis determined by corneal topography.

Following the cataract surgery, the CH did not significantly change during the study visits (p = 0.109) (Table 2, Figure 1A). However, there was a significant change in the CRF from baseline during the study visits (per protocol set) in 40 study eyes (p = 0.002) (Table 2, Figure 1B). According to the post hoc analysis, the mean CRF decreased significantly from the first (V1) to the second postoperative visit (V2) (10.49 ± 3.22 vs. 9.31 ± 1.87, p = 0.049), after a slight but insignificant increase from baseline (V0) to the first postoperative visit (V1) (p = 0.761). However, no substantial change in the mean CRF was observed from the second (V2) to the third postoperative visit (V3) (p = 0.933).

Table 2. Changes in the analyzed characteristics from baseline during the study visits (per protocol set) in 40 study patients (eyes).

Characteristics	V0	V1	V2	V3	p
CH (mmHg) *	8.86 ± 2.44	7.73 ± 2.91	8.26 ± 1.73	8.30 ± 2.04	0.109 [a]
CRF (mmHg) *	10.04 ± 2.32	10.49 ± 3.22	9.31 ± 1.87	9.03 ± 1.99	0.002 [a]
BCVA (decimal) *	0.29 ± 0.18	0.49 ± 0.19	0.83 ± 0.12	0.92 ± 0.09	<0.001 [a]
Refraction (SE) **	−0.75 (−6.0, 3.5)	−0.37 (−1.5, 1.0)	−0.5 (−1.0, 0.5)	−0.2 (−0.75, 0.75)	0.033 [b]
Astigmatism (D) **	0.4 (−4.5, 2.4)	0.8 (−1.4, 2.9)	0.7 (−1.8, 3.0)	0.5 (−1.9, 3.0)	0.009 [b]
Axis (°) **	78.2 (1.6, 177.3)	67.9 (1.4, 175.2)	72.2 (1.3, 178.7)	68.0 (2.6, 178.8)	0.861 [b]
SIA (D) **	-	0.79 (0.11, 4.24)	0.69 (0.1, 3.76)	0.63 (0.1, 4.06)	0.741 [b]
SIA (°) **	-	132.0 (3, 177)	125.5 (3, 174)	113.5 (1.7, 177)	0.312 [b]

* mean ± SD. ** median (min, max). [a] Repeated measures ANOVA test. [b] Friedman ANOVA test Abbreviations: CH—corneal hysteresis, CRF—corneal resistance factor, BCVA—best-corrected visual acuity, SE—spherical equivalent, Astigmatism (D)—diopter of corneal astigmatism determined by corneal topography, Axis (°)—degrees of astigmatism axis, SIA (D)—diopter of surgically induced astigmatism, SIA (°)—degree of surgically induced astigmatism axis.

BCVA increased significantly from baseline during the study visits (per protocol set) (p < 0.001) (Table 2). The post hoc analysis also showed a significant increase in BCVA between each study visit (V0–V1 p < 0.001, V1–V2 p < 0.001, V2–V3 p = 0.019). The spherical equivalent (SE) refraction decreased significantly during the study period (p = 0.033). However, the post hoc analysis found a marginal decrease in the SE between V0 and V1 (p = 0.058) and a significant decline between V2 and V3 (p < 0.001).

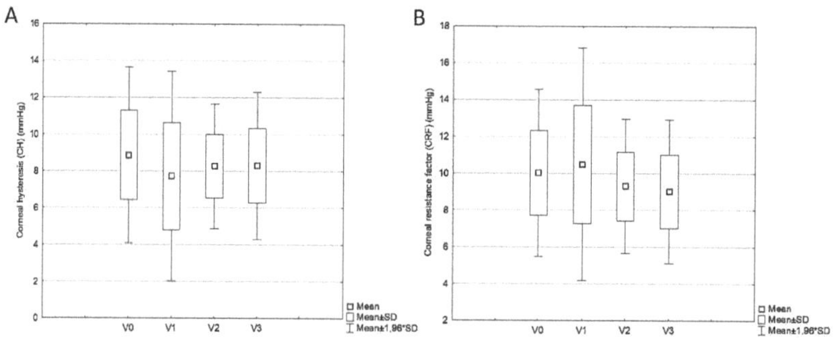

Figure 1. Change in corneal hysteresis (**A**) and corneal resistance factor (**B**) from baseline during the study visits in 40 study eyes.

As with the CRF, the diopter of corneal astigmatism determined by corneal topography significantly changed in 40 eyes from baseline to the study visits (as planned) ($p = 0.009$) (Table 2, Figure 2A). However, according to the post hoc analysis, the median diopter of astigmatism changed significantly only from the baseline (V0) to the first postoperative visit (V1) (0.4 D vs. 0.8 D, $p = 0.001$). In contrast, there were no significant changes in the median diopter of astigmatism from the first (V0) to the second (V2) ($p = 0.139$) or from the second (V2) to the third postoperative visit (V3) ($p = 0.863$). The median degree of the corneal astigmatism axis determined by corneal topography did not significantly change from the study's baseline to each visit in 40 study eyes (Table 2, Figure 2B). However, the amplitudes of corneal astigmatism diopter and axis changes were the highest between baseline (V0) and the first postoperative visit (V1), decreasing gradually until the study's end (Figure 2C,D). In contrast to the diopter of corneal astigmatism determined by corneal topography, the SIA diopter did not significantly differ throughout the study ($p = 0.741$) (Table 2). Also, no differences in the SIA axis were observed during the study period ($p = 0.312$) (Table 2).

Significantly positive, moderate to very good, or excellent correlations were seen between the CH and CRF at the beginning of the study, before cataract surgery, and at all other study visits (Table 3).

Nevertheless, no significant relation was found between corneal characteristics (CH and CRF) and the diopter and axis of corneal astigmatism at baseline and all other study visits ($p > 0.05$) (data not shown in table). Also, no relationships were observed between the baseline preoperative and all postoperative study visit values of CH, CRF, SIA diopter, and SIA axis (($p > 0.05$) (data not shown in table).

The diopter of corneal astigmatism at the final visit was significantly positive or very good to excellent and associated with its values at baseline before cataract surgery and other study visits ($p < 0.001$) (Table 4). However, the amplitude of corneal astigmatism change from baseline (V0) to the final visit (V3) related significantly positively only to the amplitude of the astigmatism change between baseline (V0) and the first postoperative visit (V1) ($p < 0.001$), while the other relations were not significant ($p > 0.05$) (Table 5).

The main predictors for the final diopter of corneal astigmatism ($R^2 = 0.898$) obtained by stepwise regression analysis were its values at baseline before cataract surgery (V0), the first (V1), and the seventh postoperative day (V2) (Table 6). Besides all those listed, the CRF at the first postoperative day (V1) was found to be marginally significant, with the negative parameter estimate of -0.098303 ($p = 0.0623$) influencing the final astigmatism diopter value relative to its one-unit change and representing the marginal impact of the weaker corneal characteristic (weaker resistance of the cornea to stress) on postoperative astigmatism.

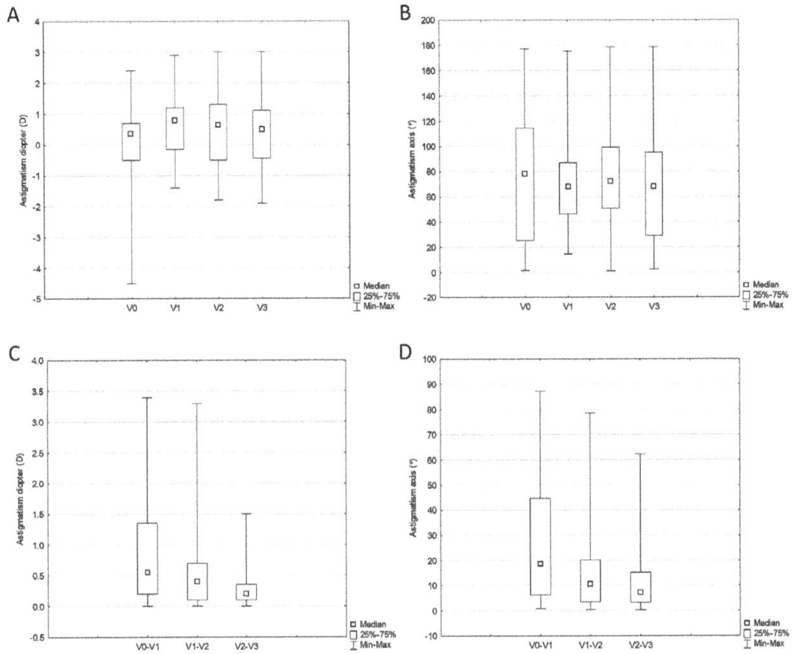

Figure 2. Change in astigmatism diopter (**A**) and axis (**B**) from baseline during the study visits in 40 study eyes and the amplitudes of their changes (**C**,**D**) between study visits.

Table 3. Correlations between corneal hysteresis and corneal resistance factor from baseline during the study visits (per protocol set) in 40 study eyes.

		Corneal Hysteresis				**Corneal Resistance Factor**			
		V0	**V1**	**V2**	**V3**	**V0**	**V1**	**V2**	**V3**
Corneal hysteresis	V0	1	0.046	0.348 *	0.498 *	0.889 **	0.217	0.441 *	0.595 **
	V1		1	0.247	0.177	0.103	0.499 *	0.345 *	0.239
	V2			1	0.560 **	0.451 *	0.223	0.809 **	0.643 **
	V3				1	0.445 *	0.175	0.506 **	0.864 **
Corneal resistance factor	V0					1	0.349 *	0.620 **	0.631 **
	V1						1	0.399 *	0.318 *
	V2							1	0.708 **
	V3								1

* $p < 0.05$. ** $p < 0.001$. Spearman rank correlation test.

Table 4. Correlations between the diopter of corneal astigmatism at final (V3), baseline (V0), and other study visits (V1, V2) in 40 study eyes.

		Diopter of Corneal Astigmatism at V3		
		Spearman R	**t (N-2)**	***p***
Diopter of corneal astigmatism	V0	0.736	6.7	<0.001
	V1	0.639	5.133	<0.001
	V2	0.894	12.267	<0.001

Table 5. Correlations between the amplitude of corneal astigmatism change from V0 to V3 and the amplitude of astigmatism changes at intermediate times during the study.

		Amplitude of Corneal Astigmatism Change between V0 and V3		
		Spearman R	t (N-2)	*p*
Amplitude of corneal astigmatism changes	V0–V1	0.525	3.803	<0.001
	V1–V2	0.203	1.276	0.209
	V2–V3	−0.062	−0.381	0.705

Table 6. Results of stepwise regression analysis for the final diopter of corneal astigmatism as a dependent variable.

Variable	Estimate	Standard Error	F	*p*	Adjusted R^2	R^2
CRF—V1	−0.098	1.028	3.69	0.0623	0.0645	
Astigmatism—V0	0.504	0.759	38.55	0.0000	0.4905	0.898
Astigmatism—V1	0.497	0.764	37.49	0.0000	0.4834	
Astigmatism—V2	0.898	0.345	333.07	0.0000	0.8949	

Abbreviations: CRF—corneal resistance factor.

4. Discussion

Cataract surgery with sophisticated intraocular lens implantation requires the most accurate prediction of postoperative refractive results. The present study tried to establish whether the biomechanical properties of the cornea influence these results and to determine which other factors have a role in postoperative astigmatism after cataract surgery.

Only a few studies have examined the association between the cornea's biomechanical properties and SIA. The first published study was by Denoyer et al. [20]. They found a positive correlation between incision size and SIA and a negative correlation between preoperative CH, CRF, and SIA values. The present study did not find a correlation between the cornea's biomechanical properties (CH and CRF) and the diopter and axis of corneal astigmatism and SIA. However, this study's results indicate that CH and CRF values changed after cataract surgery. The CH decreased marginally, and the CRF increased marginally from baseline to the first postoperative day, while both variables gradually recovered in the following days. The CH recovered better than the CRF on the 30th postoperative day, but both returned to near-preoperative values.

Denoyer et al., in their study, monitored changes in CH and CRF after cataract surgery in two groups of patients [20]. In one group, cataract surgery was performed through a small incision (2.75 mm), while in the other group, it was performed through a microincision (≤2.2 mm). In their study, CH and CRF decreased postoperatively. As in the present study, CH recovers entirely on the 30th postoperative day. However, regarding CRF, there are some discrepancies between the present study and the study of Denoyer et al. Denoyer et al. found a recovery of CRF to preoperative values in the microincision group. In the small incision group, when a step-constructed triplanar incision was performed, the CRF recovered rapidly, while when other uniplanar and biplanar incisions were completed, the CRF was significantly reduced. Based on these results, the authors suggested that the stepped triplanar construction of the incision is a better choice in cataract surgery because it does not weaken the corneal resistance [20].

Zheng et al., in their study, examined the changes in CH and CRF after cataract surgery performed through 2.2 mm and 3.0 mm incisions. The incisions were made biplanarly at the 10 o'clock position with a distance of 0.5 mm from the limbus. While CH values fluctuated, as in the study of Denoyer et al., CRF values did not change significantly during the four weeks after surgery [21].

Pniakowska et al. analyzed the changes in CH and CRF after cataract surgery through a 2 mm incision at the 12 o'clock position without specifying the architectural type of the incision in two groups of patients: group 1 with corneal astigmatism values of less than +1.0 dcyl and group 2 with values between +1.0 dcyl and +2.25 dcyl. Their results showed a postoperative decrease in CH and CRF values in the first group of patients. The CH recovered to preoperative values, and the CRF remained significantly reduced one month after surgery. In the second group, the CH and CRF remained significantly lowered one month after cataract surgery [22].

In the present study, cataract surgery was performed through a 2.75 mm biplanar incision, and as previously mentioned, we noted a slight but statistically insignificant increase in CRF values in the 1st postoperative day, with a significant decrease till the 7th, and a gradual insignificant reduction toward the 30th postoperative day. This decrease in CRF values on the 30th postoperative day contradicts the results of Zheng et al. but coincides with the results of the studies by Denoyer et al. and Pniakowska et al. Following Denoyer et al.'s thinking about the influence of the architecture of the incision on corneal resistance, it might be stated that the small biplanar incision leads to a certain degree of weakening of the corneal resistance.

Usually, SIA positively correlates with incision size, and larger incisions induce more astigmatism. An incision width of 1.8–2.2 mm has a relatively small SIA [23]. Astigmatic effects have been reduced after decreasing the incision size from 3.2 mm to 2.2 mm or 1.8 mm. A study that included 146 eyes found that a corneal incision of 2.75 mm for cataract surgery, using either a temporal or superior approach, induces little astigmatism change in eyes [24]. Another study that included 100 eyes of 50 patients who underwent bilateral intraocular lens implantation through a 2.2 mm or 2.75 mm corneal incision found that a lower incision size of 2.2 mm compared to 2.75 mm did not result in less SIA [25]. In addition, a study that investigated the changes in incision sizes after implantation of an intraocular lens with a mean incision size of 2.27 mm found that the CH and CRF values were not correlated with the final incision size, and the CH was more predictive of postoperative surgically induced astigmatism than incision size [26].

The present study did not find a correlation between corneal biomechanical properties and postoperative astigmatism after cataract surgery. However, as in the CRF value, there was a significant change in the diopter of corneal astigmatism from baseline during the study visits (per protocol set). These two variables changed similarly; the mean CRF and the median diopter of corneal astigmatism increased from baseline to the first postoperative day, while after that, they both decreased in the 7th and 30th postoperative days.

The increase in median diopter of corneal astigmatism after cataract surgery is because of a corneal shape change due to wounds at the incision site and postoperative corneal edema [27]. Regarding CRF, while in most studies, it decreases postoperatively or remains the same, in this study, we note a slight increase on the first postoperative day. Similar behavior of the cornea was described in the study of Alió et al. [28]. They registered a postoperative increase in CRF, followed by its decrease, after cataract surgery in the group with microincision, while in the group with coaxial phacoemulsification, they did not find a significant change.

Postoperative astigmatism can also be influenced by corneal thickness [29]. The cornea is thicker in the vertical than the horizontal direction, so the posterior cornea surface is more astigmatic than the anterior corneal surface. The cornea is also thinner in older age [30]. However, pericentral corneal thickness is significantly greater in the superior quadrant and not affected by aging compared to the inferior, nasal, and temporal quadrants [29]. In this study, we did not measure the corneal thickness, and the surgery was performed through a 2.75 mm corneal incision at 12 o'clock in the superior position. This area has the thickest cornea compared to other places, and corneal thickness is negatively related to corneal astigmatism [31].

Different corneal incision positions have different risks of SIA because of the different distances of each position to the central visual axis [32]. Common incision positions include temporal, superior, and nasal. In the present study, we used a corneal incision positioned at 12 o'clock in the superior position. Temporal and nasal incisions postoperatively have similar corneal and astigmatic changes and induce a lower degree of SIA compared to the superior position. Superior positions have longer proximity of the superior limbus to the central visual axis and are recommended for with-the-rule and negligible astigmatism [33].

Several limitations of the present study must be mentioned. Similar changes in median diopter of corneal astigmatism and CRF observed in this study could be explained by postoperative changes in corneal thickness. A corneal pachymeter measures corneal thickness, a sensitive indicator of endothelial physiology that correlates well with functional measurements. However, this study did not monitor corneal thickness, which is a limiting factor. Second, the operation was performed only through a 2.75 mm corneal incision, so we could not compare the impact on CH and CRF values with different incision sizes. Third, different corneal incision positions (superior used in this study, temporal) have different risks of postoperative astigmatism. Finally, the sample size in this study was small, reducing the study's power.

5. Conclusions

Postoperative astigmatism is a significant cause of poor visual acuity after cataract surgery. In this short-term follow-up of one month postoperatively, there was no correlation between preoperative CH and CRF and postoperative astigmatism using 2.75 mm superior incision cataract surgery. However, the main predictors for the final diopter of astigmatism were its values at baseline before cataract surgery, the first, and the seventh postoperative day. The discrepancy with the results of several studies conducted so far points to the need for additional research on a larger number of patients in order to better understand the cornea's reaction to cataract surgery and thus achieve more precise postoperative results.

Author Contributions: K.Č. designed the trial and wrote the study protocol; she was responsible for regulatory authority, ethics committee approval, patient recruitment, examinations, and original draft writing. M.T. was responsible for statistical analysis, interpretation of data, and results writing, and T.B. was responsible for correspondence and critically reviewing and editing the manuscript. A.M., I.Š. and K.I. were liable for collecting medical records and documentation, reviewing, and editing. T.J. performed the cataract surgery and supervised the study protocol. All authors have read and agreed to the published version of the manuscript.

Funding: This research received no specific grant from public, commercial, or not-for-profit funding agencies.

Institutional Review Board Statement: The study was conducted according to the Declaration of Helsinki and approved by the Eye Clinic's Ethics Committee (protocol number 09/137-22, approval date: 5 December 2022).

Informed Consent Statement: Informed consent was obtained from all subjects included in the study.

Data Availability Statement: The data presented in this study are available on a specific request from the corresponding author.

Conflicts of Interest: All authors declare no competing interests.

References

1. Liang, J.L.; Xing, X.L.; Yang, X.T.; Jiang, Y.F.; Zhang, H. Clinical comparison analysis in surgically induced astigmatism of the total, anterior and posterior cornea after 2.2-mm versus 3.0-mm clear corneal incision cataract surgery. *Zhonghua Yan Ke Za Zhi* **2019**, *55*, 495–501. [CrossRef] [PubMed]
2. Pattanayak, S.; Mathur, S.; Nanda, A.K.; Subudhi, B.N.R. Postoperative astigmatic considerations in manual small-incision cataract surgery—A review. *Indian J. Ophthalmol.* **2022**, *70*, 3785–3790. [CrossRef] [PubMed]
3. Sonmez, S.; Karaca, C. The effect of tunnel length and position on postoperative corneal astigmatism: An optical coherence tomographic study. *Eur. J. Ophthalmol.* **2020**, *30*, 104–111. [CrossRef] [PubMed]
4. Hashemi, H.; Khabazkhoob, M.; Soroush, S.; Shariati, R.; Miraftab, M.; Yekta, A. The location of incision in cataract surgery and its impact on induced astigmatism. *Curr. Opin. Ophthalmol.* **2016**, *27*, 58–64. [CrossRef] [PubMed]
5. Barequet, I.S.; Yu, E.; Vitale, S.; Cassard, S.; Azar, D.T.; Stark, W.J. Astigmatism outcomes of horizontal temporal versus nasal clear corneal incision cataract surgery. *J. Cataract Refract. Surg.* **2004**, *30*, 418–423. [CrossRef] [PubMed]

6. Borasio, E.; Mehta, J.S.; Maurino, V. Surgically induced astigmatism after phacoemulsification in eyes with mild to moderate corneal astigmatism: Temporal versus on-axis clear corneal incisions. *J. Cataract Refract. Surg.* **2006**, *32*, 565–572. [CrossRef] [PubMed]
7. Altan-Yaycioglu, R.; Akova, Y.A.; Akca, S.; Gur, S.; Oktem, C. Effect on astigmatism of the location of clear corneal incision in phacoemulsification of cataract. *J. Refract. Surg.* **2007**, *23*, 515–518. [CrossRef] [PubMed]
8. Roman, S.; Givort, G.; Ullern, M. Choice of the site of incision for cataract surgery without suture according to preoperative astigmatism. *J. Fr. Ophtalmol.* **1997**, *20*, 673–679.
9. Archana, S.; Khurana, A.K.; Chawla, U. A comparative study of sclero-corneal and clear corneal tunnel incision in manual small-incision cataract surgery. *Nepal. J. Ophthalmol.* **2011**, *3*, 19–22. [CrossRef]
10. Taban, M.; Rao, B.; Reznik, J.; Zhang, J.; Chen, Z.; McDonnell, P.J. Dynamic morphology of sutureless cataract wounds—Effect of incision angle and location. *Surv. Ophthalmol.* **2004**, *49* (Suppl. S2), S62–S72. [CrossRef]
11. Simşek, S.; Yaşar, T.; Demirok, A.; Cinal, A.; Yilmaz, O.F. Effect of superior and temporal clear corneal incisions on astigmatism after sutureless phacoemulsification. *J. Cataract Refract. Surg.* **1998**, *24*, 515–518. [CrossRef] [PubMed]
12. Ernest, P.; Hill, W.; Potvin, R. Minimizing surgically induced astigmatism at the time of cataract surgery using a square posterior limbal incision. *J. Ophthalmol.* **2011**, *2011*, 243170. [CrossRef] [PubMed]
13. Glass, D.H.; Roberts, C.J.; Litsky, A.S.; Weber, P.A. A viscoelastic biomechanical model of the cornea describing the effect of viscosity and elasticity on hysteresis. *Investig. Ophthalmol. Vis. Sci.* **2008**, *49*, 3919–3926. [CrossRef] [PubMed]
14. Kotecha, A. What biomechanical properties of the cornea are relevant for the clinician? *Surv. Ophthalmol.* **2007**, *52* (Suppl. S2), S109–S114. [CrossRef] [PubMed]
15. Chong, J.; Dupps, W.J., Jr. Corneal biomechanics: Measurement and structural correlations. *Exp. Eye. Res.* **2021**, *205*, 108508. [CrossRef] [PubMed]
16. Chylack, L.T., Jr.; Wolfe, J.K.; Singer, D.M.; Leske, M.C.; Bullimore, M.A.; Bailey, I.L.; Friend, J.; McCarthy, D.; Wu, S.Y. The Lens Opacities Classification System III. *Arch. Ophthalmol.* **1993**, *111*, 831–836. [CrossRef] [PubMed]
17. Koch, D.D.; Wang, L. Surgically induced astigmatism. *J. Refract. Surg.* **2015**, *31*, 565. [CrossRef] [PubMed]
18. Luce, D.A. Determining in vivo biomechanical properties of the cornea with an ocular response analyzer. *J. Cataract. Refract. Surg.* **2005**, *31*, 156–162. [CrossRef] [PubMed]
19. Kaushik, S.; Pandav, S.S. Ocular response analyzer. *J. Curr. Glaucoma Pract.* **2012**, *6*, 17–19. [CrossRef]
20. Denoyer, A.; Ricaud, X.; Van Went, C.; Labbé, A.; Baudouin, C. Influence of corneal biomechanical properties on surgically induced astigmatism in cataract surgery. *J. Cataract Refract. Surg.* **2013**, *39*, 1204–1210. [CrossRef]
21. Zhang, Z.; Yu, H.; Dong, H.; Wang, L.; Jia, Y.D.; Zhang, S.H. Corneal biomechanical properties changes after coaxial 2.2-mm microincision and standard 3.0-mm phacoemulsification. *Int. J. Ophthalmol.* **2016**, *9*, 230–234. [CrossRef]
22. Pniakowska, Z.; Jurowski, P. Influence of preoperative astigmatism on corneal biomechanics and accurate intraocular pressure measurement after micro-incision phacoemulsification. *Int. J. Ophthalmol.* **2019**, *12*, 587–591. [CrossRef]
23. Yang, J.; Wang, X.; Zhang, H.; Pang, Y.; Wei, R.H. Clinical evaluation of surgery-induced astigmatism in cataract surgery using 2.2 mm or 1.8 mm clear corneal micro-incisions. *Int. J. Ophthalmol.* **2017**, *10*, 68–71. [CrossRef] [PubMed]
24. Giansanti, F.; Rapizzi, E.; Virgili, G.; Mencucci, R.; Bini, A.; Vannozzi, L.; Menchini, U. Clear corneal incision of 2.75 mm for cataract surgery induces little change of astigmatism in eyes with low preoperative corneal cylinder. *Eur. J. Ophthalmol.* **2006**, *16*, 385–393. [CrossRef]
25. Karmiris, E.; Chalkiadaki, E.; Papakonstantinou, E.; Georgalas, I. Long-term clinical outcomes obtained with bilateral implantation of a multifocal intraocular lens through two different-sized corneal incisions. *Saudi J. Ophthalmol.* **2022**, *36*, 207–212. [CrossRef] [PubMed]
26. Guarnieri, A.; Moreno-Montañés, J.; Sabater, A.; Gosende-Chico, I.; Bonet-Farriol, E. Final incision size after cataract surgery with toric intraocular lens implantation using 2 techniques. *J. Cataract Refract. Surg.* **2013**, *39*, 1675–1681. [CrossRef] [PubMed]
27. Alió, J.L.; Agdeppa, M.C.; Rodríguez-Prats, J.L.; Amparo, F.; Piñero, D.P. Factors influencing corneal biomechanical changes after microincision cataract surgery and standard coaxial phacoemulsification. *J. Cataract. Refract. Surg.* **2010**, *36*, 890–897. [CrossRef]
28. Sheoran, K.; Arya, S.K.; Bansal, R.K.; Jinagal, J.; Jha, U.P. Surgically induced astigmatism and posterior corneal curvature changes following phacoemulsification. *Indian J. Ophthalmol.* **2022**, *70*, 406–412. [CrossRef]
29. Ueno, Y.; Hiraoka, T.; Miyazaki, M.; Ito, M.; Oshika, T. Corneal thickness profile and posterior corneal astigmatism in normal corneas. *Ophthalmology* **2015**, *122*, 1072–1078. [CrossRef]
30. Ueno, Y.; Hiraoka, T.; Beheregaray, S.; Miyazaki, M.; Ito, M.; Oshika, T. Age-related changes in anterior, posterior, and total corneal astigmatism. *J. Refract. Surg.* **2014**, *30*, 192–197. [CrossRef]
31. Zhu, L.; Yuan, Z.; Liang, S.; Zhao, D.; Zhou, C. Relationship between corneal astigmatism and the distribution of corneal thickness along different principal meridians. *Res. Square* 2019. *preprint*. [CrossRef]

32. Nikose, A.S.; Saha, D.; Laddha, P.M.; Patil, M. Surgically induced astigmatism after phacoemulsification by temporal clear corneal and superior clear corneal approach: A comparison. *Clin. Ophthalmol.* **2018**, *12*, 65–70. [CrossRef] [PubMed]
33. Hayashi, K.; Sato, T.; Yoshida, M.; Yoshimura, K. Corneal shape changes of the total and posterior cornea after temporal versus nasal clear corneal incision cataract surgery. *Br. J. Ophthalmol.* **2019**, *103*, 181–185. [CrossRef] [PubMed]

life

MDPI

Article

Oxidative Stress, Persistent Inflammation and Blood Coagulation Alterations in Serum Proteome of Patients with Neovascular Age-Related Macular Degeneration

Mateusz Winiarczyk [1,*], Bernd Thiede [2], Tor Paaske Utheim [3,4], Kai Kaarniranta [5,6,7], Dagmara Winiarczyk [8], Katarzyna Michalak [9] and Jerzy Mackiewicz [1]

1 Department of Vitreoretinal Surgery, Medical University of Lublin, 20-079 Lublin, Poland; jerzymackiewicz@umlub.pl
2 Department of Biosciences, University of Oslo, 0371 Oslo, Norway; bernd.thiede@ibv.uio.no
3 Department of Medical Biochemistry, Oslo University Hospital, 0372 Oslo, Norway; uxutto@ous-hf.no
4 Department of Ophthalmology, Oslo University Hospital, 0450 Oslo, Norway
5 Department of Ophthalmology, University of Eastern Finland, 70211 Kuopio, Finland; kai.kaarniranta@uef.fi
6 Department of Ophthalmology, Kuopio University Hospital, 70200 Kuopio, Finland
7 Department of Molecular Genetics, University of Lodz, 90-136 Lodz, Poland
8 Department and Clinic of Animal Internal Diseases, Faculty of Veterinary Medicine, University of Life Sciences, 20-612 Lublin, Poland; dagmara.winiarczyk@up.lublin.pl
9 Department of Epizootiology and Clinic of Infectious Diseases, University of Life Sciences, 20-612 Lublin, Poland; katarzyna.michalak@up.lublin.pl
* Correspondence: mateuszwiniarczyk@umlub.pl

Abstract: Neovascular age-related macular degeneration (AMD) is a major cause of irreversible blindness in elderly populations in developed countries. AMD's etiopathology is multifactorial, with strong environmental and genetic components, but the exact molecular pathomechanisms underlying the disease are still unknown. In this study, we analyzed blood serum collected from 74 neovascular AMD patients and 58 healthy controls to identify proteins that may serve as potential biomarkers and expand our knowledge about the etiopathogenesis of the disease. The study revealed 17 differentially expressed proteins—11 up-regulated and 6 down-regulated—in neovascular AMD, which are involved in the biological processes previously linked with the disease—oxidative stress and persistent inflammation, impaired cellular transport, lipid metabolism and blood coagulation. In conclusion, the differences in the expressions of the proteins identified in this study may contribute to our understanding of the mechanisms underlying AMD and possibly serve in future as promising biomarkers.

Keywords: AMD proteome; proteomics; serum biomarkers; age-related macular degeneration

1. Introduction

Age-related macular degeneration (AMD) is a progressive, usually bilateral disease affecting the macula—the central part of the retina that is responsible for central, high-quality vision in good-lighting conditions. AMD is usually divided into its atrophic (dry) form, where retinal pigment epithelium (RPE) cells suffer progressive loss, and neovascular (wet, nAMD), with the creation of the pathological choroidal neovascularization (CNV) sprouting from the choroid into the subretinal or retinal tissue, with a tendency to leakage and evoking detrimental oedema. Both the atrophic and neovascular forms share some hallmarks, like the presence of the drusen—subretinal debris deposits. While numerous clinical trials are ongoing, there is currently no effective treatment for dry AMD. In nAMD, anti-vascular endothelial growth factor (anti-VEGF) intravitreal injections are the main line of treatment, yet their effect is usually limited to stopping or slowing down the disease, less often to significant visual improvement, especially if the treatment is introduced in the advanced form of the disease.

According to the WHO, the global population is rapidly aging, and the prevalence of AMD is therefore expected to rise. The estimated global prevalence of AMD in a population aged between 45 and 85 is 8.69%, and an increase from 196 to 288 million cases is expected from 2020 to 2040 [1]. Early diagnosis enables adequate treatment and a better prognosis. As such, there is a strong need for early screening strategies and better understanding of the disease on the molecular level.

The etiology of AMD is not fully understood, yet it is known to be a multifactorial disease, with strong genetic and environmental risk factors, where chronic oxidative stress, impaired clearance and prolonged inflammation result in pathological choroidal neovascularization [2,3]. A number of proteomic studies on AMD have already been conducted, with sometimes conflicting results, yet there are some patterns in the identified proteins and the metabolic pathways that they are involved in that support our current knowledge of the disease's etiology [4–7]. In our previous studies, we focused on the tear film proteome, providing interesting findings [8–10]. In this study, we aim to characterize the serum proteome of nAMD patients and discuss the potential clinical value of the obtained results.

2. Materials and Methods

After fulfilling the inclusion criteria, 132 age- and gender-matched patients were included in the study. The control group consisted of 58 people, and the AMD group consisted of 74 patients. The control group consisted of patients scheduled for cataract surgery who showed no other ocular pathology. The AMD group consisted of advanced neovascular AMD patients receiving ant-VEGF treatment, all in the active phase of the disease. The control group consisted of 28 men and 30 women, with a mean age of 73.51 (SD = 7.99) years, while the study group consisted of 34 men and 40 women, with a mean age of 73.91 (SD = 9.36). The inclusion criteria for the AMD group were as follows: an active form of disease featuring choroidal neovascularization (CNV) on fluorescein angiography or angio-OCT in at least one eye and the presence of subretinal or intraretinal fluid.

The exclusion criteria were any ocular diseases that would disturb the results, e.g., diabetic retinopathy, glaucoma and previous ocular surgery except for cataract extraction. Additionally, any moderately advanced or advanced stage of any systemic disease, such as diabetes, hyperlipidemia, uncontrolled hypertension, cardiovascular disease or autoimmune disorder, was an exclusion criterion.

2.1. In-Solution Digestion

To start, 50 µL 25 mM ammonium bicarbonate, pH 7.8, was added to a 3 µL serum sample. For the reduction and alkylation of cysteines, 2.5 µL of 200 mM DTT in 100 mM Tris-HCl, pH 8, was added, and the samples were incubated at 37 °C for 1 h, followed by the addition of 7.5 µL 200 mM iodoacetamide for 1 h at room temperature in the dark. The alkylation reaction was quenched by adding 10 µL 200 mM DTT at 37 °C for 1 h. Subsequently, the proteins were digested with 5 µg trypsin GOLD (Promega, Madison, WI, USA) for 16 h at 37 °C. The digestion was stopped by adding 5 µL 50% formic acid, and the generated peptides were purified using a 10 µL OMIX C18 micro-SPE pipette tip (Agilent, Santa Clara, CA, USA) and dried using a Speed Vac concentrator (Concentrator Plus, Eppendorf, Hamburg, Germany).

2.2. LC-MS Analysis

The samples were analyzed by LC-MS using a timsTOF Pro (Bruker Daltonik, Bremen, Germany) which was coupled online to a nanoElute nanoflow liquid chromatography system (Bruker Daltonik, Bremen, Germany) via a CaptiveSpray nanoelectrospray ion source. The dried peptides were dissolved in 4 µL 0.1% formic acid, and 2 µL of sample was injected. The peptides were separated on a reversed-phase C18 column (25 cm × 75 μm, 1.5 μm, PepSep (Bruker Daltonics, Bremen, Germany)). Mobile phase A contained water with 0.1% formic acid, and acetonitrile with 0.1% formic acid was used as mobile phase B. The peptides were separated by a gradient from 0 to 35% mobile phase B over 30 min at a flow rate of 300 nl/min at a column temperature of 50 °C. MS acquisition was performed in DDA-PASEF mode. The capillary voltage was set to 1.5 kV, with a mass range of 100 to 1700 m/z. The number of PASEF ranges was set to 20, with a total cycle time of 1.16 s, charge up to 5, target intensity of 20,000, intensity threshold of 1750, and active exclusion with release after 0.4 min. An inversed reduced TIMS mobility ($1/k_0$) of 0.85–1.40 Vs/cm^2 was used with a time range of 100 ms, an accumulation time of 100 ms, a duty cycle of 100%, and a ramp rate of 9.51 Hz. Precursors for data-dependent acquisition were fragmented with an ion-mobility-dependent collision energy, which was linearly increased from 20 to 59 eV.

2.3. Database Search

The LC/MS data were searched against the human Uniprot database (20,384 entries) using PEAKS X+ software version 10.5 (Bioinformatics Solutions, Waterloo, ON, Canada). The following parameters were used: digestion enzyme, trypsin; maximum missed cleavage, 2; fragment ion mass error tolerance, 0.03 Da; and parent ion error tolerance, 15 ppm. The oxidation of methionine and acetylation of the N-terminus were specified as variable modifications and carbamidomethylation of cysteines as a fixed modification. The maximum number of PTMs per peptide was set to 2. A false discovery rate of 1% was applied to the datasets.

2.4. Label-Free Quantification

For label-free quantification (LFQ) using PEAKS, ID-directed LFQ with outlier removal was applied. The following parameters were used on the peptide features: quality ≥ 3, peptide ID count per group ≥ 1, detected in at least ten samples per group. The following parameters were applied for the protein: FDR ≤ 1%, fold change ≥ 2, significance method ANOVA with at least 2 peptides.

3. Results

Blood serum collected from 74 late-stage, neovascular AMD patients and 58 healthy controls were analyzed by liquid chromatography coupled with mass spectrometry (LC-MS)-based proteomics. In total, 748 protein groups were identified (Figure 1). The label-free quantification revealed 17 differentially expressed proteins comparing the blood serum of both groups. There were 11 up-regulated proteins in the AMD group (Table 1 and Figure 2), whereas 6 were down-regulated (Table 2). The main functions and common pathways of different proteins were determined using the STRING database, powered by the Swiss Institute of Bioinformatics, Novo Nordisk Foundation Center for Protein Research and European Molecular Biology Laboratory [11]. This application allows us to predict and check direct (physical) and indirect (functional) associations between proteins and to predict protein–protein interactions. The gene-of-interest co-expression is presented in Figure 3, while the protein–protein association network is visualized in Figure 4. The main functions of the identified proteins according to the STRING database are summarized in Table 3.

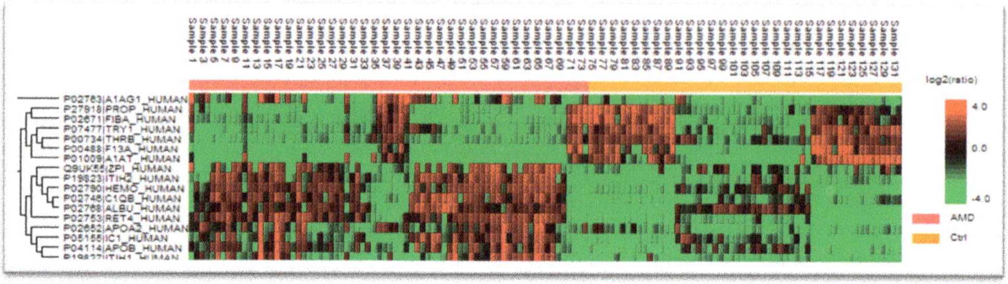

Figure 1. Distribution of proteins in groups with given ratio.

Table 1. Up-regulated serum proteins. Ratio (Rt)—a parameter indicating the overexpression or suppression of a protein. Rt shows how many times the protein content is up- or down-regulated compared to the control group. Score is the probability that the result is not random. A higher score indicates a more confident match. Accession number refers to the Uniprot human database.

Name	Accession Number	Entry Name	Ratio	Score
RET4_HUMAN	P02753	Retinol-binding protein 4	1.00:0.27	200
ITIH2_HUMAN	P19823	Inter-alpha-trypsin inhibitor heavy chain H2	1.00:0.27	137.34
C1QB_HUMAN	P02746	Complement C1q subcomponent subunit B	1.00:0.36	118.75
APOA2_HUMAN	P02652	Apolipoprotein A-II	1.00:0.36	117.69
ITIH1_HUMAN	P19827	Inter-alpha-trypsin inhibitor heavy chain H1	1.00:0.26	101.39
HEMO_HUMAN	P02790	Hemopexin	1.00:0.40	84.1
APOB_HUMAN	P04114	Apolipoprotein B-100	1.00:0.40	71.24
A1AG1_HUMAN	P02763	Alpha-1-acid glycoprotein 1	1.00:0.26	70.02
IC1_HUMAN	P05155	Plasma protease C1 inhibitor	1.00:0.44	61.55
ALBU_HUMAN	P02768	Albumin	1.00:0.49	59.92
ZPI_HUMAN	Q9UK55	Protein Z-dependent protease inhibitor	1.00:0.46	48.72

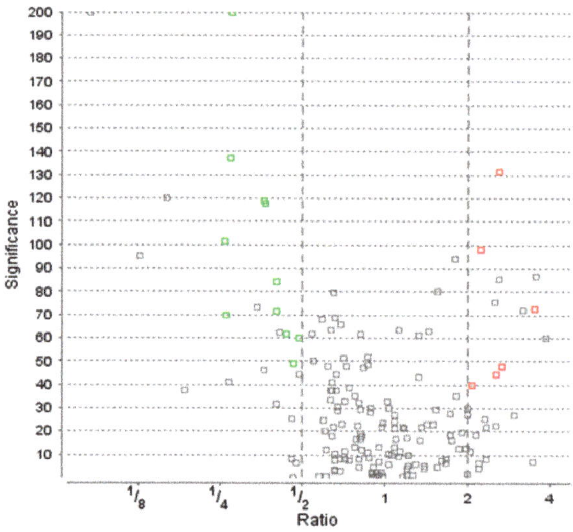

Figure 2. Protein distribution with ratio and significance according to ANOVA analysis of Variance. AMD—age-related macular degeneration study group; Ctrl—control group. Green squares represent the significantly upregulated proteins in AMD group while red the downregulated ones. Grey color means the proteins did not satisfy other conditions.

Table 2. Down-regulated serum proteins. Ratio (Rt)—a parameter indicating the overexpression or suppression of a protein. Rt shows how many times the protein content is up- or down-regulated compared to the control group. Score is the probability that the result is not random. A higher score indicates a more confident match. Accession number refers to the Uniprot human database.

Name	Accession Number	Entry Name	Ratio	Score
THRB_HUMAN	P00734	Prothrombin	1.00:2.61	131.67
PROP_HUMAN	P27918	Properdin	1.00:2.23	98.24
F13A_HUMAN	P00488	Coagulation factor XIII A chain	1.00:3.51	72.72
A1AT_HUMAN	P01009	Alpha-1-antitrypsin	1.00:2.66	48.01
TRY1_HUMAN	P07477	Trypsin-1	1.00:2.52	44.2
FIBA_HUMAN	P02671	Fibrinogen alpha chain	1.00:2.07	39.49

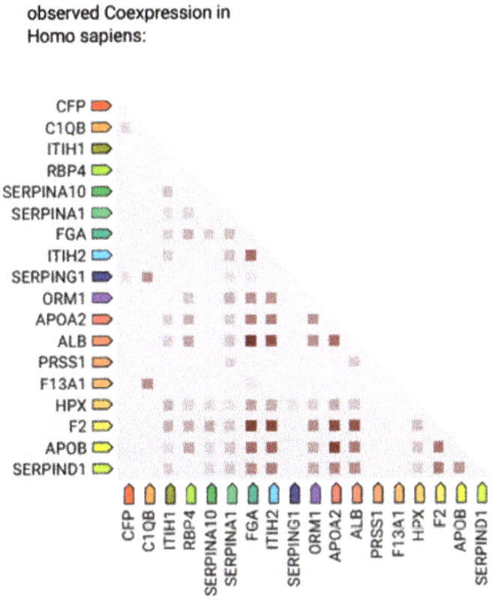

Figure 3. Gene-of-interest co-expression, created using STRING. Lighter and darker marks represent weaker and stronger co-expression scores, based on RNA expression patterns and protein coregulation given by ProteomeHD.

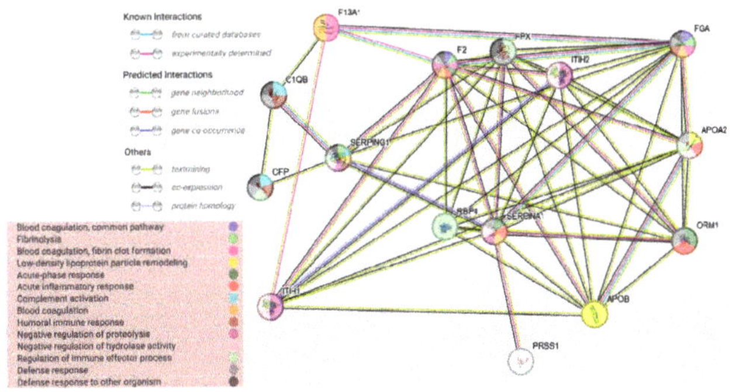

Figure 4. Protein–protein association networks, determined using STRING database. Abbreviations refer to protein names in Uniprot database.

Table 3. Main functions of significantly differing proteins according to STRING database. Protein name refers to the Uniprot human database.

Protein Name	STRING Abbreviation	Function According to STRING
RET4_HUMAN	RBP4	Transporting retinol from liver to tissues
ITIH2_HUMAN	ITIH2	Binding agent between hyaluronan and serum proteins
ITIH1_HUMAN	ITIH1	Binding agent between hyaluronan and serum proteins
C1QB_HUMAN	C1QB	Cooperation with the proenzymes C1r and C1s to yield C1
APOA2_HUMAN	APOA2	Taking part in HDL metabolism and its stabilization
APOB_HUMAN	APOB	Recognition signal for the cellular binding and internalization of LDL particles by the apo-B/E receptor
HEMO_HUMAN	HPX	Taking part in heme binding and transporting it to the liver
A1AG1_HUMAN	ORM1	Transporting numerous ligands in the blood stream
IC1_HUMAN	IC1	Probably taking part in blood coagulation, fibrinolysis and the generation of kinins
ALBU_HUMAN	ALB	Binding ions such as Ca(II), Na(I), K(I) and also particles like fatty acids, hormones, bilirubin and drugs
ZPI_HUMAN	SERPINA10	Together with PROZ, calcium and phospholipids, blocking coagulation protease factor Xa
THRB_HUMAN	F2	Active in inflammation and wound healing
PROP_HUMAN	CFP	Taking part in CFI-CFH-mediated degradation of Complement C3 beta chain (C3b)
F13A_HUMAN	F13A1	Stabilizing the fibrin clot
A1AT_HUMAN	SERPINA 1	Inactivating of serine proteases
TRY1_HUMAN	PRSS1	Belongs to the peptidase S1 family
FIBA_HUMAN	FGA	Basic component of blood clots

4. Discussion

In this study, we identified 17 different proteins, 11 up-regulated and 6 down-regulated, in neovascular AMD. They were categorized into groups depending on their involvement in metabolic pathways and biological processes, as further described below.

In the course of the STRING connection analysis between the identified proteins, 72 edges were observed, representing a variety of protein–protein interactions, including gene fusion or structural homology (Figure 3). Additionally, the functionalities of proteins were also determined and presented by color (Figure 4, Table 3). The main biological process that was represented by the majority of proteins relates to the defense response, correlated with the immune status, or binding and transporting particles such as ligands, small proteins or ions. To observe more correlations between proteins, a diagram representing co-expression was created to capture the relationships between proteins that do not physically interact or colocalize. Their genes correlated in expression across a large number of experiments [12]. The various types of interrelationships between the proteins may be a valuable starting point for to further research on the proteins identified in this publication.

4.1. Impaired Cellular Transportation

Maintaining homeostasis in retinal tissue is extremely demanding for the RPE cells, as they are some of the most metabolically active cells in the human organism [13]. A constant need to excrete the waste material is supported by a highly complex system of influx–outflux transportation and energy delivery [14]. With aging, this system starts to collapse, resulting in the accumulation of waste material in the form of drusen on the border of Bruch's Membrane (BM) and RPE [15–17]. Disruptions in the communication between cells and the breakdown of cellular waste removal systems, particularly autophagy, have been observed in AMD. RPE cells deteriorate with age, reducing their capability to clear metabolic by-products, resulting in the buildup of clumped, misfolded proteins outside cells due to the failure of autophagy—a recurring theme across various neurodegenerative disorders like Parkinson's disease or Alzheimer's disease [2,18,19].

In this study, we found the altered levels of proteins involved in the transportation process, which may reflect its breakdown in AMD.

Retinol-binding protein 4 (RBP4) was the most profoundly up-regulated protein in our study, with a 4:1 ratio in AMD patients. This low molecular protein creates a complex with transthyretin (TTR), maintaining the serum retinol (vitamin A form) in the bloodstream, and is solely responsible for delivering it into the RPE cells. Meanwhile, in RPE cells, all-trans retinol accelerates the formation of drusen with lipofuscin formed by A2E accretion. There are reports of up-regulation of RBP4 in serum in the course of AMD, and drugs being developed to limit its expression, leading to a lower RBP4-mediated lipofuscin bisretinoid distribution into the retina, where they are involved in lipofuscin aggregation in RPE cells [20].

RBP4 has mostly been linked in ophthalmology with the atrophic form of AMD and Stargardt disease [20–22]. There are preliminary data on a phase 1b/2 clinical trial of Tinlarebant—an oral RBP4 antagonist, showing its potential in slowing or preventing new lesions in Stargardt disease [23]. Given the natural course of the disease, with a formation of the atrophic scar also occurring in the neovascular form, it can be hypothesized that RBP4 is also involved in late-stage nAMD.

Other transportation proteins, described in more detail below, were albumin, alpha-1- acid glycoprotein 1, hemopexin, apolipoprotein A-II and B and Inter-alpha-trypsin inhibitors 1 and 2.

4.2. Trypsin Metabolism

Trypsin is a serine protease secreted by the pancreas, with the main function of proteolysis in the small intestine. It has three major isoenzymes (Trypsin-1, Trypsin-2, Trypsin-3), each with a different preference for cleavage of lysine and arginine [24]. Its alterations have not been previously linked to the development of AMD.

Alpha-1-antitrypsin, a serpin and one of the major trypsin inhibitors, was previously found to be up-regulated in the vitreous body of nAMD patients [25], as well as in the aqueous and blood of patients with glaucoma [26]. It is an acute phase protein inhibiting numerous proteases and therefore playing a protective role in the inflammatory process.

Inter-alpha-trypsin inhibitors (ITIs) consist of proteins with high inhibitory action against trypsin. ITI heavy chain 2 was previously found to be up-regulated in dry AMD, where its role as a hyaluronan carrier in serum was underlined. As hyaluronan is involved in extracellular matrix (ECM) remodeling and inflammation, the up-regulation of ITIH2 was seen as a risk factor for AMD progression [27,28]. ITIH2 was also proposed as a potential biomarker of tuberculosis and was considered as a tumor growth inhibitor when overexpressed [29,30].

We noticed ITIH1 and ITIH2 to be almost three- and four-fold up-regulated in the nAMD patients, with simultaneous down-regulation of Alpha-1-antitrypsin and Trypsin-1. These findings may suggest suppression in the trypsin metabolism in the course of AMD.

4.3. Coagulation Balance

Although previous studies have shown that coagulation factors probably do not play a significant role in AMD [31–33], there are conflicting data on anti-VEGF injections' effect on the coagulation parameters [34].

Prothrombin is a serum glycoprotein, an inactive thrombin form. Prothrombin time (PT) is a parameter that is used clinically for the evaluation of the clotting time. Coagulation factor XIII A (F13A1) is converted into an active form by thrombin, being involved in the coagulation balance by stabilizing the thrombus [35]. Fibrinogen in the final stage of coagulation is converted into fibrin via thrombin-mediated proteolytic cleavage. It is also an acute phase protein (APP), elevated in previous studies concerning AMD [3,36–39].

Both PT and F13A1 gene polymorphisms were previously associated with the response to photodynamic therapy (PDT) in nAMD [40]. As PDT is currently almost completely displaced by anti-VEGF therapy, no follow-up study has been performed.

Protein Z-dependent protease inhibitor (ZPI) is a protein from the serpin family, with a major anti-coagulation effect by the inhibition of factor Xa in the presence of protein Z (PZ). In healthy subjects, ZPI and ZP usually circulate as a complex [41,42]. Elevated levels of protein Z were found in central retinal and vein occlusion [43], and ZPI was expressed with a significant difference in nAMD in another plasma proteomic study [44].

All the coagulation balance proteins were significantly down-regulated in our study, except for protein Z-dependent protease inhibitor, which is in line with the findings of the study by Altinkaynak et al. [34], probably being the effect of numerous intravitreal aflibercept injections. Blood coagulation is still being investigated in nAMD, as hemorrhagic events usually dramatically worsen the course of the disease, leaving large retinal scars, with no prognosis for functional improvement. Whether the disturbance of the coagulation protein levels in our study is a part of the etiopathology of nAMD, or the effect of anti-VEGF injections, is unclear. Either way, it seems that proper regulation of coagulation disorders would be beneficial in AMD patients, especially in the group at high risk of developing hemorrhagic events.

4.4. Lipid Metabolism

Lipid metabolism is crucial for the pathogenesis of AMD. It is hypothesized that the activity and composition of high-density lipoproteins (HDLs), together with other lipid disorders, are factors in AMD's pathogenesis, as lipids are a major component in drusen. Similarities were suggested in the pathophysiology of AMD and cardiovascular disease [45]. Also, as was established by the AREDS reports, a number of available dietary supplements are rich in omega 3, 6 and polyunsaturated fatty acids (PUFAs), and it seems as though it is not the high total lipids that are responsible for AMD, but more so the prevalence of the "bad" lipids (TG, LDLs) and an impaired metabolism on the cellular level of RPE, especially given that RPE cells are the most metabolically active body cells—thus, even minor alterations on a cellular level can cause serious detrimental effects [46]. Also, as elevated total lipids are generally known to increase the risk of cardiovascular diseases, patients are usually aware of the need for lipid control. There is also a new concept of ferroptosis being one of the crucial mechanisms of cell death in AMD [47]. It is initiated by lipid peroxidation and iron-dependent accumulation in RPE cells. This can be linked with higher hemopexin levels in our AMD group, as discussed further.

APOA2 mediates the cholesterol transferring into high-density lipid C (HDL-C), together with apolipoprotein A-I (APOA1), helping the RPE cells eliminate the lipidic debris. Both APOA1 and APOA2 are discussed as biomarkers and treatment targets in diabetic retinopathy (DR), polypoidal choroidal vasculopathy (PCV), and AMD, although there is no consistency in studies regarding the mechanism of action [48–51].

ApoB-100 is a protein that is secreted by the RPE cells, and it was found to be a major early component in drusen formation [52,53]. It was recently suggested that apoB100 plays a protective role in the development of CNV [54]. In the study by Cao et al., ApoB-100 was more up-regulated in the aqueous humor of patients with early and intermediate non-neovascular AMD and lower in neovascular AMD. Authors interpret that as what they call a "paradoxical" protective role of ApoB-100—as the nAMD patients with higher ApoB levels respond better to the anti-VEGF therapy and have smaller CNVs in general, the authors suspect that higher ApoB levels lead to the formation of drusen and non-neovascular AMD but protect from progression to nAMD. In another study by Curcio et al., ApoB-100 was associated with the progression of dry AMD to its neovascular form in a response-to-retention pattern that was similar to that of coronary artery disease [55,56]. In a large genome-wide association study (GWAS), the ApoB level was associated with a lower risk of intermediate and geographic atrophy (GA) AMD, but not with the presence of CNV [57].

APOA2 and apoB-100 were both up-regulated in the AMD group in our study, which is in line with other studies, where elevated levels of APOA were also observed in serum [58] or in Bruch's membrane (BM) (apoB-100) [49,59].

4.5. Inflammation and Complement Proteins

The concept of a prolonged inflammatory process and its detrimental effect on the ability of RPE cells to "self-clean" have been well documented in numerous studies. With aging, the RPE cells lose their ability to eliminate the metabolic products, which leads to the accumulation of the multicomponent debris between the BM and the RPE cells. Both the toxic debris itself and the sheer physical pressure that it exerts on the RPE cells lead to increased local inflammation. While a transient inflammatory process is beneficial for the tissue, when prolonged, it overpowers the cells' ability to regenerate and leads to the collapse of the regenerative process [3,60–62]. This, in turn, results in cell death and the distortion of the natural blood–retinal barrier, choroidal neovascularization ingrowth and exudation with a hemorrhage—the hallmarks of nAMD. Inflammation, together with retinal autoantibodies, seems to play an important role in neovascularization, as has been discussed in great detail in a paper by Heloterä et al. [3]. In this study, we identified numerous alterations in the inflammatory-related proteins, associated mainly with complement activation and reactive oxygen species. Also, we noticed significant alterations in the levels of acute phase proteins (APPs). APPs can be roughly divided into positive (increasing inflammation) and negative (decreasing inflammation). The positive APPs that we identified were fibrinogen (down-regulated), complement factors (up-regulated), alpha-1-antitrypsin (down-regulated), and alpha-1-acid glycoprotein 1 (up-regulated), while the negative APPs were albumin (up-regulated) and RBP4 (up-regulated). This is somewhat contrary to the concept of AMD as a disease where persistent inflammation occurs. On the other hand, all the patients were receiving anti-VEGF injections, which may have altered their blood parameters, similarly to the down-regulation of the coagulation cascade proteins.

Properdin is a potent inflammation mediator, an activator of an alternative complement pathway of complement, which is commonly linked with AMD's pathogenesis. Properdin is also a pattern-recognition protein, involved in apoptotic and necrotic pathways [63]. It seems that the over-activation of complementation plays a crucial role in AMD's development and progression [64,65]. One of the factors in the alternative pathway that is most commonly associated with AMD is complement factor H (CFH) [60,66,67]. Properdin was down-regulated in our study in the AMD group.

Hemopexin (HPX) acts as a protective protein by binding heme—an inflammation-amplifying enzyme originating from hemoglobin after erythrocyte lysis [68,69]. Heme toxicity is a serious issue, especially in large subretinal hemorrhages, resulting in irreversible macular scarring [70]. HPX is also associated with CFH and thus complements activation. The HPX plasma levels corresponded with three loci of CFH genes in pQTL analysis [71], but these findings were not confirmed in the following study by Lauwen et al., where no correlation with CFH, nor the up-regulation of HPX in the blood plasma of AMD patients, was observed [72]. In our study, HPX showed more than two-fold up-regulation in the AMD group. Higher HPX levels can be related to the lowered coagulation balance proteins in the AMD group, acting in a counterbalancing protective manner.

Plasma protease C1 inhibitor (C1INH) is a potent anti-inflammatory protein from the serpin family. Its anti-inflammatory effect, besides from the protease inhibition, also derives from interaction with endothelial cells end leukocytes, mitigating leukocyte migration [73]. In a large study focused on this particular protein, C1INH was significantly up-regulated in the plasma of AMD patients [74], which correlates with our findings of over two-fold up-regulation of C1INH.

AGP is a plasma protein involved in binding and transportation processes. It is also one of the acute phase proteins [75]. AGP was previously described in proteomic studies concerning AMD as being up-regulated in dry AMD [27] and identified in both the vitreous body and aqueous humor in neovascular AMD [25,76].

Complement C1q subcomponent subunit B was also up-regulated almost three-fold in our study.

Albumin, the most abundant circulatory protein, which was found to be two-fold up-regulated in the AMD group, lately became a target in the anti-inflammatory treatment of AMD. The heme–albumin complex was recently proven to reduce the detrimental effect of reactive oxygen species on the retina in the ARPE-19 cell culture [77].

4.6. Limitations of the Study

Our study has several limitations. Most notably, the relatively small sample size of our study group should be mentioned. However, given the lack of similar studies concerning the Central European population, we contribute some further data to the field of proteomics. Another limitation to consider is the uncertainty regarding the health status of the patients in our study. The presence of co-existing diseases was excluded based on medical records and by patients' family doctors, but a full medical examination was not conducted before collecting the samples for the study. This is particularly important due to the potential disturbances in the proteomic study's results caused by common systemic diseases such as diabetes or hyperlipidemia [78–80].

5. Conclusions

In this study, we identified 17 different proteins in the blood serum of nAMD patients. In addition to local tissue alterations, our results indicate that systemic biomarkers link nAMD to a changed cellular transport mechanism, lipid metabolism, extracellular matrix re-organization, coagulation processes and inflammatory responses. Thus, proteomics, together with other omic analysis, may open new ways to understand AMD's pathology and its progression and to analyze treatment responses.

Author Contributions: Conceptualization, M.W.; Data curation, D.W. and K.M.; Formal analysis, T.P.U. and K.M.; Funding acquisition, M.W., B.T., T.P.U. and K.K.; Investigation, M.W.; Methodology, M.W. and B.T.; Project administration, M.W. and J.M.; Resources, M.W.; Validation, M.W.; Visualization, B.T. and K.M.; Writing—original draft, M.W.; Writing—review and editing, M.W., B.T., T.P.U., K.K., D.W. and K.M. All authors have read and agreed to the published version of the manuscript.

Funding: Mass spectrometry-based proteomic analyses were performed by the Proteomics Core Facility, Department of Biosciences, University of Oslo. This facility is a member of the National Network of Advanced Proteomics Infrastructure (NAPI), which is funded by the Research Council of Norway INFRASTRUKTUR-program (project number: 295910).

Institutional Review Board Statement: The study was conducted in accordance with the Declaration of Helsinki and approved by the Bioethics Committee of Medical University of Lublin (protocol code KE-0254/108/2020 and 28 May 2020 of approval).

Informed Consent Statement: Informed consent was obtained from all subjects involved in the study.

Data Availability Statement: All data are available from the corresponding author.

Conflicts of Interest: The authors declare no conflicts of interest.

References

1. Wong, W.L.; Su, X.; Li, X.; Cheung, C.M.G.; Klein, R.; Cheng, C.-Y.; Wong, T.Y. Global Prevalence of Age-Related Macular Degeneration and Disease Burden Projection for 2020 and 2040: A Systematic Review and Meta-Analysis. *Lancet Glob. Health* **2014**, *2*, e106–e116. [CrossRef] [PubMed]
2. Kaarniranta, K.; Blasiak, J.; Liton, P.; Boulton, M.; Klionsky, D.J.; Sinha, D. Autophagy in Age-Related Macular Degeneration. *Autophagy* **2023**, *19*, 388–400. [CrossRef] [PubMed]
3. Heloterä, H.; Kaarniranta, K. A Linkage between Angiogenesis and Inflammation in Neovascular Age-Related Macular Degeneration. *Cells* **2022**, *11*, 3453. [CrossRef] [PubMed]

4. Ahmad, M.T.; Zhang, P.; Dufresne, C.; Ferrucci, L.; Semba, R.D. The Human Eye Proteome Project: Updates on an Emerging Proteome. *Proteomics* **2018**, *18*, 1700394. [CrossRef] [PubMed]
5. Rinsky, B.; Beykin, G.; Grunin, M.; Amer, R.; Khateb, S.; Tiosano, L.; Almeida, D.; Hagbi-Levi, S.; Elbaz-Hayoun, S.; Chowers, I. Analysis of the Aqueous Humor Proteome in Patients with Age-Related Macular Degeneration. *Investig. Ophthalmol. Vis. Sci.* **2021**, *62*, 18. [CrossRef] [PubMed]
6. Cehofski, L.J.; Honoré, B.; Vorum, H. A Review: Proteomics in Retinal Artery Occlusion, Retinal Vein Occlusion, Diabetic Retinopathy and Acquired Macular Disorders. *Int. J. Mol. Sci.* **2017**, *18*, 907. [CrossRef] [PubMed]
7. García-Quintanilla, L.; Rodríguez-Martínez, L.; Bandín-Vilar, E.; Gil-Martínez, M.; González-Barcia, M.; Mondelo-García, C.; Fernández-Ferreiro, A.; Mateos, J. Recent Advances in Proteomics-Based Approaches to Studying Age-Related Macular Degeneration: A Systematic Review. *Int. J. Mol. Sci.* **2022**, *23*, 14759. [CrossRef]
8. Winiarczyk, M.; Kaarniranta, K.; Winiarczyk, S.; Adaszek, Ł.; Winiarczyk, D.; Mackiewicz, J. Tear Film Proteome in Age-Related Macular Degeneration. *Graefe's Arch. Clin. Exp. Ophthalmol.* **2018**, *256*, 1127–1139. [CrossRef] [PubMed]
9. Winiarczyk, M.; Winiarczyk, D.; Michalak, K.; Kaarniranta, K.; Adaszek, Ł.; Winiarczyk, S.; Mackiewicz, J. Dysregulated Tear Film Proteins in Macular Edema Due to the Neovascular Age-Related Macular Degeneration Are Involved in the Regulation of Protein Clearance, Inflammation, and Neovascularization. *J. Clin. Med.* **2021**, *10*, 3060. [CrossRef]
10. Winiarczyk, M.; Biela, K.; Michalak, K.; Winiarczyk, D.; Mackiewicz, J. Changes in Tear Proteomic Profile in Ocular Diseases. *Int. J. Environ. Res. Public Health* **2022**, *19*, 13341. [CrossRef]
11. Szklarczyk, D.; Kirsch, R.; Koutrouli, M.; Nastou, K.; Mehryary, F.; Hachilif, R.; Gable, A.L.; Fang, T.; Doncheva, N.T.; Pyysalo, S.; et al. The STRING Database in 2023: Protein-Protein Association Networks and Functional Enrichment Analyses for Any Sequenced Genome of Interest. *Nucleic Acids Res.* **2023**, *51*, D638–D646. [CrossRef] [PubMed]
12. Kustatscher, G.; Grabowski, P.; Schrader, T.A.; Passmore, J.B.; Schrader, M.; Rappsilber, J. Co-Regulation Map of the Human Proteome Enables Identification of Protein Functions. *Nat. Biotechnol.* **2019**, *37*, 1361–1371. [CrossRef] [PubMed]
13. Strauss, O. The Retinal Pigment Epithelium in Visual Function. *Physiol. Rev.* **2005**, *85*, 845–881. [CrossRef] [PubMed]
14. Fisher, C.R.; Ferrington, D.A. Perspective on AMD Pathobiology: A Bioenergetic Crisis in the RPE. *Invest Ophthalmol Vis Sci* **2018**, *59*, AMD41–AMD47. [CrossRef] [PubMed]
15. Curcio, C.A. Soft Drusen in Age-Related Macular Degeneration: Biology and Targeting Via the Oil Spill Strategies. *Investig. Ophthalmol. Vis. Sci.* **2018**, *59*, AMD160–AMD181. [CrossRef] [PubMed]
16. Ban, N.; Lee, T.J.; Sene, A.; Choudhary, M.; Lekwuwa, M.; Dong, Z.; Santeford, A.; Lin, J.B.; Malek, G.; Ory, D.S.; et al. Impaired Monocyte Cholesterol Clearance Initiates Age-Related Retinal Degeneration and Vision Loss. *JCI Insight* **2018**, *3*, e120824. [CrossRef] [PubMed]
17. Lee, Y.; Hussain, A.A.; Seok, J.-H.; Kim, S.-H.; Marshall, J. Modulating the Transport Characteristics of Bruch's Membrane with Steroidal Glycosides and Its Relevance to Age-Related Macular Degeneration (AMD). *Investig. Ophthalmol. Vis. Sci.* **2015**, *56*, 8403–8418. [CrossRef] [PubMed]
18. Pinelli, R.; Bertelli, M.; Scaffidi, E.; Fulceri, F.; Busceti, C.L.; Biagioni, F.; Fornai, F. Measurement of Drusen and Their Correlation with Visual Symptoms in Patients Affected by Age-Related Macular Degeneration. *Arch. Ital. Biol.* **2020**, *158*, 82–104. [CrossRef]
19. Kaarniranta, K.; Salminen, A.; Haapasalo, A.; Soininen, H.; Hiltunen, M. Age-Related Macular Degeneration (AMD): Alzheimer's Disease in the Eye? *J. Alzheimers Dis.* **2011**, *24*, 615–631. [CrossRef]
20. Cioffi, C.L.; Dobri, N.; Freeman, E.E.; Conlon, M.P.; Chen, P.; Stafford, D.G.; Schwarz, D.M.C.; Golden, K.C.; Zhu, L.; Kitchen, D.B.; et al. Design, Synthesis, and Evaluation of Nonretinoid Retinol Binding Protein 4 Antagonists for the Potential Treatment of Atrophic Age-Related Macular Degeneration and Stargardt Disease. *J. Med. Chem.* **2014**, *57*, 7731–7757. [CrossRef]
21. Cioffi, C.L.; Racz, B.; Freeman, E.E.; Conlon, M.P.; Chen, P.; Stafford, D.G.; Schwarz, D.M.C.; Zhu, L.; Kitchen, D.B.; Barnes, K.D.; et al. Bicyclic [3.3.0]-Octahydrocyclopenta[c]Pyrrolo Antagonists of Retinol Binding Protein 4: Potential Treatment of Atrophic Age-Related Macular Degeneration and Stargardt Disease. *J. Med. Chem.* **2015**, *58*, 5863–5888. [CrossRef] [PubMed]
22. Kim, N.; Priefer, R. Retinol Binding Protein 4 Antagonists and Protein Synthesis Inhibitors: Potential for Therapeutic Development. *Eur. J. Med. Chem.* **2021**, *226*, 113856. [CrossRef] [PubMed]
23. Grigg, J.R.; Chen, F.K.; Chen, T.-C.; Jamieson, R.V.; Scholl, H.P.; Mata, N.L.; Nguyen, Q.D. A Phase 1b/2 Study of the Safety and Tolerability of Tinlarebant in Adolescent Patients Affected by Stargardt Disease– 15 Month Preliminary Data. *Investig. Ophthalmol. Vis. Sci.* **2023**, *64*, 2597.
24. Schilling, O.; Biniossek, M.L.; Mayer, B.; Elsässer, B.; Brandstetter, H.; Goettig, P.; Stenman, U.-H.; Koistinen, H. Specificity Profiling of Human Trypsin-Isoenzymes. *Biol. Chem.* **2018**, *399*, 997–1007. [CrossRef] [PubMed]
25. Koss, M.J.; Hoffmann, J.; Nguyen, N.; Pfister, M.; Mischak, H.; Mullen, W.; Husi, H.; Rejdak, R.; Koch, F.; Jankowski, J.; et al. Proteomics of Vitreous Humor of Patients with Exudative Age-Related Macular Degeneration. *PLoS ONE* **2014**, *9*, e96895. [CrossRef]
26. Boehm, N.; Wolters, D.; Thiel, U.; Lossbrand, U.; Wiegel, N.; Pfeiffer, N.; Grus, F.H. New Insights into Autoantibody Profiles from Immune Privileged Sites in the Eye: A Glaucoma Study. *Brain Behav. Immun.* **2012**, *26*, 96–102. [CrossRef] [PubMed]
27. Qu, S.-C.; Xu, D.; Li, T.-T.; Zhang, J.-F.; Liu, F. iTRAQ-Based Proteomics Analysis of Aqueous Humor in Patients with Dry Age-Related Macular Degeneration. *Int. J. Ophthalmol.* **2019**, *12*, 1758–1766. [CrossRef] [PubMed]
28. Petrey, A.; de la Motte, C. Hyaluronan, a Crucial Regulator of Inflammation. *Front. Immunol.* **2014**, *5*, 101. [CrossRef] [PubMed]

29. Paris, S.; Sesboüé, R.; Delpech, B.; Chauzy, C.; Thiberville, L.; Martin, J.-P.; Frébourg, T.; Diarra-Mehrpour, M. Inhibition of Tumor Growth and Metastatic Spreading by Overexpression of Inter-Alpha-Trypsin Inhibitor Family Chains. *Int. J. Cancer* **2002**, *97*, 615–620. [CrossRef]
30. Cuvelier, A.; Muir, J.F.; Martin, J.P.; Sesboüé, R. Proteins of the inter-alpha trypsin inhibitor (ITI) family. A major role in the biology of the extracellular matrix. *Rev. Mal. Respir.* **2000**, *17*, 437–446.
31. Haas, P.; Aggermann, T.; Steindl, K.; Krugluger, W.; Pühringer, H.; Oberkanins, C.; Frantal, S.; Binder, S. Genetic Cardiovascular Risk Factors and Age-Related Macular Degeneration. *Acta Ophthalmol.* **2011**, *89*, 335–338. [CrossRef] [PubMed]
32. Rudnicka, A.R.; MacCallum, P.K.; Whitelocke, R.; Meade, T.W. Circulating Markers of Arterial Thrombosis and Late-Stage Age-Related Macular Degeneration: A Case–Control Study. *Eye* **2010**, *24*, 1199–1206. [CrossRef] [PubMed]
33. Georgakopoulos, C.D.; Makri, O.E.; Pallikari, A.; Kagkelaris, K.; Plotas, P.; Grammenou, V.; Emmanuil, A. Effect of Intravitreal Injection of Aflibercept on Blood Coagulation Parameters in Patients with Age-Related Macular Degeneration. *Ophthalmol. Eye Dis.* **2020**, *12*, 2515841420903929. [CrossRef] [PubMed]
34. Altinkaynak, H.; Kars, M.E.; Kurkcuoglu, P.Z.; Ugurlu, N. Blood Coagulation Parameters after Intravitreal Injection of Aflibercept in Patients with Neovascular Age-Related Macular Degeneration. *Int. Ophthalmol.* **2018**, *38*, 2397–2402. [CrossRef] [PubMed]
35. Ząbczyk, M.; Natorska, J.; Undas, A. Factor XIII and Fibrin Clot Properties in Acute Venous Thromboembolism. *Int. J. Mol. Sci.* **2021**, *22*, 1607. [CrossRef] [PubMed]
36. Serra, R.; Rallo, V.; Pinna, A.; Steri, M.; Piras, M.G.; Marongiu, M.; Coscas, F.; Gorospe, M.; Schlessinger, D.; Fiorillo, E.; et al. Polygenic Risk Score and Biochemical/Environmental Variables Predict a Low-Risk Profile of Age-Related Macular Degeneration in Sardinia. *Graefes Arch. Clin. Exp. Ophthalmol.* **2023**, *261*, 691–698. [CrossRef] [PubMed]
37. Chakravarthy, U.; Wong, T.Y.; Fletcher, A.; Piault, E.; Evans, C.; Zlateva, G.; Buggage, R.; Pleil, A.; Mitchell, P. Clinical Risk Factors for Age-Related Macular Degeneration: A Systematic Review and Meta-Analysis. *BMC Ophthalmol.* **2010**, *10*, 31. [CrossRef] [PubMed]
38. Smith, W.; Mitchell, P.; Leeder, S.R.; Wang, J.J. Plasma Fibrinogen Levels, Other Cardiovascular Risk Factors, and Age-Related Maculopathy: The Blue Mountains Eye Study. *Arch. Ophthalmol.* **1998**, *116*, 583–587. [CrossRef] [PubMed]
39. Sridevi Gurubaran, I.; Heloterä, H.; Marry, S.; Koskela, A.; Hyttinen, J.M.T.; Paterno, J.J.; Urtti, A.; Chen, M.; Xu, H.; Kauppinen, A.; et al. Oxidative Stress and Mitochondrial Damage in Dry Age-Related Macular Degeneration Like NFE2L2/PGC-1α -/- Mouse Model Evoke Complement Component C5a Independent of C3. *Biology* **2021**, *10*, 622. [CrossRef]
40. Parmeggiani, F.; Costagliola, C.; Gemmati, D.; D'Angelo, S.; Perri, P.; Scapoli, G.L.; Catozzi, L.; Federici, F.; Sebastiani, A.; Incorvaia, C. Predictive Role of Coagulation-Balance Gene Polymorphisms in the Efficacy of Photodynamic Therapy with Verteporfin for Classic Choroidal Neovascularization Secondary to Age-Related Macular Degeneration. *Pharmacogenetics Genom.* **2007**, *17*, 1039. [CrossRef]
41. Al-Shanqeeti, A.; Vlieg, A.v.H.; Berntorp, E.; Rosendaal, F.; Broze, G.J., Jr. Protein Z and Protein Z-Dependent Protease Inhibitor. *Thromb. Haemost.* **2005**, *93*, 411–413. [CrossRef] [PubMed]
42. Han, X.; Fiehler, R.; Broze, G.J., Jr. Characterization of the Protein Z–Dependent Protease Inhibitor. *Blood* **2000**, *96*, 3049–3055. [CrossRef] [PubMed]
43. Koren-Michowitz, M.; Eting, E.; Rahimi-Levene, N.; Garach-Jehoshua, O.; Volcheck, Y.; Kornberg, A. Protein Z Levels and Central Retinal Vein or Artery Occlusion. *Eur. J. Haematol.* **2005**, *75*, 401–405. [CrossRef] [PubMed]
44. Kim, H.-J.; Woo, S.J.; Suh, E.J.; Ahn, J.; Park, J.H.; Hong, H.K.; Lee, J.E.; Ahn, S.J.; Hwang, D.J.; Kim, K.W.; et al. Identification of Vinculin as a Potential Plasma Marker for Age-Related Macular Degeneration. *Invest. Ophthalmol. Vis. Sci.* **2014**, *55*, 7166–7176. [CrossRef] [PubMed]
45. Wu, J.; Uchino, M.; Sastry, S.M.; Schaumberg, D.A. Age-Related Macular Degeneration and the Incidence of Cardiovascular Disease: A Systematic Review and Meta-Analysis. *PLoS ONE* **2014**, *9*, e89600. [CrossRef] [PubMed]
46. Jun, S.; Datta, S.; Wang, L.; Pegany, R.; Cano, M.; Handa, J.T. The Impact of Lipids, Lipid Oxidation, and Inflammation on AMD, and the Potential Role of miRNAs on Lipid Metabolism in the RPE. *Exp. Eye Res.* **2019**, *181*, 346–355. [CrossRef] [PubMed]
47. Zhao, T.; Guo, X.; Sun, Y. Iron Accumulation and Lipid Peroxidation in the Aging Retina: Implication of Ferroptosis in Age-Related Macular Degeneration. *Aging Dis.* **2021**, *12*, 529–551. [CrossRef]
48. Zhang, X.; Nie, Y.; Gong, Z.; Zhu, M.; Qiu, B.; Wang, Q. Plasma Apolipoproteins Predicting the Occurrence and Severity of Diabetic Retinopathy in Patients with Type 2 Diabetes Mellitus. *Front. Endocrinol.* **2022**, *13*, 915575. [CrossRef] [PubMed]
49. Kelly, U.L.; Grigsby, D.; Cady, M.A.; Landowski, M.; Skiba, N.P.; Liu, J.; Remaley, A.T.; Klingeborn, M.; Rickman, C.B. High-Density Lipoproteins Are a Potential Therapeutic Target for Age-Related Macular Degeneration. *J. Biol. Chem.* **2020**, *295*, 13601–13616. [CrossRef]
50. van Leeuwen, E.M.; Emri, E.; Merle, B.M.J.; Colijn, J.M.; Kersten, E.; Cougnard-Gregoire, A.; Dammeier, S.; Meester-Smoor, M.; Pool, F.M.; de Jong, E.K.; et al. A New Perspective on Lipid Research in Age-Related Macular Degeneration. *Prog. Retin. Eye Res.* **2018**, *67*, 56–86. [CrossRef]
51. Zhang, X.; Qiu, B.; Gong, Z.; Chen, X.; Wang, Y.; Nie, Y. Differentially Regulated Apolipoproteins and Lipid Profiles as Novel Biomarkers for Polypoidal Choroidal Vasculopathy and Neovascular Age-Related Macular Degeneration. *Front. Endocrinol.* **2022**, *13*, 946327. [CrossRef] [PubMed]
52. Ruberti, J.W.; Curcio, C.A.; Millican, C.L.; Menco, B.P.M.; Huang, J.-D.; Johnson, M. Quick-Freeze/Deep-Etch Visualization of Age-Related Lipid Accumulation in Bruch's Membrane. *Investig. Ophthalmol. Vis. Sci.* **2003**, *44*, 1753–1759. [CrossRef]

53. Haimovici, R.; Gantz, D.L.; Rumelt, S.; Freddo, T.F.; Small, D.M. The Lipid Composition of Drusen, Bruch's Membrane, and Sclera by Hot Stage Polarizing Light Microscopy. *Investig. Ophthalmol. Vis. Sci.* **2001**, *42*, 1592–1599.
54. Cao, X.; Sanchez, J.C.; Dinabandhu, A.; Guo, C.; Patel, T.P.; Yang, Z.; Hu, M.-W.; Chen, L.; Wang, Y.; Malik, D.; et al. Aqueous Proteins Help Predict the Response of Patients with Neovascular Age-Related Macular Degeneration to Anti-VEGF Therapy. *J. Clin. Investig.* **2022**, *132*, e144469. [CrossRef]
55. Curcio, C.A.; Johnson, M.; Huang, J.-D.; Rudolf, M. Aging, Age-Related Macular Degeneration, and the Response-to-Retention of Apolipoprotein B-Containing Lipoproteins. *Prog. Retin. Eye Res.* **2009**, *28*, 393–422. [CrossRef]
56. Tabas, I.; Williams, K.J.; Borén, J. Subendothelial Lipoprotein Retention as the Initiating Process in Atherosclerosis: Update and Therapeutic Implications. *Circulation* **2007**, *116*, 1832–1844. [CrossRef] [PubMed]
57. Han, X.; Ong, J.-S.; Hewitt, A.W.; Gharahkhani, P.; MacGregor, S. The Effects of Eight Serum Lipid Biomarkers on Age-Related Macular Degeneration Risk: A Mendelian Randomization Study. *Int. J. Epidemiol.* **2021**, *50*, 325–336. [CrossRef]
58. Paun, C.C.; Ersoy, L.; Schick, T.; Groenewoud, J.M.M.; Lechanteur, Y.T.; Fauser, S.; Hoyng, C.B.; de Jong, E.K.; den Hollander, A.I. Genetic Variants and Systemic Complement Activation Levels Are Associated With Serum Lipoprotein Levels in Age-Related Macular Degeneration. *Investig. Ophthalmol. Vis. Sci.* **2015**, *56*, 7766–7773. [CrossRef]
59. Curcio, C.A.; Johnson, M.; Huang, J.-D.; Rudolf, M. Apolipoprotein B-Containing Lipoproteins in Retinal Aging and Age-Related Macular Degeneration. *J. Lipid Res.* **2010**, *51*, 451–467. [CrossRef]
60. Armento, A.; Schmidt, T.L.; Sonntag, I.; Merle, D.A.; Jarboui, M.A.; Kilger, E.; Clark, S.J.; Ueffing, M. CFH Loss in Human RPE Cells Leads to Inflammation and Complement System Dysregulation via the NF-κB Pathway. *Int. J. Mol. Sci.* **2021**, *22*, 8727. [CrossRef]
61. Čolak, E.; Majkić-Singh, N.; Žorić, L.; Radosavljević, A.; Kosanović-Jaković, N. The Impact of Inflammation to the Antioxidant Defense Parameters in AMD Patients. *Aging Clin. Exp. Res.* **2012**, *24*, 588–594. [CrossRef] [PubMed]
62. Kauppinen, A.; Paterno, J.J.; Blasiak, J.; Salminen, A.; Kaarniranta, K. Inflammation and Its Role in Age-Related Macular Degeneration. *Cell. Mol. Life Sci.* **2016**, *73*, 1765–1786. [CrossRef] [PubMed]
63. Kemper, C.; Atkinson, J.P.; Hourcade, D.E. Properdin: Emerging Roles of a Pattern-Recognition Molecule. *Annu Rev Immunol* **2010**, *28*, 131–155. [CrossRef] [PubMed]
64. Armento, A.; Ueffing, M.; Clark, S.J. The Complement System in Age-Related Macular Degeneration. *Cell. Mol. Life Sci.* **2021**, *78*, 4487–4505. [CrossRef]
65. McHarg, S.; Clark, S.J.; Day, A.J.; Bishop, P.N. Age-Related Macular Degeneration and the Role of the Complement System. *Mol. Immunol.* **2015**, *67*, 43–50. [CrossRef] [PubMed]
66. Chen, H.; Yu, K.-D.; Xu, G.-Z. Association between Variant Y402H in Age-Related Macular Degeneration (AMD) Susceptibility Gene CFH and Treatment Response of AMD: A Meta-Analysis. *PLoS ONE* **2012**, *7*, e42464. [CrossRef] [PubMed]
67. Marazita, M.C.; Dugour, A.; Marquioni-Ramella, M.D.; Figueroa, J.M.; Suburo, A.M. Oxidative Stress-Induced Premature Senescence Dysregulates VEGF and CFH Expression in Retinal Pigment Epithelial Cells: Implications for Age-Related Macular Degeneration. *Redox Biol.* **2016**, *7*, 78–87. [CrossRef]
68. Lin, T.; Maita, D.; Thundivalappil, S.R.; Riley, F.E.; Hambsch, J.; Van Marter, L.J.; Christou, H.A.; Berra, L.; Fagan, S.; Christiani, D.C.; et al. Hemopexin in Severe Inflammation and Infection: Mouse Models and Human Diseases. *Crit. Care* **2015**, *19*, 166. [CrossRef] [PubMed]
69. Detzel, M.S.; Schmalohr, B.F.; Steinbock, F.; Hopp, M.-T.; Ramoji, A.; George, A.A.P.; Neugebauer, U.; Imhof, D. Revisiting the Interaction of Heme with Hemopexin. *Biol. Chem.* **2021**, *402*, 675–691. [CrossRef]
70. Sniatecki, J.J.; Ho-Yen, G.; Clarke, B.; Barbara, R.; Lash, S.; Papathomas, T.; Antonakis, S.; Gupta, B. Treatment of Submacular Hemorrhage with Tissue Plasminogen Activator and Pneumatic Displacement in Age-Related Macular Degeneration. *Eur. J. Ophthalmol.* **2021**, *31*, 643–648. [CrossRef]
71. Suhre, K.; Arnold, M.; Bhagwat, A.M.; Cotton, R.J.; Engelke, R.; Raffler, J.; Sarwath, H.; Thareja, G.; Wahl, A.; DeLisle, R.K.; et al. Connecting Genetic Risk to Disease End Points through the Human Blood Plasma Proteome. *Nat. Commun.* **2017**, *8*, 14357. [CrossRef] [PubMed]
72. Lauwen, S.; Bakker, B.; de Jong, E.K.; Fauser, S.; Hoyng, C.B.; Lefeber, D.J.; den Hollander, A.I. Analysis of Hemopexin Plasma Levels in Patients with Age-Related Macular Degeneration. *Mol. Vis.* **2022**, *28*, 536–543. [PubMed]
73. Iii, A.E.D.; Lu, F.; Mejia, P. C1 Inhibitor, a Multi-Functional Serine Protease Inhibitor. *Thromb. Haemost.* **2010**, *104*, 886–893. [CrossRef] [PubMed]
74. Gibson, J.; Hakobyan, S.; Cree, A.J.; Collins, A.; Harris, C.L.; Ennis, S.; Morgan, B.P.; Lotery, A.J. Variation in Complement Component C1 Inhibitor in Age-Related Macular Degeneration. *Immunobiology* **2012**, *217*, 251–255. [CrossRef] [PubMed]
75. Huang, Z.; Ung, T. Effect of Alpha-1-Acid Glycoprotein Binding on Pharmacokinetics and Pharmacodynamics. *Curr. Drug Metab.* **2013**, *14*, 226–238. [CrossRef] [PubMed]
76. Kim, T.W.; Kang, J.W.; Ahn, J.; Lee, E.K.; Cho, K.-C.; Han, B.N.R.; Hong, N.Y.; Park, J.; Kim, K.P. Proteomic Analysis of the Aqueous Humor in Age-Related Macular Degeneration (AMD) Patients. *J. Proteome Res.* **2012**, *11*, 4034–4043. [CrossRef] [PubMed]
77. Allyn, M.M.; Rincon-Benavides, M.A.; Chandler, H.L.; Higuita-Castro, N.; Palmer, A.F.; Swindle-Reilly, K.E. Sustained Release of Heme–Albumin as a Potential Novel Therapeutic Approach for Age-Related Macular Degeneration. *Biomater. Sci.* **2022**, *10*, 7004–7014. [CrossRef] [PubMed]

78. Cheema, A.K.; Kaur, P.; Fadel, A.; Younes, N.; Zirie, M.; Rizk, N.M. Integrated Datasets of Proteomic and Metabolomic Biomarkers to Predict Its Impacts on Comorbidities of Type 2 Diabetes Mellitus. *Diabetes Metab. Syndr. Obes.* **2020**, *13*, 2409–2431. [CrossRef]
79. Du, H.; Rao, Y.; Liu, R.; Deng, K.; Guan, Y.; Luo, D.; Mao, Q.; Yu, J.; Bo, T.; Fan, Z.; et al. Proteomics and Metabolomics Analyses Reveal the Full Spectrum of Inflammatory and Lipid Metabolic Abnormalities in Dyslipidemia. *Biomed. Chromatogr.* **2021**, *35*, e5183. [CrossRef]
80. Carrasco-Zanini, J.; Pietzner, M.; Lindbohm, J.V.; Wheeler, E.; Oerton, E.; Kerrison, N.; Simpson, M.; Westacott, M.; Drolet, D.; Kivimaki, M.; et al. Proteomic Signatures for Identification of Impaired Glucose Tolerance. *Nat. Med.* **2022**, *28*, 2293–2300. [CrossRef]

life

MDPI

Article

The Association between Ovarian Cancer and the Incidence of Newly Developed Dry Eye Disease: A Nationwide Population-Based Study

Chia-Yi Lee [1,2,3,†], Shun-Fa Yang [1,4,†], Yu-Ling Chang [5], Jing-Yang Huang [4] and Chao-Kai Chang [2,6,*]

1 Institute of Medicine, Chung Shan Medical University, Taichung 402, Taiwan
2 Nobel Eye Institute, Taipei 115, Taiwan
3 Department of Ophthalmology, Jen-Ai Hospital Dali Branch, Taichung 412, Taiwan
4 Department of Medical Research, Chung Shan Medical University Hospital, Taichung 402, Taiwan
5 Department of Medical Education, Cathay General Hospital, Taipei 106, Taiwan
6 Department of Optometry, Da-Yeh University, Chunghua 515, Taiwan
* Correspondence: chaokai@mail.dyu.edu.tw; Tel.: +886-2-2370-5666
† The authors contribute equally contributed equally to this work.

Abstract: We aim to investigate the potential correlation between the presence of ovarian cancer and the development of dry eye disease (DED) via the usage of the Longitudinal Health Insurance Database (LHID) of Taiwan. A retrospective cohort study was executed, and patients with ovarian cancer were selected according to the diagnostic and procedure codes. One ovarian cancer patient was matched to four non-ovarian cancer participants which served as control group, and a total of 4992 and 19,968 patients constructed the ovarian cancer and control groups, respectively. The primary outcome in the current study is the development of DED according to the diagnostic and procedure codes. Cox proportional hazard regression was utilized to produce the adjusted hazard ratio (aHR) and related 95% confidence interval (CI) of DED between the two groups. There were 542 and 2502 DED events observed in the ovarian cancer group and the control group, respectively. The ovarian cancer group illustrated a significantly higher incidence of DED development than the control group after the adjustment of several confounders (aHR: 1.10, 95% CI: 1.01–1.21, $p = 0.040$). In the subgroup analysis stratified by age, ovarian cancer patients aged older than 60 years showed a higher incidence of DED compared to the non-ovarian cancer population (aHR: 1.19, 95% CI: 1.08–1.28, $p = 0.011$). In addition, ovarian cancer patients with a disease duration longer than five years also showed higher incidence of DED formation than the non-ovarian cancer population (aHR: 1.13, 95% CI: 1.04–1.22, $p = 0.027$). In conclusion, the presence of ovarian cancer is associated with higher incidence of subsequent DED, especially in those older than 60 years and with a disease interval of more than five years.

Keywords: dry eye disease; ovarian cancer; oxidative stress; age; epidemiology

1. Introduction

Ovarian cancer is a common gynecological cancer in the world, which is the fifth leading etiology of cancer-related mortality among women in the American population [1,2]. The risk factors of the ovarian cancer involved delayed childbearing, usage of hormone replacement therapy, early menarche, oral contraceptive usage, family history of ovarian cancer, obesity, and pre-existing endometriosis [1,3,4]. The treatment options for ovarian cancer include the surgical removal and chemotherapy, and bevacizumab has gained attention in the recent years [5,6]. Despite the advance of therapy, the prognosis of ovarian cancer is still poor, with a five-year survival rate lower than 50 percent [7].

There are several pathophysiologies regarding the development of ovarian cancer in pervious research [8–10]. The steroid hormone effects of progesterone and estrogen in ovarian environment correlate to ovarian cancer formation [11], and the gene mutation, such as

BRCA1 and BRCA2 genes, elevated the risk of high-grade serous ovarian carcinoma [12]. In addition, the oxidative stress is another crucial mechanism for the development of ovarian cancer [13,14]. Higher reactive oxygen species, including inducible nitric oxide synthase and superoxide dismutase, was observed in individuals with ovarian cancer [15]. In addition, the antioxidant enzyme NAD(P)H:quinone oxidoreductase 1 could regulate the response to chemotherapy in ovarian cancer [16], and the antioxidant-related gene NRF2 has been shown to be an indicator for the prognosis of ovarian cancer [17].

Several conditions that associated with ovarian cancer were reported [18,19]. The type-2 diabetes mellitus (T2DM) revealed strong association to the poor prognosis of ovarian cancer in previous analysis [20]. Other metabolic syndromes like hyperlipidemia also correlate to increasing risk of ovarian cancer development [21]. Ovarian cancer tends to occur in patients with higher body mass index and obesity [4]. In addition, dementia is a disease related to oxidative stress [22], occurring in 2.1 percent of ovarian cancer individuals [23].

Dry eye disease (DED) is an ocular surface disorder that relates to meibomian gland dysfunction (MGD) and loss of tear film homeostasis [24–26]. Previous publications illustrated a positive relationship between DED occurrence and several diseases such as Sjogren syndrome, T2DM, and the rheumatic arthritis [27]. For further mechanisms, DED is an ocular surface disease that characterized with loss of tear film homeostasis and the increment of both inflammation and oxidative stress [28–30]. In a preceding article, both the expressions of interleukin-6 and the reactive oxygen species are significantly higher in the individuals with DED [25]. In addition, certain systemic morbidities, including Sjogren syndrome and systemic lupus erythematous, which serve as the predisposing factors for DED formation, are associated with inflammatory response [27,31]. Regarding DED and ovarian cancer, there is limited research that discusses the relationship between them. Because higher oxidative stress presents in both ovarian cancer and DED [13,32], there may be a correlation between these two diseases which need further validation.

The purpose of the current study is to evaluate the potential correlation between the presence of ovarian cancer and the development of subsequent DED events.

2. Materials and Methods

2.1. Data Resource

Females in the National Health Insurance Research Database (NHIRD) system were used for the performance of our analyses. The Taiwan NHIRD records the medical consultation documents of the 23 million people living in Taiwan from 1 January 2000 to 31 December 2020. The available medical information in Taiwan NHIRD are presented as follows: the International Classification of Diseases-Ninth Revision (ICD-9) of diagnostic code, the International Classification of Diseases-Tenth Revision (ICD-10) of diagnostic code, age, sex, occupation, income amount, urbanization intensity, education level, the image-based codes, laboratory exam-based codes, medical department-related codes, procedure/surgery codes, and finally, the international ATC codes for medicine. Only the image exam, laboratory exam, procedure/surgery, and medicine offered by the Taiwan national health insurance system are available in the NHIRD. The Taiwan Longitudinal Health Insurance Database (LHID) 2000 is a sub-database of Taiwan NHIRD, and was applied to the analysis in the current study. The LHID 2000 contains about two million people that were randomly drafted from the NHIRD using the automated software, and the available information in the LHID 2000 is the same as those in the NHIRD.

2.2. Study Population Selection

A retrospective cohort study was executed. The patients in the LHID 2000 were regarded as having ovarian cancer if completed the subsequent criteria: (1) ovarian cancer diagnosis according to corresponding ICD-9 plus ICD-10 diagnostic codes; (2) the completion of a pelvic exam before the day of the ovarian cancer diagnosis, according to the procedure/surgery codes; (3) the completion of a pelvic ultrasound exam, computed tomography, or the cancer antigen 125 test before the day of the ovarian cancer diagnosis, according to the procedure/surgery codes; and (4) the ovarian cancer was diagnosed in the gynecological department. The index date was designated as the six months after the emergence of the ovarian cancer-related diagnosis. The following exclusion criteria was adopted: (1) the ovarian cancer was diagnosed before 2001 or after 2019, to standardize the timeliness of ovarian cancer; (2) the primary outcome occurred before the index date; (3) the blindness occurred before the index date, in accordance with corresponding ICD-9 and ICD-10 diagnosis codes; (4) the ophthalmic tumor occurred before the index date, in accordance with corresponding ICD-9 and ICD-10 diagnosis codes; (5) the eye removal intervention was arranged before the index date, in accordance with corresponding intervention/surgery codes; and (6) the severe ocular injury occurred before the index date, in accordance with corresponding ICD-9 and ICD-10 diagnosis codes. For comparison, one ovarian cancer patient was age-matched to four non-ovarian cancer individuals, and the latter population constituted the control group. The reason for a 1:4 match is because we wanted to include as many cases as possible to reduce the bias from low patient numbers. However, if we matched 1 ovarian cancer patient to 8 or 10 non-ovarian cancer patients, the extreme discordance of the patient number between the two groups may have contributed to statistical bias. As a result, after discussing with our statistical specialist and consult previous publications [33,34], we decide to execute the match process with 1:4. A total of 4992 and 19,968 participants were enrolled into the ovarian cancer group and the control group, respectively. The flowchart of patient selection is available as Figure 1.

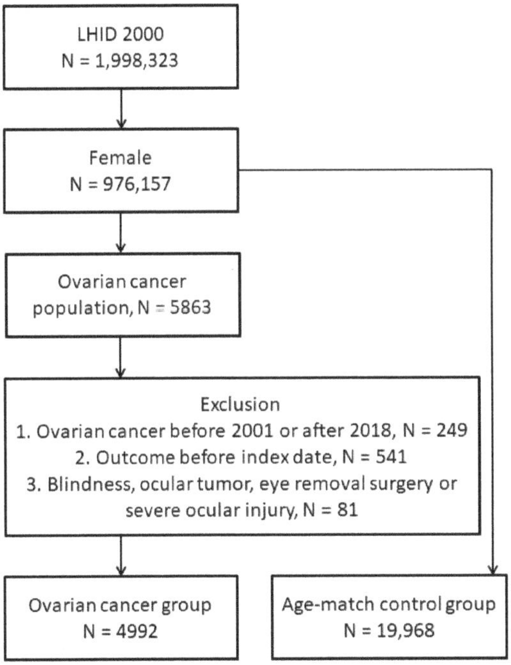

Figure 1. The flowchart of subject selection. N: number, LHID: Longitudinal Health Insurance Database.

2.3. Primary Outcome

The primary outcome of the current study is the development of DED, which is based on the following conditions: (1) a diagnosis of DED according to corresponding ICD-9 and ICD-10 diagnostic codes; (2) the arrangement of slit-lamp biomicroscope exam before the DED diagnosis according to the corresponding procedure/surgery code; (3) the arrangement of fluorescein stain test or Schirmer test before the DED diagnosis according to the corresponding procedure/surgery codes; (4) the prescription of artificial tear after the diagnosis of DED according to corresponding ATC codes; and (5) the DED diagnosis was made in the ophthalmic department. To better establish the time sequence between the ovarian cancer episode and following DED development, only the DED events found after the index date were accounted as outcome achievement. For the evaluation of primary outcome, the participants in the current study were tracked until the development of DED, discarded from the national health insurance program, or up to the deadline of NHIRD/LHID 2000, which indicate a date of 31 December 2020.

2.4. Covariates and Co-Morbidities

In addition to the primary outcome, several confounders were included in the analysis model to adjust the effect of these factors on DED development as possible: age, urbanization, hypertension, T2DM, ischemic heart diseases, hyperlipidemia, peripheral vascular disease, end-stage renal disease, rheumatoid arthritis, systemic lupus erythematosus, Sjogren syndrome, MGE/Blepharitis, and the receipt of cataract surgery. The presence of these covariates were based on the demographic codes, ICD-9 and ICD-10 diagnostic codes, and the procedure/surgery codes in the NHIRD/LHID 2000. In addition, only the diseases that diagnosed for more than two years were enrolled as the confounder to ensure the disease interval and associated effect on DED formation.

2.5. Statistical Analysis

The SAS edition 9.4 version (SAS Institute Inc., Cary, NC, USA) was adopted for all the statistical analyses in current study. Descriptive analysis were used to present the demographic data and co-morbidities of the two groups, and the normality of study population was tested and affirmed using the Shapiro–Wilk test before subsequent analysis ($p > 0.05$). The standard mean difference (SMD) was applied to compare the distribution of each parameter between the two populations, and an SMD amount > 0.1 was regarded as the significant difference. Then, the Cox proportional hazard regression analysis was executed to produce an adjusted hazard ratio (aHR) and related 95 percent confidence interval (CI) of DED development between the two populations. The effect of age, urbanization, and DED-associated co-morbidities were all adjusted in the Cox proportional hazard regression analysis. In the subgroup analyses, the ovarian cancer patients were stratified according to age (<40 years, 40–60 years, and <60 years) and duration of ovarian cancer (<2 years, 2–4 years, and >4 years). The Cox proportional hazard regression was adopted again with the adjustments of all the co-morbidities, and yielded the aHR and corresponding 95% CI. The Cox proportional hazard regression belongs to the family of survival analysis, which can present the ratio of an exposure population (the ovarian cancer group in the current study) surviving from an outcome/morbidity (which is DED in the current study). In addition to the comparison between exposure and non-exposure groups, the Cox proportional hazard regression can integrate the effect of multiple factors in the model; thus, the effect of known risk factors of DED like age, T2DM, and Sjogren syndrome can be adjusted in the analysis to elevate the accuracy of our results. When compared to other multiple regression analyses, the Cox proportional hazard regression can put the survival time (from exposure to outcome or the end of study period) in the analysis model, and the analysis can be better refined. Finally, a $p < 0.05$ was set as statistical significance in the current study, and p values underneath 0.001 were depicted as $p < 0.001$.

3. Results

The baseline characteristics are presented in Table 1. The age distributions between the two groups were not-significantly different due to the matching process (SMD = 0.002). The level of urbanization was also similar between the two groups (SMD = 0.007). Regarding the co-morbidities, the distribution of T2DM, ischemic heart disease, and blepharitis/MGD were significantly higher in the ovarian cancer group than the control group (all SMD > 0.1), while the rests of co-morbidities showed similar distribution between the two groups (all SMD < 0.1) (Table 1).

Table 1. Baseline characteristic between the study groups.

Characteristic	Control Group (N = 19,968)	Ovarian Cancer Group (N = 4992)	SMD
Age at index date			0.002
<40	5965 (29.87%)	1490 (29.85%)	
40–49	5127 (25.68%)	1267 (25.38%)	
50–59	4099 (20.53%)	1038 (20.79%)	
60–69	2369 (11.86%)	589 (11.80%)	
70–79	1567 (7.85%)	398 (7.97%)	
≥80	841 (4.21%)	210 (4.21%)	
Urbanization			0.007
1 (high)	6637 (33.24%)	1714 (34.33%)	
2	5911 (29.60%)	1524 (30.53%)	
3	3103 (15.54%)	775 (15.52%)	
4	2584 (12.94%)	604 (12.10%)	
5	365 (1.83%)	85 (1.70%)	
6	793 (3.97%)	165 (3.31%)	
7 (low)	575 (2.88%)	125 (2.50%)	
Co-morbidity			
Hypertension	3237 (16.21%)	947 (18.97%)	0.045
T2DM	1523 (7.63%)	468 (9.38%)	0.398 *
Ischemic heart diseases	755 (3.78%)	248 (4.97%)	0.117 *
Hyperlipidemia	1680 (8.41%)	448 (8.97%)	0.017
Peripheral vascular disease	92 (0.46%)	24 (0.48%)	0.005
End-stage renal disease	78 (0.39%)	42 (0.84%)	0.076
Rheumatoid arthritis	121 (0.61%)	37 (0.74%)	0.031
Systemic lupus erythematosus	23 (0.12%)	11 (0.22%)	0.009
Sjogren Syndrome	184 (0.92%)	49 (0.98%)	0.010
Blepharitis/MGD	976 (4.88%)	296 (5.92%)	0.249 *
Cataract surgery	250 (1.25%)	61 (1.22%)	0.003

T2DM: type 2 diabetes mellitus, MGD: meibomian gland dysfunction, N: number, SMD: standard mean difference.
* denotes significant difference between groups.

After the follow-up interval, there were 542 and 2502 episodes of DED found in the ovarian cancer group and the control group, respectively (Table 2). The ovarian cancer group demonstrated a significantly higher incidence of DED development than the control group, with the adjustment of several confounders (aHR: 1.10, 95% CI: 1.01–1.21, $p = 0.040$) (Table 2). In the subgroup analysis stratified by age, the ovarian cancer patients younger than 60 years did not show higher incidence of DED than the control group (both $p > 0.05$), but the ovarian cancer patients older than 60 years revealed a higher incidence of DED compared to the non-ovarian cancer population (aHR: 1.19, 95% CI: 1.08–1.28, $p = 0.011$). On the other hand, the ovarian cancer patients with disease duration more than five years showed higher chance for developing DED than the non-ovarian cancer population (aHR: 1.13, 95% CI: 1.04–1.22, $p = 0.027$). Still, the ovarian cancer individuals with disease duration lesser than five years showed similar rate of DED occurrence compared to the non-ovarian cancer population (both $p > 0.05$) (Table 3).

Table 2. Risk of dry eye disease between the two groups.

Dry Eye Event	Control Group (N = 19,968)	Ovarian Cancer Group (N = 4992)	*p* Value
Follow-up person-month	1,875,677	375,612	
Cases	2502	542	
Crude HR (95% CI)	Reference	1.08 (0.98–1.18)	
aHR (95% CI)	Reference	1.10 (1.01–1.21)	0.040 *

aHR: adjusted hazard ratio, adjusted for demographics and co-morbidities, CI: confidence interval, N: number.
* denotes significant difference between groups.

Table 3. Subgroup analysis stratified by age and duration of ovarian cancer.

Subgroup	aHR #	95% CI	*p* Value
Age			
<40 years	0.92	0.76–1.01	0.264
41–60 years	1.05	0.97–1.11	0.355
>60 years	1.19	1.08–1.28	0.011 *
Duration of ovarian cancer			
<2 years	1.04	0.92–1.14	0.319
2–5 years	1.00	0.94–1.13	0.186
>5 years	1.13	1.04–1.22	0.027 *

aHR: adjusted hazard ratio, adjusted for demographics and co-morbidities, CI: confidence interval. * Denotes significant difference between groups. # Risk of dry eye in ovarian cancer population compared to non-ovarian cancer population.

4. Discussion

Briefly, the current study demonstrated a higher incidence of later DED in the patients diagnosed with ovarian cancer. Moreover, the incidence of DED was even higher in the ovarian cancer patients older than 60 years. On the other hand, the patients diagnosed with ovarian cancer for more than five years presented with a significantly higher risk of developing DED than the non-ovarian cancer population.

The patients diagnosed with ovarian cancer associated with a higher incidence of subsequent DED in the current study. In a previous study, the existence of ovarian cancer showed a significant relationship to several diseases like the obesity and T2DM [4,20]. Still, no evidence for the correlation between ovarian cancer and eye disease was proposed previously. In some experimental research, oxidative stress on the ocular surface was significantly elevated in the individuals with moderate DED [25,35]. Regarding the correlation between antioxidant and DED development, a previous study demonstrated that the higher amount of antioxidant may decrease the severity of DED signs and symptoms [36]. Since both the ovarian cancer and DED share similar mechanism of elevated oxidative stress [15,25,37], the presence of ovarian cancer may indicate a higher baseline oxidative stress, and the incidence of DED may be elevated in such condition. This concept was supported by the results of the current study. To our knowledge, this may be a preliminary experience to demonstrate the positive correlation between the ovarian cancer and the following DED development. Moreover, we excluded the patients diagnosed with DED before or within 6 months after the diagnosis of ovarian cancer; thus, the time sequence between the two diseases was be established. In addition, we adjusted the effect of several predisposing factors of DED including age, T2DM, Sjogren syndrome, MGD, and cataract surgery in the Cox proportional hazard regression [38,39]. Consequently, the ovarian cancer may be an independent risk factor for the development of DED. Oxidative stress possibly served as the main mechanism for the ovarian cancer-to-DED relationship because inflammation and elevated oxidative stress were regarded as the major pathophysiologies for many eye diseases including DED [25,40]. On the other hand, ovarian cancer did not raise systemic inflammation prominently, but could contribute to the increasing serum oxidative stress [15], which can circulate to the whole body involve the orbital and ocular region. As a consequence, elevated oxidative stress could be the reason for the increasing DED incidence in the ovarian cancer population. In addition to oxidative stress, serum sex hormones level like estrogen are crucial for the onset of DED during in vitro fertilization [41], and both the elevation of estrogen and progesterone are associated with the development of DED, despite a few papers demonstrating contrary results [42]. Since ovarian cancer featured with increased estrogen and progesterone [11], this may be another mechanism for DED development in individuals with ovarian cancer.

On the other hand, the percentage of DED was numerically higher in the control group compared to the ovarian cancer group, which is theoretically contrary to the results of Cox proportional hazard regression. Still, the follow-up person-month per patient was also higher in the control group than that in the ovarian cancer group. Consequently, it may be reasonable that the percentage of DED is slightly higher in the population with longer follow up period. Because the Cox proportional hazard regression can consider the effect of exposure-to-event time on the incidence of outcome, the incidence of DED became significantly higher in the ovarian cancer group after the adjustment. The longer follow-up person-per-month in the control group may result from the fact that the population with ovarian cancer experiences a higher mortality rate than the normal population, and the mean age of ovarian cancer patients was significantly shorter in the previous study.

In the subgroup analysis, ovarian cancer patients aged older than 60 years showed a higher incidence of DED compared to the non-ovarian-cancer individuals, and the aHR of DED in the ovarian cancer subgroups toward non-ovarian-cancer subgroups numerically decreased with younger age. Age is a known risk factor for DED, in which the prevalence of DED elevates every five years in the population older than 50 years [43]. Also, the tear volume was significantly lower in patients older than 40 years [44]. On the other hand, ovarian cancer tends to occur in the female population older than 50 years old, which shows an incidence rate higher than 25 per 100,000 women [3]. In addition to the role in the development of the two diseases, age is also related to increased oxidative stress [44]. Due to the metabolism, the reactive oxygen species expression was significantly increased in the elderly population [45]. Consequently, old age may lead to higher rate of ovarian cancer, and both of these factors are associated with higher oxidative stress; thus, DED occurred much easier in this situation. Regarding the influence of disease duration, the ovarian cancer patient with a disease period longer than five years showed a higher chance for developing DED. There was sparse research which reported this phenomenon. The moderate oxidative stress level can promote the proliferation of ovarian cancer [15]; thus, we speculate that the persistent oxidative stress that accompanies prolonged ovarian cancer course could cause more damage to the human body, including the ocular surface. In addition, ovarian cancer progresses over time, and the advanced stage of ovarian cancer may contribute to a higher level of oxidative stress. Nevertheless, further study is needed to confirm this hypothesis.

Concerning the epidemiology, the ovarian cancer is the second most frequent gynecological cancer worldwide, just after breast cancer [7]. There were more than 200,000 patients diagnosed with ovarian cancer in 2018 [7], and more than 100,000 women die of ovarian cancer annually throughout the world [1]. North America, Europe, and Oceania showed the highest mortality rate from ovarian cancer [46]. DED, similarly to ovarian cancer, affects numerous people, with an annual incidence of more than five percent in men and women older than 40 years [27,47]. In specific situations, like the population using a visual display terminal frequently, the incidence of DED can reach a rate as high as 60 percent [48]. Advanced DED can not only damage the ocular surface, but can also contribute to significant visual impairment and depressive conditions [27]. Because both DED and ovarian cancer affects a huge number of people and would contribute to tremendous cost and disability, any correlation between them may be demonstrated to better prevent the development of these two prevalent diseases.

There are several major limitations in the current study. Firstly, both the NHIRD and LHID 2000 are claimed databases which only preserve the codes for diagnosis, examination, procedure, and medication prescription. As a consequence, much crucial information, including the severity of co-morbidities, the site of ovarian cancer, the laterality of ovarian cancer, the detailed pathological report of ovarian cancer, the results of image and laboratory exam for ovarian cancer, the TNM stage for ovarian cancer, the treatment response of ovarian cancer, the detail of surgery for ovarian cancer if arranged, the recurrence of ovarian cancer, the type of DED, the external eye image of DED, the results of DED-related examination, the severity of DED, the grade of MGD in DED population, the treatment response of DED, and the subjective symptom of DED, cannot be accessed or cannot be accessed with enough accuracy. Similarly, we cannot obtain the serum sex hormones level in the Taiwan NHIRD because it only contained claimed data. In addition, the contact lens wear and the receipt of refractive surgery are prominent risk factors for the development of DED [38], but the two covariates cannot be evaluated via the NHIRD and LHID 2000 because both managements are self-paid in Taiwan, which will not be recorded in the national health insurance system. In addition, nearly all the participants in the current study are Taiwanese, and thus the external validity of our results is limited. Finally, the ovarian cancer group showed a higher ratio of T2DM, ischemic heart disease, and MGD, which leads to a high heterogeneity between the two groups concerning the evaluation of DED risk. However, we applied the Cox proportional hazard regression to adjust the effect of these parameters. As a result, the influence of heterogeneity on the accuracy of our analysis might not be prominent.

5. Conclusions

In conclusion, the existence of ovarian cancer is associated with higher incidence of subsequent DED after the adjustments of multiple risk factors. Furthermore, the risk of DED in the ovarian cancer population increase with the aging and prolonged disease course. Consequently, the routine ophthalmic examination for the ovarian cancer patients older than 60 years or diagnosed for more than five years could be recommended. A further large-scale prospective study to reveal whether the presence of ovarian cancer would influence the therapeutic outcome of DED is necessary.

Author Contributions: Conceptualization, C.-Y.L. and C.-K.C.; methodology, C.-Y.L., C.-K.C. and S.-F.Y.; software, C.-K.C. and Y.-L.C.; formal analysis, C.-K.C.; data curation, J.-Y.H.; writing—original draft preparation, C.-Y.L.; writing—review and editing, S.-F.Y. and C.-K.C.; revision, C.-K.C.; validation, C.-K.C.; supervision, C.-K.C. All authors have read and agreed to the published version of the manuscript.

Funding: This research received no external funding.

Institutional Review Board Statement: The current study adhered to the declaration of Helsinki in 1964 and its late amendments. In addition, the current study was also approved by the Taiwan National Health Insurance Administration and the Institutional Review Board of Chung Shan Medical University (Project code: CS1-20108, approval date: 16 June 2020).

Informed Consent Statement: The essentiality of written informed consent obtain was abandoned by the institutions described above due to the retrospective design.

Data Availability Statement: The original data used in the current study are not available due to the policy of Taiwan National Health Insurance Administration.

Conflicts of Interest: The authors declare no conflicts of interest.

References

1. Penny, S.M. Ovarian Cancer: An Overview. *Radiol. Technol.* **2020**, *91*, 561–575. [PubMed]
2. Zhang, R.; Siu, M.K.Y.; Ngan, H.Y.S.; Chan, K.K.L. Molecular Biomarkers for the Early Detection of Ovarian Cancer. *Int. J. Mol. Sci.* **2022**, *23*, 12041. [CrossRef] [PubMed]
3. Roett, M.A.; Evans, P. Ovarian cancer: An overview. *Am. Fam. Phys.* **2009**, *80*, 609–616. [PubMed]
4. La Vecchia, C. Ovarian cancer: Epidemiology and risk factors. *Eur. J. Cancer Prev.* **2017**, *26*, 55–62. [CrossRef] [PubMed]
5. Rooth, C. Ovarian cancer: Risk factors, treatment and management. *Br. J. Nurs.* **2013**, *22*, S23–S30. [CrossRef] [PubMed]
6. Eisenhauer, E.A. Real-world evidence in the treatment of ovarian cancer. *Ann. Oncol.* **2017**, *28*, viii61–viii65. [CrossRef]
7. Stewart, C.; Ralyea, C.; Lockwood, S. Ovarian Cancer: An Integrated Review. *Semin. Oncol. Nurs.* **2019**, *35*, 151–156. [CrossRef] [PubMed]
8. Orr, B.; Edwards, R.P. Diagnosis and Treatment of Ovarian Cancer. *Hematol. Oncol. Clin. N. Am.* **2018**, *32*, 943–964. [CrossRef] [PubMed]
9. Tossetta, G.; Inversetti, A. Ovarian Cancer: Advances in Pathophysiology and Therapies. *Int. J. Mol. Sci.* **2023**, *24*, 8930. [CrossRef]
10. Hou, D.; Liu, Z.; Xu, X.; Liu, Q.; Zhang, X.; Kong, B.; Wei, J.J.; Gong, Y.; Shao, C. Increased oxidative stress mediates the antitumor effect of PARP inhibition in ovarian cancer. *Redox Biol.* **2018**, *17*, 99–111. [CrossRef]
11. Nezhat, F.R.; Apostol, R.; Nezhat, C.; Pejovic, T. New insights in the pathophysiology of ovarian cancer and implications for screening and prevention. *Am. J. Obstet. Gynecol.* **2015**, *213*, 262–267. [CrossRef] [PubMed]
12. Kroeger, P.T., Jr.; Drapkin, R. Pathogenesis and heterogeneity of ovarian cancer. *Curr. Opin. Obstet. Gynecol.* **2017**, *29*, 26–34. [CrossRef] [PubMed]

13. Jelic, M.D.; Mandic, A.D.; Maricic, S.M.; Srdjenovic, B.U. Oxidative stress and its role in cancer. *J. Cancer Res. Ther.* **2021**, *17*, 22–28. [CrossRef] [PubMed]
14. Song, C.; Yu, B.; Wang, J.; Ji, X.; Zhang, L.; Tian, X.; Yu, X.; Feng, C.; Wang, X.; Zhang, X. Moderate Static Magnet Fields Suppress Ovarian Cancer Metastasis via ROS-Mediated Oxidative Stress. *Oxid. Med. Cell Longev.* **2021**, *2021*, 7103345. [CrossRef] [PubMed]
15. Ding, D.N.; Xie, L.Z.; Shen, Y.; Li, J.; Guo, Y.; Fu, Y.; Liu, F.Y.; Han, F.J. Insights into the Role of Oxidative Stress in Ovarian Cancer. *Oxid. Med. Cell Longev.* **2021**, *2021*, 8388258. [CrossRef] [PubMed]
16. Tossetta, G.; Fantone, S.; Goteri, G.; Giannubilo, S.R.; Ciavattini, A.; Marzioni, D. The Role of NQO1 in Ovarian Cancer. *Int. J. Mol. Sci.* **2023**, *24*, 7839. [CrossRef] [PubMed]
17. Batista, L.; Gruosso, T.; Mechta-Grigoriou, F. Ovarian cancer emerging subtypes: Role of oxidative stress and fibrosis in tumour development and response to treatment. *Int. J. Biochem. Cell Biol.* **2013**, *45*, 1092–1098. [CrossRef] [PubMed]
18. Mallen, A.R.; Townsend, M.K.; Tworoger, S.S. Risk Factors for Ovarian Carcinoma. *Hematol. Oncol. Clin. N. Am.* **2018**, *32*, 891–902. [CrossRef] [PubMed]
19. Geng, S.; Zhang, X.; Zhu, X.; Wang, Y.; Wang, Y.; Sun, Y. Psychological factors increase the risk of ovarian cancer. *J. Obstet. Gynaecol.* **2023**, *43*, 2187573. [CrossRef]
20. Slavchev, S.; Kornovski, Y.; Yordanov, A.; Ivanova, Y.; Kostov, S.; Slavcheva, S. Survival in Advanced Epithelial Ovarian Cancer Associated with Cardiovascular Comorbidities and Type 2 Diabetes Mellitus. *Curr. Oncol.* **2021**, *28*, 3668–3682. [CrossRef]
21. Zhang, D.; Xi, Y.; Feng, Y. Ovarian cancer risk in relation to blood lipid levels and hyperlipidemia: A systematic review and meta-analysis of observational epidemiologic studies. *Eur. J. Cancer Prev.* **2021**, *30*, 161–170. [CrossRef] [PubMed]
22. Chen, Z.; Zhong, C. Oxidative stress in Alzheimer's disease. *Neurosci. Bull.* **2014**, *30*, 271–281. [CrossRef] [PubMed]
23. Vranes, C.; Zhao, H.; Noer, M.C.; Fu, S.; Sun, C.C.; Harrison, R.; Ramirez, P.T.; Høgdall, C.K.; Giordano, S.H.; Meyer, L.A. Secondary validation of an ovarian cancer-specific comorbidity index in a US population. *Int. J. Gynecol. Cancer* **2023**, *33*, 749–754. [CrossRef] [PubMed]
24. Lee, C.Y.; Yang, K.L.; Sun, C.C.; Huang, J.Y.; Chen, H.C.; Chen, H.C.; Yang, S.F. The Development of Dry Eye Disease After Surgery-Indicated Chronic Rhinosinusitis: A Population-Based Cohort Study. *Int. J. Environ. Res. Public Health* **2020**, *17*, 3829. [CrossRef] [PubMed]
25. Bron, A.J.; de Paiva, C.S.; Chauhan, S.K.; Bonini, S.; Gabison, E.E.; Jain, S.; Knop, E.; Markoulli, M.; Ogawa, Y.; Perez, V.; et al. TFOS DEWS II pathophysiology report. *Ocul. Surf.* **2017**, *15*, 438–510. [CrossRef] [PubMed]
26. O'Neil, E.C.; Henderson, M.; Massaro-Giordano, M.; Bunya, V.Y. Advances in dry eye disease treatment. *Curr. Opin. Ophthalmol.* **2019**, *30*, 166–178. [CrossRef] [PubMed]
27. Rouen, P.A.; White, M.L. Dry Eye Disease: Prevalence, Assessment, and Management. *Home Healthc. Now* **2018**, *36*, 74–83. [CrossRef] [PubMed]
28. Kojima, T.; Dogru, M.; Kawashima, M.; Nakamura, S.; Tsubota, K. Advances in the diagnosis and treatment of dry eye. *Prog. Retin. Eye Res.* **2020**, *78*, 100842. [CrossRef]
29. Seen, S.; Tong, L. Dry eye disease and oxidative stress. *Acta Ophthalmol.* **2018**, *96*, e412–e420. [CrossRef]
30. Dammak, A.; Pastrana, C.; Martin-Gil, A.; Carpena-Torres, C.; Peral Cerda, A.; Simovart, M.; Alarma, P.; Huete-Toral, F.; Carracedo, G. Oxidative Stress in the Anterior Ocular Diseases: Diagnostic and Treatment. *Biomedicines* **2023**, *11*, 292. [CrossRef]
31. Generali, E.; Cantarini, L.; Selmi, C. Ocular Involvement in Systemic Autoimmune Diseases. *Clin. Rev. Allergy Immunol.* **2015**, *49*, 263–270. [CrossRef] [PubMed]
32. Dogru, M.; Kojima, T.; Simsek, C.; Tsubota, K. Potential Role of Oxidative Stress in Ocular Surface Inflammation and Dry Eye Disease. *Investig. Ophthalmol. Vis. Sci.* **2018**, *59*, Des163–Des168. [CrossRef] [PubMed]
33. Kok, V.C.; Tsai, H.J.; Su, C.F.; Lee, C.K. The Risks for Ovarian, Endometrial, Breast, Colorectal, and Other Cancers in Women with Newly Diagnosed Endometriosis or Adenomyosis: A Population-Based Study. *Int. J. Gynecol. Cancer* **2015**, *25*, 968–976. [CrossRef] [PubMed]
34. Ding, D.C.; Chen, W.; Wang, J.H.; Lin, S.Z. Association between polycystic ovarian syndrome and endometrial, ovarian, and breast cancer: A population-based cohort study in Taiwan. *Medicine* **2018**, *97*, e12608. [CrossRef] [PubMed]
35. Navel, V.; Sapin, V.; Henrioux, F.; Blanchon, L.; Labbé, A.; Chiambaretta, F.; Baudouin, C.; Dutheil, F. Oxidative and antioxidative stress markers in dry eye disease: A systematic review and meta-analysis. *Acta Ophthalmol.* **2022**, *100*, 45–57. [CrossRef] [PubMed]
36. Aldaas, K.M.; Ismail, O.M.; Hakim, J.; Van Buren, E.D.; Lin, F.C.; Hardin, J.S.; Meyer, J.J. Association of Dry Eye Disease with Dyslipidemia and Statin Use. *Am. J. Ophthalmol.* **2020**, *218*, 54–58. [CrossRef] [PubMed]
37. Li, H.; Sun, K.; Zhao, R.; Hu, J.; Hao, Z.; Wang, F.; Lu, Y.; Liu, F.; Zhang, Y. Inflammatory biomarkers of coronary heart disease. *Front. Biosci. (Schol. Ed.)* **2018**, *10*, 185–196. [CrossRef] [PubMed]
38. Qian, L.; Wei, W. Identified risk factors for dry eye syndrome: A systematic review and meta-analysis. *PLoS ONE* **2022**, *17*, e0271267. [CrossRef] [PubMed]
39. Wang, M.T.M.; Vidal-Rohr, M.; Muntz, A.; Diprose, W.K.; Ormonde, S.E.; Wolffsohn, J.S.; Craig, J.P. Systemic risk factors of dry eye disease subtypes: A New Zealand cross-sectional study. *Ocul. Surf.* **2020**, *18*, 374–380. [CrossRef]
40. Hsueh, Y.J.; Chen, Y.N.; Tsao, Y.T.; Cheng, C.M.; Wu, W.C.; Chen, H.C. The Pathomechanism, Antioxidant Biomarkers, and Treatment of Oxidative Stress-Related Eye Diseases. *Int. J. Mol. Sci.* **2022**, *23*, 1255. [CrossRef]
41. Boga, A.; Stapleton, F.; Chapman, M.; Golebiowski, B. Effects of elevated serum estrogen on dry eye in women undergoing in vitro fertilisation. *Ocul. Surf.* **2023**, *29*, 511–520. [CrossRef] [PubMed]

42. Gorimanipalli, B.; Khamar, P.; Sethu, S.; Shetty, R. Hormones and dry eye disease. *Indian J. Ophthalmol.* **2023**, *71*, 1276–1284. [CrossRef] [PubMed]
43. de Paiva, C.S. Effects of Aging in Dry Eye. *Int. Ophthalmol. Clin.* **2017**, *57*, 47–64. [CrossRef] [PubMed]
44. Kawashima, M. Systemic Health and Dry Eye. *Investig. Ophthalmol. Vis. Sci.* **2018**, *59*, Des138–Des142. [CrossRef]
45. Bolduc, J.A.; Collins, J.A.; Loeser, R.F. Reactive oxygen species, aging and articular cartilage homeostasis. *Free Radic. Biol. Med.* **2019**, *132*, 73–82. [CrossRef] [PubMed]
46. Webb, P.M.; Jordan, S.J. Epidemiology of epithelial ovarian cancer. *Best Pract. Res. Clin. Obstet. Gynaecol.* **2017**, *41*, 3–14. [CrossRef] [PubMed]
47. McCann, P.; Abraham, A.G.; Mukhopadhyay, A.; Panagiotopoulou, K.; Chen, H.; Rittiphairoj, T.; Gregory, D.G.; Hauswirth, S.G.; Ifantides, C.; Qureshi, R.; et al. Prevalence and Incidence of Dry Eye and Meibomian Gland Dysfunction in the United States: A Systematic Review and Meta-analysis. *JAMA Ophthalmol.* **2022**, *140*, 1181–1192. [CrossRef]
48. Uchino, M.; Yokoi, N.; Uchino, Y.; Dogru, M.; Kawashima, M.; Komuro, A.; Sonomura, Y.; Kato, H.; Kinoshita, S.; Schaumberg, D.A.; et al. Prevalence of dry eye disease and its risk factors in visual display terminal users: The Osaka study. *Am. J. Ophthalmol.* **2013**, *156*, 759–766. [CrossRef]

life

Article

Longitudinal Changes of Cornea Volume Measured by Means of Anterior Segment-Optical Coherence Tomography in Patients with Stable and Progressive Keratoconus

Sabrina Vaccaro [1], Chiara Vivarelli [2,3], Angeli Christy Yu [2,3], Nicolò Pecora [1], Giovanna Lionetti [1], Raffaella Gioia [1], Vincenzo Scorcia [1] and Giuseppe Giannaccare [4,*]

1 Department of Ophthalmology, University Magna Græcia of Catanzaro, 88100 Catanzaro, Italy; sabrina_vaccaro@libero.it (S.V.); nicolo.pecora@studenti.unicz.it (N.P.); lionettigiovanna@libero.it (G.L.); raffaella.gioia@studenti.unicz.it (R.G.); vscorcia@unicz.it (V.S.)
2 Department of Translational Medicine, University of Ferrara, 44121 Ferrara, Italy; chiara.vivarelli@edu.unife.it (C.V.); angelichristy.yu@unife.it (A.C.Y.)
3 Department of Ophthalmology, Ospedali Privati Forlì "Villa Igea", 47122 Forlì, Italy
4 Eye Clinic, Department of Surgical Sciences, University of Cagliari, Via Università 40, 09124 Cagliari, Italy
* Correspondence: giuseppe.giannaccare@unica.it; Tel.: +39-3317186201

Abstract: Keratoconus is a corneal disease which results in progressive thinning and protrusion of the cornea leading to irregular astigmatism. The purpose of this study was to evaluate longitudinal changes in corneal volume (CV) occurring over time in keratoconus eyes. Consecutive patients affected by keratoconus were evaluated by means of anterior segment-optical coherence tomography (AS-OCT) at two different time points: baseline (T0) and after 1 year (T1). Anterior and posterior refractive value; corneal thickness at the thinnest point (TP) and corneal volume (CV) calculated within discs of 3, 5 and 8 mm of diameter; anterior chamber depth (ACD); and anterior chamber volume (ACV) were obtained. Enrolled patients were divided into 3 groups (groups 1, 2, 3) according to the increasing disease severity and into 2 groups (groups A, B) according to the progression or stability of the disease. Overall, 116 eyes of 116 patients (76 males and 40 females, mean age 34.76 ± 13.99 years) were included. For the entire group of keratoconus patients, in comparison with T0, mean TP decreased at T1 from 458.7 ± 52.2 µm to 454.6 ± 51.6 µm (p = 0.0004); in parallel, mean value of CV calculated at 5 mm and 8 mm decreased significantly (from 10.78 ± 0.8 at T0 to 10.75 ± 0.79 at T1 (p = 0.02), and from 32.03 ± 2.01 mm^3 at T0 to 31.95 ± 1.98 at T1 (p = 0.02), respectively). Conversely, there were no statistically significant differences in CV at 3 mm from T0 to T1 (p = 0.08), as well as for ACD and ACV. Regarding the course of the disease, patients belonging to group A showed statistically significant differences from T0 to T1 for TP, and for CV at 3 mm, 5 mm and 8 mm ($p < 0.0001$, $p < 0.0001$, $p < 0.001$ and p = 0.0058 respectively). There were no statistically significant differences for ACD (p = 0.6916) and ACV calculated at 3, 5 and 8 mm (p = 0.7709, p = 0.3765, p = 0.2475, respectively) in group A. At the same time, no statistically significant differences for ACD (p = 0.2897) and ACV calculated at 3, 5 and 8 mm (p = 0.9849, p = 0.6420, p = 0.8338, respectively) were found in group B. There were statistically significant positive correlations between changes of TP and CV at 3 mm (r = 0.6324, $p < 0.0001$), 5 mm (r = 0.7622, $p < 0.0001$) and 8 mm (r = 0.5987 $p < 0.0001$). In conclusion, given the strong correlation with TP, CV might be considered an additional AS-OCT parameter to be used in association with conventional parameters when detecting longitudinal changes in keratoconic eyes.

Keywords: keratoconus; cornea; AS-OCT; corneal volume; corneal thickness

1. Introduction

Keratoconus is a complex corneal disease, associated with both genetic and environmental factors [1,2]. Once considered non-inflammatory, its etiopathogenesis has now been related to pro-inflammatory pathways [3–5]. It is characterized by central corneal thinning and protrusion that lead to progressive irregular astigmatism [1,2]. The majority cases, accounting for 90% of the total, are binocular, often characterized by asymmetrical progression in both eyes [6,7]. The alteration in the curvature of the cornea results in the generation of substantial levels of higher order aberrations, leading to a significant reduction in visual quality [8]. In 2015, the Global Consensus on Keratoconus and Ectatic Diseases highlighted the role of changes occurring in the posterior corneal surface and in corneal thickness for the diagnosis of keratoconus [9]. Alterations of both disposition and composition of collagen lamellae have been shown in eyes with keratoconus. This alteration leads to loss of corneal rigidity and, consequently, corneal protrusion and thinning [10,11]. It has been proposed that several factors, including localized changes in proteolitic enzyme activity and pro-inflammatory citokines and a reduced production of collagen I, are associated with breaks in Bowman's layer and may simultaneously also promote the unraveling of collagen fibrils, lamellar slippage and the disinsertion of lamellae from their anchoring sites in Bowman's layer [12–16]. When comparing keratoconus with normal corneas, the collagen fibrillar mass is unevenly distributed, particularly at the apex of the cone, and the organization of the stromal lamellae is drastically altered [12].

The diagnosis of keratoconus is reached thanks to corneal imaging that is able to provide different levels of details, from corneal topography and pachymetry to anterior segment-optical coherence tomography (AS-OCT). These instruments are essential when assessing the course of the pathology. Corneal topography facilitates a comprehensive evaluation of the precise shape, size and location of keratoconus. The analysis of corneal ectasia involves the assessment of corneal thickness through the use of corneal pachymetry [9,17]. Furthermore, the identification of keratoconus has undergone progressive improvements in recent years, passing from basic assessments of the anterior corneal surface to precise three-dimensional structural analysis of the entire cornea [18]. The concept of considering the cornea as a solid entity possessing a distinct volume has been put forth as a prospective and valuable clinical parameter for the identification and monitoring of frank keratoconus, as well as for patients with subclinical manifestations [19,20]. The clinical application of AS-OCT, a non-contact technique that follows the principles of low-coherence interferometry, has enabled the determination of structural corneal changes that occur in keratoconus as the disease progresses [21]. Through the examination of the alteration that occurs in the corneal microarchitecture of eyes affected by keratoconus, the disease's severity can be determined [22].

Though corneal volume (CV) measured by means of AS-OCT is sometimes used in clinical and research practice to provide additional information about changes involving posterior cornea, the real clinical impact of this parameter is not known [23,24]. Several studies have reported a reduction in the corneal thinnest point (TP) in patients with keratoconus compared with normal eyes, which is associated with the increase of corneal curvature and the progression of the disease [19,25–27]. However, the reduction of CV was shown only in advanced stages. In particular, Morishige et al. have demonstrated that loss of CV occurs after the reduction of TP, suggesting that it is affected by the stromal degradation that occurs only in the advanced stage of keratoconus [28].

Since longitudinal changes of CV in keratoconus eyes have yet to be investigated, we sought to evaluate, over time, these modifications in patients with both stable and progressive keratoconus.

2. Materials and Methods

This institutional retrospective cohort study reviewed the medical records of all keratoconus eyes followed at a tertiary referral center (Department of Ophthalmology, University of Magna Graecia, Catanzaro, Italy) from April 2012 to December 2021. The study followed the principles of the 1964 Declaration of Helsinki and was approved by the local ethics committee (Comitato Etico Regione Calabria—Sezione Area Centro). A detailed informed consent form for study participation was signed by all patients during a routine control visit.

Inclusion criteria were a diagnosis of keratoconus and the presence of two examinations with good quality corneal imaging one year apart. Data from each subject were examined at least twice by different ophthalmologists to confirm the diagnosis. The presence of keratoconus was determined by a slit lamp examination, which included signs such as stromal thinning, Vogt's streaks, Fleischer's rings, and tomographic findings suggestive of keratoconus. The exclusion criteria for this study included any history of ocular surgery, particularly eyes that had undergone keratoplasty; systemic or ocular disease (excluding keratoconus); or use of ocular medications (excluding antihistamines). Patients who were wearing contact lenses were instructed to discontinue their use 48 h prior to their scheduled visit. Tomographic maps for keratometry and pachymetry values and AS-OCT scans for CV at different diameters, namely 3 mm (Figure 1), 5 mm (Figure 2) and 8 mm (Figure 3) centered on the corneal apex, were obtained using Casia 1 (Tomey Corp., Nagoya, Japan) at baseline (T0), and after 1 year (T1) and 2 years (T2).

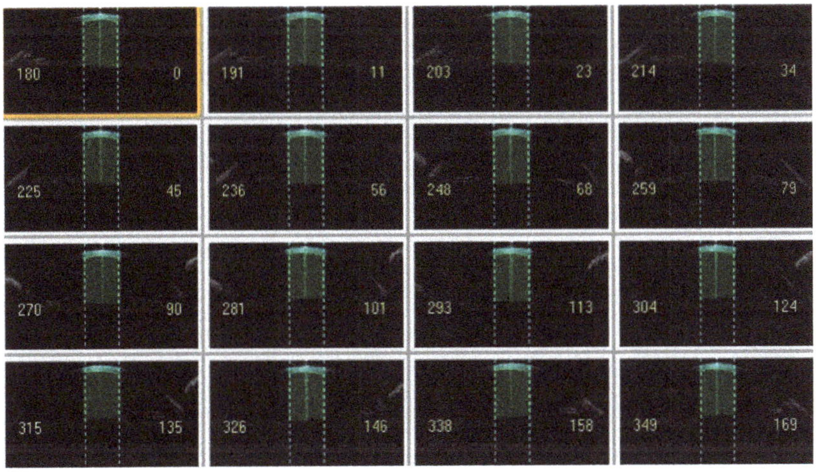

Figure 1. Anterior segment-optical coherence tomography showing cornea volume at 3 mm (light green) and anterior chamber volume at 3 mm (dark green).

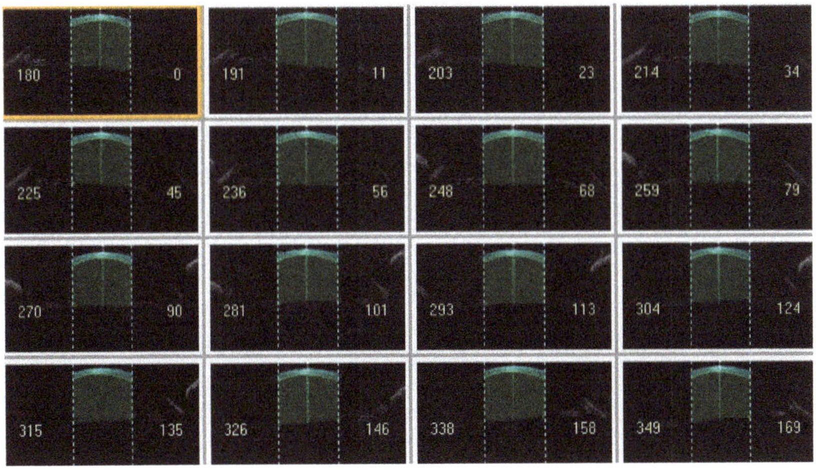

Figure 2. Anterior segment-optical coherence tomography showing cornea volume at 5 mm (light green) and anterior chamber volume at 5 mm (dark green).

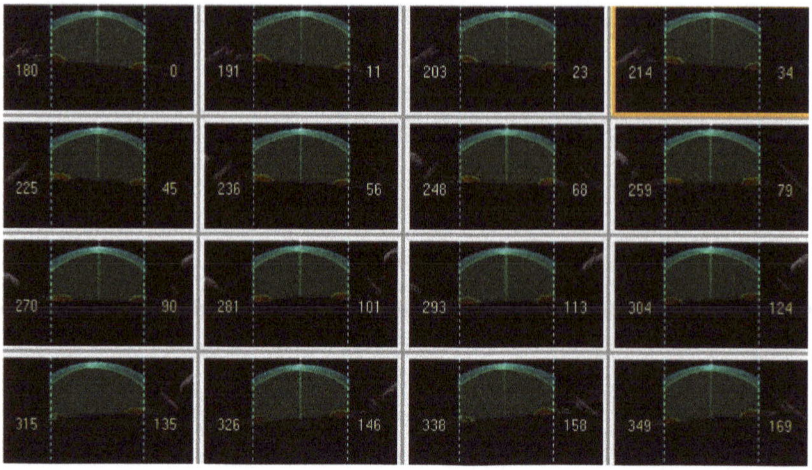

Figure 3. Anterior segment-optical coherence tomography showing cornea volume at 8 mm (light green) and anterior chamber volume at 8 mm (dark green).

Thanks to the three-dimensional image of the anterior segment, the calculations of anterior chamber depth (ACD) and anterior chamber volume (ACV) were also performed. Data were collected by the same examiner (NP) and analyzed independently by an additional operator (SV).

Each eye with keratoconus was staged in terms of severity of the disease according to the steepest keratometry (K) values, using a simple keratoconus classification, and according to the progression of the disease evaluated as a reduction of TP in 1 year. With regard to the former classification, eyes with a steepest K value lower than 45 D were classified as mild (group 1), those with a K value between 45 and 52 D as moderate (group 2) and those with K value higher than 52 D as severe (group 3) [25]. With regard to the latter classification, eyes with an increase of K values > 1 D and/or pachymetry with a ≥2% decrease in TP in 1 year were classified as progressive keratoconus (group A) while those with no/lower increase were classified as stable (group B) [29,30]. During the period of observation, keratoplasty was not necessary for any of the eyes that were examined.

Statistical Methods

Statistical analyses were performed using Prism version 9.4.0 (GraphPad Software Inc., San Diego, CA, USA) and Jamovi version 2.4.1.0 (The jamovi project, Sidney, Australia). Normally distributed data were expressed as mean ± standard deviation (SD), otherwise as median values with interquartile range (IQR). Parametric and nonparametric tests were chosen based on data normality. The Anderson–Darling and Kolmogorov–Smirnov tests were applied to assess whether data were normally distributed. Student's *t* test, Mann–Whitney U test, Dunnett's multiple comparison test and Friedman test were used to compare variables, when appropriate. The Pearson correlation test was used to evaluate the correlation of parameters. A *p*-value less than 0.05 was considered statistically significant.

3. Results

The study included 116 eyes of 116 patients (76 males and 40 females, mean age 34.76 ± 13.99 years) who received two consecutive annual examinations. At baseline, 72 eyes were classified as affected by mild keratoconus (group 1), 34 as moderate (group 2) and 10 as severe (group 3). There were no statistically significant differences among groups for age, sex or eye distribution. The mean ± SD steep K values for mild, moderate and severe cases were 45.70 ± 1.60 D, 50.78 ± 1.42 D and 56.86 ± 1.86 D, respectively.

The mean ± SD values for CV at the different diameter discs (3, 5, and 8 mm) are shown in Table 1.

Table 1. Baseline corneal volume at three diameters.

	All (n = 116)	Group 1 (n = 72)	Group 2 (n = 34)	Group 3 (n = 10)
Corneal volume 3 mm Ø (mm^3) mean ± SD	3.67 ± 0.29	3.77 ± 0.25	3.53 ± 0.27	3.24 ± 0.28
Corneal volume 5 mm Ø (mm^3) mean ± SD	10.79 ± 0.75	11.01 ± 0.70	10.55 ± 0.73	9.92 ± 0.90
Corneal volume 8 mm Ø (mm^3) mean ± SD	32.05 ± 1.90	32.38 ± 1.89	31.70 ± 2.01	30.68 ± 2.31

SD: standard deviation.

For the entire group of keratoconus patients, in comparison with T0, mean TP decreased at T1 from 458.7 ± 52.2 µm to 454.6 ± 51.6 µm (p = 0.0004); in the same period, statistically significant differences were detected regarding CV at 5 mm and 8 mm (from 10.78 ± 0.8 mm^3 to 10.75 ± 0.79 mm^3, p = 0.02, and from 32.03 ± 2.01 mm^3 to 31.95 ± 1.98 mm^3, p = 0.02, respectively). Conversely, there were no statistically significant differences in CV at 3 mm from T0 (3.66 ± 0.31 mm^3) to T1 (3.64 ± 0.31 mm^3) (p = 0.08) (Figure 4), or for ACD (p = 0.2568) and ACV calculated at 3, 5 and 8 mm (p = 0.8464, p = 0.4627, p = 0.3714 respectively).

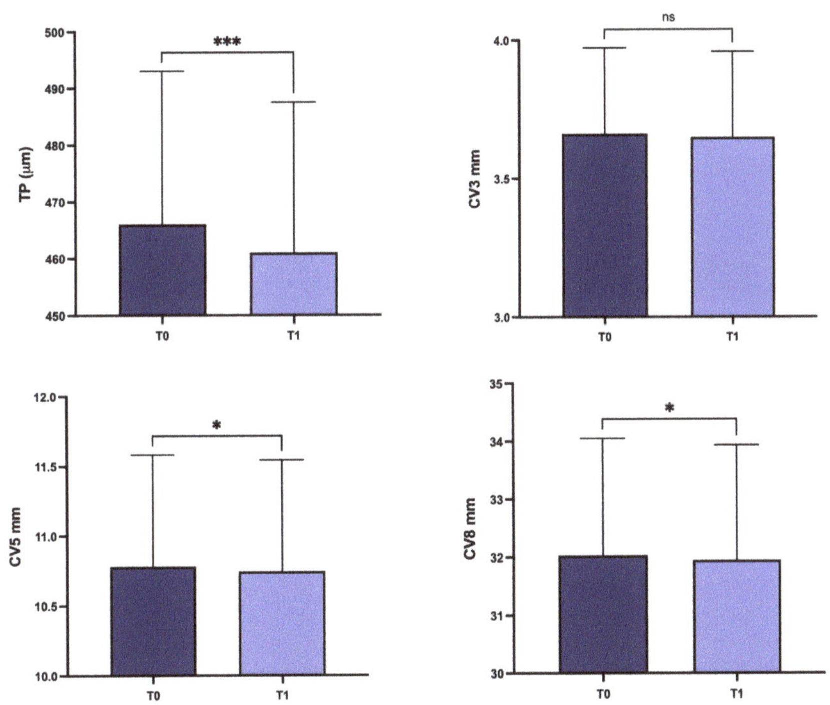

Figure 4. Values of corneal thickness at the thinnest point, and corneal volume at baseline and 1 year later in the overall study population. TP: corneal thickness at the thinnest point; CV3: corneal volume at 3 mm diameter; CV5: corneal volume at 5 mm diameter; CV8: corneal volume at 8 mm diameter; T0: baseline; T1: 1 year later; ns, not significant; * $p < 0.05$; *** $p < 0.001$.

There were positive correlations that were statistically significant between the average TP and the CV at 3 mm (r = 0.918; $p < 0.001$), 5 mm (r = 0.891; $p < 0.001$) and 8 mm (r = 0.788; $p < 0.001$) (Table 2).

Table 2. Correlation matrix among corneal thickness at the thinnest point, and corneal volume at different diameters.

Correlation Matrix					
		TP	**CV 3 mm**	**CV 5 mm**	**CV 8 mm**
TP	Pearson's r	-			
	df	-			
	p-value	-			
CV 3 mm	Pearson's r	0.918	-		
	df	114	-		
	p-value	<0.001	-		
CV 5 mm	Pearson's r	0.891	0.971	-	
	df	114	114	-	
	p-value	<0.001	<0.001	-	
CV 8 mm	Pearson's r	0.788	0.888	0.960	-
	df	114	114	114	-
	p-value	<0.001	<0.001	<0.001	-

TP: Corneal thickness at the thinnest point; CV3: Corneal volume at 3 mm diameter; CV5: Corneal volume at 5 mm diameter; CV8: Corneal volume at 8 mm diameter.

There were statistically significant positive correlations between changes of TP and CV at 3 mm (r = 0.6324, $p < 0.0001$), 5 mm (r = 0.7622, $p < 0.0001$) and 8 mm (r = 0.5987, $p < 0.0001$) (Figure 5).

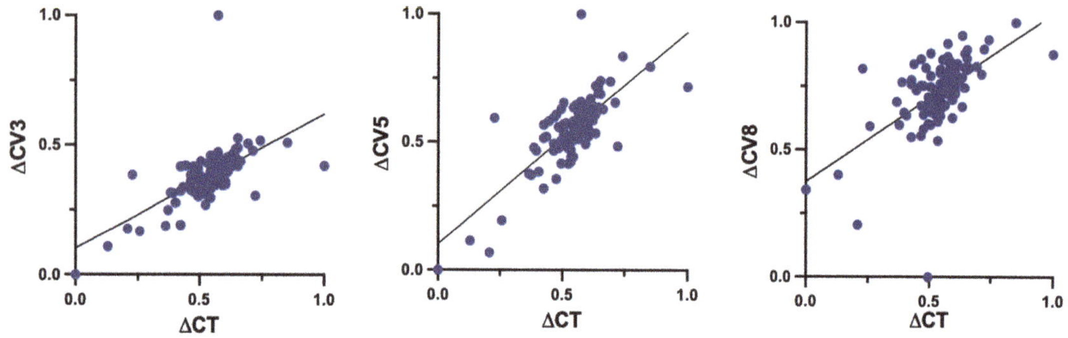

Figure 5. Correlations between changes (Δ) of TP and CV at 3 mm, 5 mm and 8 mm. TP: corneal thickness at the thinnest point; CV3: corneal volume at 3 mm diameter; CV5: corneal volume at 5 mm diameter; CV8: corneal volume at 8 mm diameter.

Concerning patients with stable (group B; $n = 86$) or progressive (group A; $n = 30$) disease, there were statistically significant differences in group A for TP, CV at 3 mm, 5 mm and 8 mm ($p < 0.0001$, $p < 0.0001$, $p < 0.001$ and $p = 0.0058$ respectively) (Figure 6).

In patients belonging to group B, there were no statistically significant differences in TP or in CV at 3 mm, 5 mm and 8 mm ($p = 0.4601$, $p = 0.3275$, $p = 0.8482$ and $p = 0.5574$ respectively). There were no statistically significant differences for ACD ($p = 0.6916$) or for ACV calculated at 3, 5 and 8 mm ($p = 0.7709$, $p = 0.3765$, $p = 0.2475$ respectively) in group A. At the same time, no statistically significant differences for ACD ($p = 0.2897$) or for ACV calculated at 3, 5 and 8 mm ($p = 0.9849$, $p = 0.6420$, $p = 0.8338$ respectively) were found in group B.

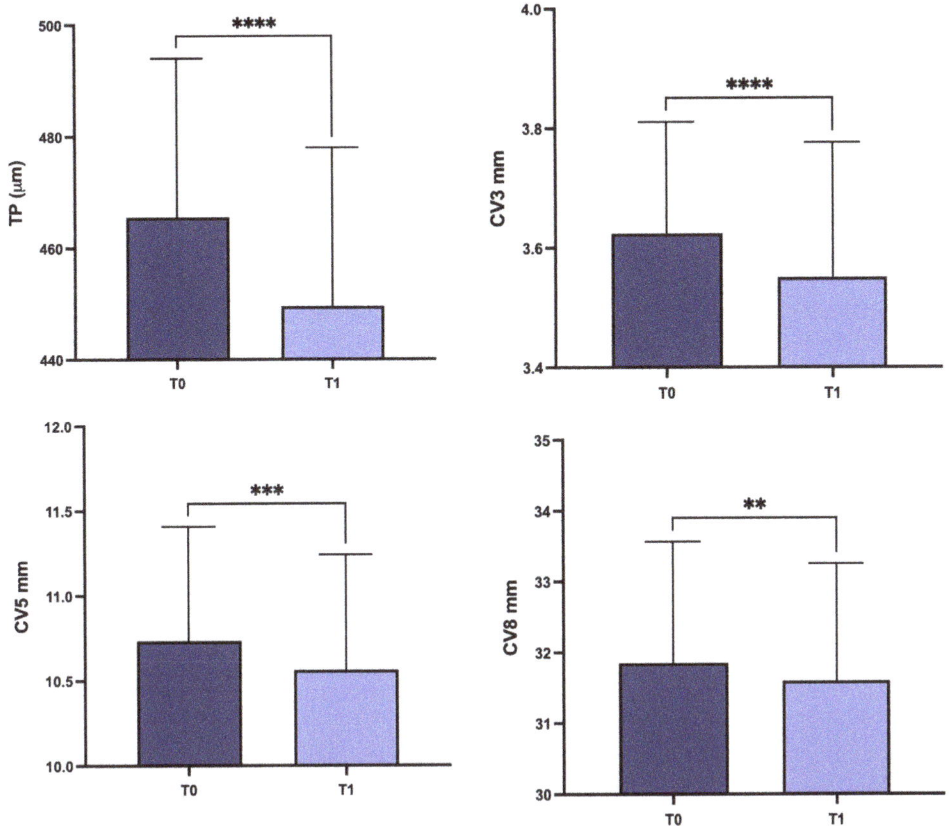

Figure 6. Values of TP, CV3, CV5 and CV8 values at T0 and in the subgroup A. TP: corneal thickness at the thinnest point; CV3: corneal volume at 3 mm diameter; CV5: corneal volume at 5 mm diameter; CV8: corneal volume at 8 mm diameter; T0: baseline; T1: 1 year later; ** $p < 0.01$, *** $p < 0.001$, **** $p < 0.0001$.

4. Discussion

The Global Consensus on Keratoconus and Ectatic Diseases highlighted the important role of the assessment of alterations in the posterior corneal surface and corneal thickness when diagnosing keratoconus [8]. The recent adoption of AS-OCT for the assessment of CV might offer additional insights into alterations affecting the cornea [20,23]. AS-OCT has the advantage of acquiring three-dimensional images of the anterior segment of the eyes, in addition to cross-sectional images [21]. Significant changes in TP and CV have been reported between patients with subclinical and clinical keratoconus in comparison with a control group [23]. The combined use of pachymetric and volumetric data has been shown to offer a more effective assessment of corneal structure in patients with keratoconus, exhibiting favorable levels of sensitivity and specificity when identifying both clinical and subclinical cases [24–28,31]. A previous study has documented a considerable reduction in CV in patients with moderate and severe keratoconus, with the most pronounced decrease observed in the central and para-central regions. This implies that the decrease in CV could be a result of stromal degradation, a process that happens in the later stages of the disease [32]. A recent study created a quantitative staging method for keratoconus using AS-OCT and demonstrated a robust concordance with the already established classification systems. This staging method, named STEP is determined by the stromal overall minimum thickness (ST) and epithelium overall standard deviation (EP). Integrating stromal and corneal epithelial data with the use of AS-OCT has the potential to further improve the treatment and management of keratoconus [33]. Cavas-Martínez et al. conducted a study that provided evidence of a notable decrease in CV during the early stages of keratoconus. Furthermore, the study revealed that the extent of this loss becomes more pronounced as the severity of the disease increases, as determined by the Amsler–Krumeich grading system [32,34].

In accordance with these findings, our study demonstrates a statistically significant decrease over time of TP in patients with keratoconus. At the same time, statistically significant differences were detected regarding CV at 5 mm and 8 mm (but not at 3 mm) from T0 to T1. This discrepancy may be attributed to the fact that a larger diameter allows for a higher likelihood of analyzing the corneal area in which the cone is typically located, which is situated in the middle periphery rather than the central region [35]. Similarly, Cui et al. analyzed 48 patients, a control group of 29 individuals with myopic astigmatism and 19 patients who had subclinical keratoconus. The corneal assessment was conducted using the Pentacam Scheimpflug system, in addition to central corneal thickness they considered CV at 3 mm, 5 mm and 7 mm. They found that subclinical keratoconus and normal corneas differed significantly with regard to all parameters, with the exception of CV3 and CV5. The study utilized partial least squares (PLS) analysis to develop models, taking into account thickness and corneal volume values. The resulting model had a sensitivity of 79.3% and a specificity of 94.7%. It appears that the combination of corneal thickness and volume parameters distinguishes keratoconus corneas from normal corneas more effectively than a single parameter [31]. In a previous study Ambrósio et al., in order to investigate corneal architecture, presented novel corneal tomography parameters obtained from the Pentacam Comprehensive Eye Scanner. Specifically, they analyzed the distribution of corneal volume and the spatial profile of corneal thickness, calculated at different diameters of CV from 1.0 to 7.0 mm with 0.5 mm steps, in order to distinguish keratoconic from healthy corneas. Keratoconic eyes are characterized by thinner diameter and volume, with a more abrupt increase in these parameters from the thinnest point to the periphery, compared with normal eyes [24]. A recent study assessed the precision of various corneal parameters in identifying keratoconus by employing a dual Scheimpflug–Placido system. The study found that the corneal volume at 10 mm did not show any significant differences between the keratoconus group and the healthy group [36].

In contrast with prior investigations, our research exclusively focused on patients diagnosed with keratoconus. Within the subgroup of patients with progressive disease (group A), there were statistically significant differences observed in either thickness or volume measurements over time. On the contrary, no differences were detected in patients with stable disease (group B). Furthermore, strong correlations have been demonstrated between TP (both mean values and changes from T0 to T1) and all of the types of CV (3 mm, 5 mm and 8 mm) in the entire population of patients irrespective of the progression of the disease.

Knowing the cornea's volume could be useful to assess the progression of the KC. However, it is important to note that CV has been measured through the utilization of several clinical examination methods, such as a Scheimpflug camera and anterior segment-optical coherence tomography (AS-OCT). In particular, Ambrósio et al. employed the Pentacam Comprehensive Eye Scanner. Corneal thickness measurements were taken at the point of minimum thickness for each eye. The mean thickness values of the points on 22 hypothetical circles, centered on the thinnest point, were computed. These calculations were used to generate the spatial profile of corneal thickness for the creation of the corneal volume distribution. The percentage increase in volume was determined for each position by applying a mathematical formula to the initial volume of 1 mm [24]. Cervin õ et al. used a software to precisely simulate a surface using the collected data points obtained from corneal topography and ultrasonic topographic pachymetry. The volume underneath both the front and back sides of the cornea was then calculated [20]. Another study utilized raw topographic data from the Sirius system to enable morphogeometric modeling of the cornea with the assistance of CAD tools [32]. All of these studies used different software to obtain CV as, without the utilization of these programs, incorporating the parameter into clinical practice becomes challenging. In our study the calculation of CV was performed using the SS-OCT Viewer program developed by Tomey. The area corresponding to the cornea was automatically delineated in the 16 AS-OCT pictures, and the volume of interest was then determined. This method had been used by Morishige et al., who found that stromal degradation, which only happens in the advanced stage of keratoconus, has an impact on the loss of CV [28]. The primary limitation of this method is the imprecise automated segmentation. The AS-OCT software (Tomey Link Exam Viewer Version 6P.1) independently generates the demarcated area. Therefore, it is of greatest importance to have control over segmentation. Simultaneously, it is crucial to verify that the examination is centered on the corneal apex in order to establish a standardized assessment.

Furthermore, OCT provides evaluation of the changes in advanced cases of keratoconus, when the accuracy of corneal topography for reliability is reduced. In particular, when severe stromal lesions are present and a patient is undergoing keratoplasty for KC, the AS-OCT analysis is critical for determining the optimal strategy, particularly with regard to the surgical approach and methodology utilized during deep anterior lamellar keratoplasty (DALK) [17]. A previous study into the predictors that influence the formation and type of big bubbles (BB) during DALK revealed that the existence of posterior scars signifies a noteworthy risk factor for type 2 BB formation; in these cases, manual techniques should be considered to reduce the risk of penetrating keratoplasty (PK) conversion and prevent intraoperative complications [17].

Although our study is the first to investigate the longitudinal changes of CV in a large keratoconus population, it is important to acknowledge the inherent limitations of our study that deserve mentioning. Firstly, a control group of healthy subjects without corneal abnormalities has not been included in the analysis. Secondly, in order to obtain a sufficiently wide group of patients with progressive keratoconus, a cut-off value that is lower than is typical was used for the reduction of TP in 1 year to identify patient belonging to this group.

In conclusion, AS-OCT is progressively assuming a crucial role in the examination of corneal modifications among patients diagnosed with keratoconus. Given the positive correlations between TP and CV, the latter could be a useful parameter, but further research is required to elucidate the diagnostic performance of CV when evaluating patients affected by keratoconus.

Author Contributions: Conceptualization, V.S. and G.G.; methodology, G.G.; software, S.V., A.C.Y. and N.P.; validation, S.V., G.L., R.G., V.S. and A.C.Y.; formal analysis, S.V., A.C.Y. and C.V.; investigation, R.G., G.L. and N.P.; resources, S.V. and G.L.; data curation, N.P. and R.G.; writing—original draft preparation, S.V. and C.V.; writing—review and editing, G.G. and S.V.; visualization, C.V., R.G. and V.S.; supervision, G.G. and A.C.Y.; project administration, G.G. and V.S. All authors have read and agreed to the published version of the manuscript.

Funding: This research received no external funding.

Institutional Review Board Statement: The study was conducted in accordance with the Declaration of Helsinki and approved by the local ethics committee (Calabria Region Ethics Committee, Central Area Section, ethic code (0186-2022), 20 October 2022).

Informed Consent Statement: Informed consent was obtained from all subjects involved in the study.

Data Availability Statement: Data are contained within the article.

Conflicts of Interest: The authors declare no conflicts of interest.

References

1. Rabinowitz, Y.S.; Galvis, V.; Tello, A.; Rueda, D.; García, J.D. Genetics vs chronic corneal mechanical trauma in the etiology of keratoconus. *Exp. Eye Res.* **2021**, *202*, 108328. [CrossRef]

2. Bui, A.D.; Truong, A.; Pasricha, N.D.; Indaram, M. Keratoconus Diagnosis and Treatment: Recent Advances and Future Directions. *Clin. Ophthalmol.* **2023**, *17*, 2705–2718. [CrossRef] [PubMed]
3. Galvis, V.; Tello, A.; Barrera, R.; Niño, C.A. Inflammation in Keratoconus. *Cornea* **2015**, *34*, e22–e23. [CrossRef]
4. Elbeyli, A.; Kurtul, B.E. Systemic immune-inflammation index, neutrophil-to-lymphocyte ratio, and platelet-to-lymphocyte ratio levels are associated with keratoconus. *Indian J. Ophthalmol.* **2021**, *69*, 1725–1729.
5. Loh, I.P.; Sherwin, T. Is Keratoconus an Inflammatory Disease? The Implication of Inflammatory Pathways. *Ocul. Immunol. Inflamm.* **2022**, *30*, 246–255. [CrossRef] [PubMed]
6. Wei, R.H.; Zhao, S.Z.; Lim, L.; Tan, D.T. Incidence and characteristics of unilateral keratoconus classified on corneal topography. *J. Refract. Surg.* **2011**, *10*, 745–751. [CrossRef]
7. McMahon, T.T.; Szczotka-Flynn, L.; Barr, J.T.; Anderson, R.J.; Slaughter, M.E.; Lass, J.H.; Iyengar, S.K. CLEK Study Group. A new method for grading the severity of keratoconus: The Keratoconus Severity Score (KSS). *Cornea* **2006**, *7*, 794–800. [CrossRef]
8. Krachmer, J.H.; Feder, R.S.; Belin, M.W. Keratoconus and related noninflammatory corneal thinning disorders. *Surv. Ophthalmol.* **1984**, *28*, 293–322. [CrossRef] [PubMed]
9. Gomes, J.A.; Tan, D.; Rapuano, C.J.; Belin, M.W.; Ambrósio, R., Jr.; Guell, J.L.; Malecaze, F.; Nishida, K.; Sangwan, V.S. Group of Panelists for the Global Delphi Panel of Keratoconus and Ectatic Diseases. Global consensus on keratoconus and ectatic diseases. *Cornea* **2015**, *34*, 359–369. [CrossRef]
10. Andreassen, T.T.; Simonsen, A.H.; Oxlund, H. Biomechanical properties of keratoconus and normal corneas. *Exp. Eye Res.* **1980**, *31*, 435–441. [CrossRef]
11. Morishige, N.; Shin-Gyou-Uchi, R.; Azumi, H.; Ohta, H.; Morita, Y.; Yamada, N.; Kimura, K.; Takahara, A.; Sonoda, K.H. Quantitative analysis of collagen lamellae in the normal and keratoconic human cornea by second harmonic generation imaging microscopy. *Investig. Ophthalmol. Vis. Sci.* **2014**, *55*, 8377–8385. [CrossRef] [PubMed]
12. Meek, K.M.; Tuft, S.J.; Huang, Y.; Gill, P.S.; Hayes, S.; Newton, R.H.; Bron, A.J. Changes in collagen orientation and distribution in keratoconus corneas. *Investig. Ophthalmol. Vis. Sci.* **2005**, *46*, 1948–1956. [CrossRef] [PubMed]
13. Hayes, S.; Boote, C.; Tuft, S.J.; Quantock, A.J.; Meek, K.M. A study of corneal thickness, shape and collagen organisation in keratoconus using videokeratography and X-ray scattering techniques. *Exp. Eye Res.* **2007**, *84*, 423–434. [CrossRef] [PubMed]
14. Balasubramanian, S.A.; Pye, D.C.; Willcox, M.D. Are proteinases the reason for keratoconus? *Curr. Eye Res.* **2010**, *35*, 185–191. [CrossRef]
15. Foster, J.W.; Parikh, R.N.; Wang, J.; Bower, K.S.; Matthaei, M.; Chakravarti, S.; Jun, A.S.; Eberhart, C.G.; Soiberman, U.S. Transcriptomic and Immunohistochemical Analysis of Progressive Keratoconus Reveal Altered WNT10A in Epithelium and Bowman's Layer. *Investig. Ophthalmol. Vis. Sci.* **2021**, *62*, 16. [CrossRef] [PubMed]
16. Akoto, T.; Cai, J.; Nicholas, S.; McCord, H.; Estes, A.J.; Xu, H.; Karamichos, D.; Liu, Y. Unravelling the Impact of Cyclic Mechanical Stretch in Keratoconus-A Transcriptomic Profiling Study. *Int. J. Mol. Sci.* **2023**, *24*, 7437. [CrossRef] [PubMed]
17. Giannaccare, G.; Murano, G.; Carnevali, A.; Yu, A.C.; Vaccaro, S.; Scuteri, G.; Maltese, L.; Scorcia, V. Comparison of Amsler–Krumeich and Sandali Classifications for Staging Eyes with Keratoconus. *Appl. Sci.* **2021**, *11*, 4007. [CrossRef]
18. Piñero, D.P.; Nieto, J.C.; Lopez-Miguel, A. Characterization of corneal structure in keratoconus. *J. Cataract. Refract. Surg.* **2012**, *38*, 2167–2183. [CrossRef]
19. Ahmadi Hosseini, S.M.; Mohidin, N.; Abolbashari, F.; Mohd-Ali, B.; Santhirathelagan, C.T. Corneal thickness and volume in subclinical and clinical keratoconus. *Int. Ophthalmol.* **2013**, *33*, 139–145. [CrossRef]
20. Cerviño, A.; Gonzalez-Meijome, J.M.; Ferrer-Blasco, T.; Garcia-Resua, C.; Montes-Mico, R.; Parafita, M. Determination of corneal volume from anterior topography and topographic pachymetry: Application to healthy and keratoconic eyes. *Ophthalmic Physiol. Opt.* **2009**, *29*, 652–660. [CrossRef]
21. Yadav, R.; Kottaiyan, R.; Ahmad, K.; Yoon, G. Epithelium and Bowman's layer thickness and light scatter in keratoconic cornea evaluated using ultrahigh resolution optical coherence tomography. *J. Biomed. Opt.* **2012**, *11*, 116010. [CrossRef] [PubMed]
22. Sandali, O.; El Sanharawi, M.; Temstet, C.; Hamiche, T.; Galan, A.; Ghouali, W.; Goemaere, I.; Basli, E.; Borderie, V.; Laroche, L. Fourier-domain optical coherence tomography imaging in keratoconus: A corneal structural classification. *Ophthalmology* **2013**, *120*, 2403–2412. [CrossRef]
23. Fukuda, R.; Usui, T.; Miyai, T.; Mori, Y.; Miyata, K.; Amano, S. Corneal thickness and volume measurements by swept source anterior segment optical coherence tomography in normal subjects. *Curr. Eye Res.* **2013**, *38*, 531–536. [CrossRef] [PubMed]
24. Ambrósio, R., Jr.; Alonso, R.S.; Luz, A.; Coca Velarde, L.G. Corneal-thickness spatial profile and corneal-volume distribution: Tomographic indices to detect keratoconus. *J. Cataract. Refract. Surg.* **2006**, *32*, 1851–1859. [CrossRef]
25. Mannion, L.S.; Tromans, C.; O'Donnell, C. Reduction in corneal volume with severity of keratoconus. *Curr. Eye Res.* **2011**, *36*, 522–527. [CrossRef]
26. Piñero, D.P.; Alió, J.L.; Alesón, A.; Escaf Vergara, M.; Miranda, M. Corneal volume, pachymetry, and correlation of anterior and posterior corneal shape in subclinical and different stages of clinical keratoconus. *J. Cataract. Refract. Surg.* **2010**, *36*, 814–825. [CrossRef]
27. Fontes, B.M.; Ambrósio, R., Jr.; Jardim, D.; Velarde, G.C.; Nosé, W. Corneal biomechanical metrics and anterior segment parameters in mild keratoconus. *Ophthalmology* **2010**, *117*, 673–679. [CrossRef]

28. Morishige, N.; Magome, K.; Ueno, A.; Matsui, T.A.; Nishida, T. Relations Among Corneal Curvature, Thickness, and Volume in Keratoconus as Evaluated by Anterior Segment-Optical Coherence Tomography. *Investig. Ophthalmol. Vis. Sci.* **2019**, *60*, 3794–3802. [CrossRef]
29. Chatzis, N.; Hafezi, F. Progression of keratoconus and efficacy of pediatric [corrected] corneal collagen cross-linking in children and adolescents. *J. Refract. Surg.* **2012**, *28*, 753–758. [CrossRef]
30. Gore, D.M.; Shortt, A.J.; Allan, B.D. New clinical pathways for keratoconus. *Eye* **2013**, *27*, 329–339. [CrossRef] [PubMed]
31. Cui, J.; Zhang, X.; Hu, Q.; Zhou, W.Y.; Yang, F. Evaluation of Corneal Thickness and Volume Parameters of Subclinical Keratoconus Using a Pentacam Scheimflug System. *Curr. Eye Res.* **2016**, *41*, 923–926. [CrossRef]
32. Cavas-Martínez, F.; Bataille, L.; Fernández-Pacheco, D.G.; Cañavate, F.J.F.; Alio, J.L. Keratoconus Detection Based on a New Corneal Volumetric Analysis. *Sci. Rep.* **2017**, *7*, 15837. [CrossRef]
33. Lu, N.J.; Hafezi, F.; Koppen, C.; Alió Del Barrio, J.L.; Aslanides, I.M.; Awwad, S.T.; Ní Dhubhghaill, S.; Pineda, R., 2nd; Torres-Netto, E.A.; Wang, L.; et al. New keratoconus staging system based on OCT. *J. Cataract. Refract. Surg.* **2023**, *49*, 1098–1105. [CrossRef]
34. Hu, P.; Lin, L.; Wu, Z.; Jin, X.; Ni, H. Kayser-Fleischer ring with keratoconus: A coincidence? A case report. *BMC Ophthalmol.* **2020**, *20*, 190. [CrossRef] [PubMed]
35. Steinwender, G.; Kollenc, A.; Shajari, M.; Sommer, M.; Borenich, A.; Horwath-Winter, J.; Lindner, E.; Woltsche, N.; List, W.; Wedrich, A. Determining the center of a keratoconus: Comparison of different tomographic parameters and impact of disease severity. *Front. Med.* **2022**, *9*, 968318. [CrossRef] [PubMed]
36. Heidari, Z.; Jafarzadehpour, E.; Mohammadpour, M.; Hashemi, H. Best indices of dual Scheimpflug/Placido tomographer for keratoconus detection. *Int. Ophthalmol.* **2023**, *43*, 1353–1362. [CrossRef] [PubMed]

life

MDPI

Article

The Effect of Myopic Control between the Dual-Focus Contact Lenses and High-Concentration Atropine in an Asian Population

Chia-Yi Lee [1,2,3,†], Shun-Fa Yang [1,4,†], Yu-Ling Chang [5], Jing-Yang Huang [4], Ie-Bin Lian [6] and Chao-Kai Chang [2,7,*]

1 Institute of Medicine, Chung Shan Medical University, Taichung 402, Taiwan
2 Nobel Eye Institute, Taipei 115, Taiwan
3 Department of Ophthalmology, Jen-Ai Hospital Dali Branch, Taichung 412, Taiwan
4 Department of Medical Research, Chung Shan Medical University Hospital, Taichung 402, Taiwan
5 Department of Medical Education, Cathay General Hospital, Taipei 106, Taiwan
6 Institute of Statistical and Information Science, National Changhua University of Education, Changhua 500, Taiwan
7 Department of Optometry, Da-Yeh University, Chunghua 515, Taiwan
* Correspondence: chaokai@mail.dyu.edu.tw; Tel.: +886-2-2370-5666
† These authors contributed equally to this work.

Abstract: We aim to investigate the myopic control effect of high-concentration atropine (ATR) and dual-focus contact lenses (DFCLs). A retrospective cohort study was conducted. A total of 182 eyes in 91 individuals who used high-concentration ATR (0.125%) and another 70 eyes in 35 individuals who used DFCLs were enrolled in the ATR and DFCL groups, respectively. The primary outcomes were spherical equivalent refraction (SER) progression and axial length (AXL) elongation. The generalized estimate equation was utilized to yield the adjusted odds ratio (aOR) and 95% confidence interval (CI) of cycloplegic SER progression and AXL elongation between groups. According to the multivariable analysis, the change in cycloplegic SER progression was similar between the DFCL and ATR groups (aOR: 1.305, 95% CI: 0.247–2.515, $p = 0.803$). The DFCL group demonstrated a numerically higher rate of AXL elongation compared to the ATR group (aOR: 1.530, 95% CI: 0.980–1.894, $p = 0.051$). In the subgroup analysis, cycloplegic SER progression was insignificant between ATR and DFCL users in different subgroups (all $p > 0.05$). The DFCL patients with moderate astigmatism and high AXL (both $p < 0.001$) presented a high risk of AXL elongation. In conclusion, DFCL usage demonstrated similar myopic control of cycloplegic SER and AXL compared to high-concentration ATR, while DFCLs showed lower AXL control, mainly in patients with moderate astigmatism and high AXL.

Keywords: atropine; dual-focus contact lenses; spherical equivalent refraction; axial length; astigmatism

1. Introduction

Myopia, which has recently shown increased occurrence, is a disease in which images focus in front of the retinal plane, causing blurry vision [1,2]. Normally, rays enter the eye and hit the center of the retina, and the photoreceptors on the retina collect the light signals. Then, the light signals are converted to electrical signals and pass through the retina to reach the optic nerve. The optic nerve then transports these signals into the occipital lobe, where visual signals are managed, producing vision. In patients with myopia, light enters the eye and focuses on a spot in front of the retina, and the photoreceptors cannot produce sufficient signals, thus causing blurry vision.

The etiologies of the formation of myopia, or the reasons for light focusing in front of the retina rather than on the retina, are axial myopia and refractive myopia [1,2]. Axial myopia is caused by the eyeball growing too long compared to the eye's refractive power, which is the most common type of childhood/acquired myopia. The axial length of the eyeball is the distance from the cornea to the retina, and light will focus in front of the retina rather than directly hit it if the eyeball is too long, causing distant images to appear blurry [1,2]. In comparison, refractive myopia develops if the curve of the cornea or the crystalline lens is extremely steep. The prevalence of refractive myopia is not as common as axial myopia [1,2]. In rare episodes, refractive myopia can also occur if the lens is located too close to the cornea. It is also possible to possess myopia that combines both the axial and refractive pathophysiologies.

Concerning the rate of myopia, the annual prevalence of myopia is nearly 44 percent in the Caucasian population and about 80 percent in the Eastern Asian region due to differences in lifestyle [3]. The main etiologies for the development of myopia include the steepening of the corneal curvature and the elongation of the eyeball, the latter of which tends to progress after birth [4]. High myopia, which is regarded as a sphere power over −5.00 diopter (D), contributes to higher rates of optic nerve damage and myopic maculopathy, and the importance of preventing the development of high myopia cannot be overemphasized [5].

Different methods of myopia control have previously been evaluated and applied [1,6]. Atropine (ATR) is a medication used for cycloplegic refraction, or dilating the pupil, for the examination of the retina and the execution of cataract and retinal surgery [2,7], and the application of ATR in children can also slow myopia progression. The usage of ATR for myopia control can be traced back to the 1990s when no spectacle-related myopia-control products were available. The mechanism of ATR's myopia control effect is due to the retardation of axial length elongation rather than the cycloplegic function that relieves the pupil sphincter [2,7]. The application of high-concentration ATR reduces the degree of myopia progression effectively, but complications, including photophobia, blurry vision at reading distance, and ocular allergies, may occur [2,7]. The elevation of intraocular pressure after ATR utilization has been reported, but its incidence is extremely rare, and thus, the safety of ATR can be guaranteed with regard to ocular hypertension and subsequent glaucoma [2,7].

In addition, orthokeratology contact lenses can contribute to a good myopia control rate with regard to refractive status [8,9]. The orthokeratology contact lens was first proposed in the 1960s in which the initial orthokeratology contact lens resembled a rigid gas-permeable contact lens. However, the visual outcome and refractive predictability of the initial orthokeratology contact lenses were poor, and they were soon abandoned. The re-introduction of orthokeratology contact lenses occurred in the 1990s, which included the following three innovations: the reverse-geometry shape design of orthokeratology contact lenses, the emergence of high-oxygen-permeability material, and the clinical application of topography in the production of orthokeratology contact lenses [8,9]. Subsequently, orthokeratology contact lenses became a credible and effective tool for controlling myopic progression. Moreover, nearly all patients with orthokeratology contact lenses achieve spectacle independence, elevating daily convenience without a reduction in visual quality [10]. In fact, the visual quality of children wearing the orthokeratology contact lenses was shown to be numerically better than those wearing spectacle lenses [10].

When comparing the effects of ATR and orthokeratology contact lenses on myopia control, spherical equivalent refraction (SER) progression and axial length (AXL) elongation were shown to be similar between high-concentration ATR and orthokeratology contact lenses [11]. In terms of complications, irritation was observed in both the ATR and orthokeratology contact lens groups, although its severity was not enough to discard the treatments altogether [11]. Consequently, we can say that both ATR and orthokeratology contact lenses are safe and efficient tools for myopic control.

Except for the rigid design of orthokeratology contact lenses, several soft contact lenses have been produced for the purpose of controlling myopia [1,8,12,13]. Among them, dual-focus contact lenses (DFCLs) were first introduced in the mid-2010s and showed a fair myopic control effect concerning SER progression and AXL elongation compared to individuals using general soft contact lenses [14]. When considering side effects in individuals using DFCLs, only one patient was diagnosed with peripheral corneal haze, which did not interfere with visual function [14]. In addition, one patient developed uveitis during the application of DFCLs, but uveitis is less likely to be triggered by DFCLs, according to [14]. When comparing DFCLs and high-concentration ATR, previous studies have shown a numerically higher myopic control effect in high-concentration ATR [7,8,15]; however, these previous studies compared the effect of DFCLs and high-concentration ATR using different study designs and regions [7,8,15], and a comparison between DFCLs and high-concentration ATR using similar conditions has not been conducted.

Thus, the aim of the current study is to compare the myopic control effects of high-concentration ATR and DFCLs on the management of SER progression and AXL elongation in the individuals receiving these treatments. All the patients enrolled in the current study resided in the Taiwan region.

2. Materials and Methods

2.1. Participant Selection

A retrospective cohort study was performed at the Nobel Eye Institute from 1 October 2020 to 31 September 2022. The Nobel Eye Institute is a joint clinic group that owns several branches in the northern, central, and southern regions of Taiwan. The inclusion criteria of our participants were (1) age younger than 15 years, (2) use of high-concentration ATR or DFCLs in our clinics, and (3) regular follow-ups in any branch of our clinic for at least one year with a minimum of six appointments per year. One brand of high-concentration ATR (0.125% Tropine, Aseptic Innovative Medicine Co., Ltd., Taoyuan Dist, Taoyuan City, Taiwan) and one brand of DFCLs (MiSight, CooperVision, Victor, NY, USA) were used in our study. To choose the myopic control tool, the ophthalmologist proposed all types of myopic control methods, if no absolute contraindications existed (i.e., a 5-year-old child for DFCL usage), to the children and parents. Then, the ophthalmologist discussed the selection of the myopic control method with the parents (and potentially also the children), where different ophthalmologists' habits and opinions of each myopic control tool could influence the selection result. Finally, the parents chose the type of myopic control method for the children, and the ophthalmologist prescribed the tool for them if no absolute contraindication was present. In our clinics, DFCL users wore the contact lenses for 10 h per day, every day without breaks. The ATR group was given atropine between 21:00 and 23:00, just before sleep without breaks. Because this period is relatively far from the measurement intervals (15:00 to 21:00) used in our clinic, ATR instillation might not influence the SER measurement to a large extent. In addition, several exclusion criteria were applied to decrease the heterogeneity of the study population and exclude extreme visual impairment: (1) baseline best-corrected visual acuity (BCVA) lower than 20/40 on a Snellen chart, (2) high myopia with sphere power higher than −5.00 D, (3) high astigmatism with cylinder power higher than −2.50 D and (4) severe ocular defects including but not limited to corneal scars, corneal neovascularization, congenital glaucoma, congenital cataracts, advanced retinopathy of prematurity, optic nerve atrophy and color blindness. Additionally, individuals using DFCLs with any ATR application were also excluded. After the whole process, a total of 182 eyes in 91 patients and 70 eyes in 35 patients were categorized into the ATR group and DFCL group, respectively.

2.2. Primary Outcome

The basic characteristics of each individual, including age, sex, pre-treatment BCVA, sphere power, cylinder power, and AXL, were obtained from the medical documents. The BCVA was performed with a trial frame, and the optimal visual acuity was refined by our optometrists. The sphere power was tested first, followed by the cylinder axis. After that, the cylinder power was determined. With regard to the parameters of myopic progression, the primary outcomes in the current study were SER progression and AXL elongation during the one-year follow-up period. The refraction and AXL were examined with an autorefractor (KR-8900, Topcon, Itabashi-ku, Tokyo, Japan) and biometry device

(IOL Master 500, Carl Zeiss, Göschwitzer Str., Jena, Germany) in each branch of our clinic. The autorefractor measurement was performed three times, and the optical biometry was performed once for each patient. Cycloplegic refraction was performed for all the participants before beginning myopic control management and about one year after myopic control management. Refraction, including sphere and cylinder, was measured three times; the average values of the three results were entered into the dataset of the current study, and the sphere power plus half of the cylinder power was defined as the SER. All the optometry rooms in our clinics adhere to the law of optometrists in Taiwan; the room sizes, devices, light conditions, and distances between the Snellen chart and patient are the same among all the branches of our clinic. Also, the brands of Snellen chart and optical biometry are the same among all the branches of our clinic, and the time of measurement usually ranges from 15:00 to 21:00. Both SER and AXL values before management, 1 month after management, 3 months after management, 6 months after management, 9 months after management, and 12 months after management in the two groups were recorded and used in the following statistical analysis.

2.3. Statistical Analysis

SPSS version 20.0 (SPSS Inc., Chicago, IL, USA) was used for the statistical analyses of the current study. We used descriptive analysis to illustrate the basic characteristics between the two groups, and the Chi-square test and independent T-test were applied for the comparison of basic characteristics between the two groups depending on the parameters. After that, the independent T-test was executed to compare the baseline cycloplegic SER and AXL and final cycloplegic SER and AXL between the two groups, and the generalized estimate equation was adopted for analyzing the alteration of cycloplegic SER progression and AXL elongation between the two populations with adjustment of the effects of sex, age, pre-treatment BCVA, pre-treatment AXL, and pre-treatment cycloplegic SER. The adjusted odds ratio (aOR) with 95% confidence interval (CI) of the DFCL group compared to the ATR group was yielded by the generalized estimate equation. Also, we plotted a line chart for the trends of manifest SER progression and AXL elongation of the ATR and DFCL groups during the study interval. For the subgroup analysis, the total SER and AXL changes in individuals receiving high-concentration ATR or using DFCLs with moderate myopia (more than −3.00 D), moderate astigmatism (more than −1.50 D), high AXL (more than 25.00 mm) and old age (older than 12 years old) were evaluated separately using the generalized estimate equation. The statistical significance was defined as $p < 0.05$ in the current study, and a p-value lower than 0.001 was described as $p < 0.001$.

3. Results

3.1. Basic Characteristics of the Study Population

The basic characteristics of the two groups are presented in Table 1. The mean age was 10.26 ± 2.56 and 12.33 ± 2.09 years old in the ATR and DFCL groups, and the DFCL group was significantly older than the ATR group ($p < 0.001$). Also, the DFCL group showed a higher baseline sphere power than the ATR group (−1.01 ± 1.42 versus −1.43 ± 1.47, $p = 0.0028$) (Table 1). The other parameters, including sex, baseline BCVA, and baseline cylinder power, were similar between the two groups (all $p > 0.05$) (Table 1).

Table 1. Basic characteristics of the two groups.

Characteristic	ATR Group (N = 182)	DFCL Group (N = 70)	*p* Value
Age	10.26 ± 2.56	12.33 ± 2.09	<0.001 *
Sex (male:female)	45:46	15:20	0.587
Pre-treatment BCVA (LogMAR)	0.004 ± 0.007	0.008 ± 0.004	0.412
Pre-treatment sphere (D)	−1.01 ± 1.42	−1.43 ± 1.47	0.028 *
Pre-treatment cylinder (D)	−0.52 ± 0.60	−0.57 ± 0.49	0.840

ATR: atropine, BCVA: best-corrected visual acuity, D: diopter, DFCL: dual-focus contact lenses, N: number, SER: spherical equivalent refraction. * denotes significant difference between groups.

3.2. Change in Refraction and Axial Length after Treatments

The baseline cycloplegic SER was −1.28 ± 1.41 D in the ATR group and −1.71 ± 1.56 D in the DFCL group, in which DFCL showed a higher initial cycloplegic SER ($p < 0.001$). After the follow-up interval, the cycloplegic SER was −1.59 ± 1.40 D in the ATR group and −2.03 ± 1.79 D in the DFCL group. The change in cycloplegic SER (−0.31 ± 0.87 versus −0.32 ± 0.89) was similar between the ATR and DFCL groups (aOR: 1.305, 95% CI: 0.247–2.515, $p = 0.803$) after adjusting for the effects of sex, age, pre-treatment BCVA, pre-treatment AXL and pre-treatment cycloplegic SER. On the other hand, the baseline AXL was 24.06 ± 0.72 mm and 24.34 ± 0.92 mm in the ATR and DFCL groups, respectively, and the DFCL group also showed a longer baseline AXL ($p < 0.001$). One year after the treatment, the AXL was 24.10 ± 0.78 mm in the ATR group and 24.53 ± 0.96 mm in the DFCL group (Table 2), and the DFCL group presented a significantly higher AXL after treatment compared to the ATR group ($p = 0.007$) (Table 2). However, the DFCL group only demonstrated a numerically higher rate of AXL elongation than the ATR group (aOR: 1.530, 95% CI: 0.980–1.894, $p = 0.051$) according to the result of the generalized estimate equation. The trends of manifest SER progression and AXL elongation are presented in Figures 1 and 2.

Table 2. The changes in cycloplegic spherical equivalent and axial length between the two groups after the follow-up period.

Outcome	ATR Group (N = 182)	DFCL Group (N = 70)	*p* Value
SER (D)			
Pre-treatment	−1.28 ± 1.41	−1.71 ± 1.56	0.009 *
Post-treatment	−1.59 ± 1.40	−2.03 ± 1.79	0.007 *
Change	−0.31 ± 0.87	−0.32 ± 0.89	0.884
AXL (mm)			
Pre-treatment	24.06 ± 0.72	24.34 ± 0.92	<0.001 *
Post-treatment	24.10 ± 0.78	24.53 ± 0.96	0.007 *
Change	0.04 ± 0.39	0.19 ± 0.26	0.002 *

ATR: atropine, AXL: axial length, D: diopter, DFCL: dual-focus contact lenses, N: number, SER: spherical equivalent refraction. * denotes significant difference between groups.

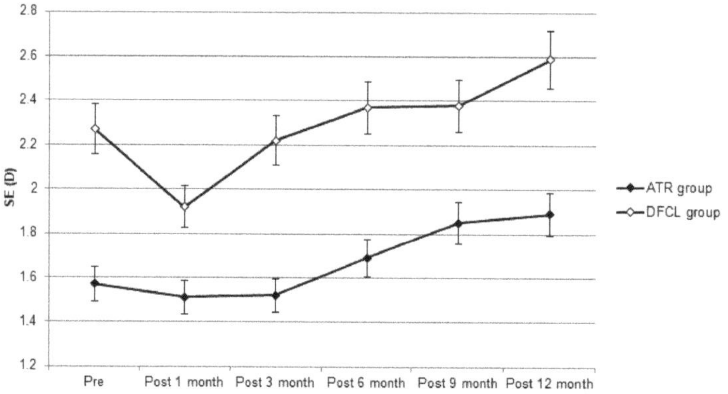

Figure 1. The trend of manifest spherical equivalent changes between the two groups. D: diopter, SE: spherical equivalent.

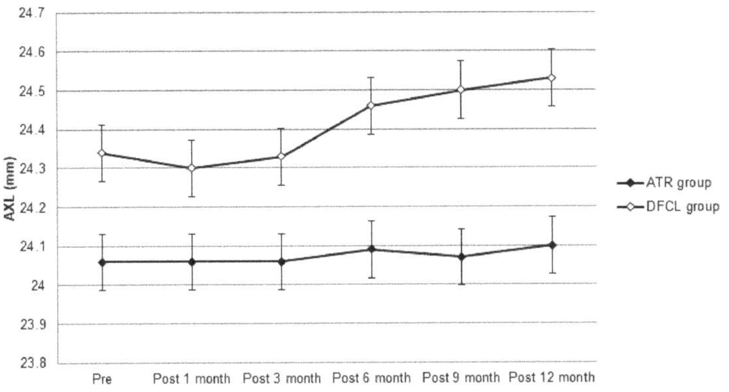

Figure 2. The trend of axial length changes between the two groups. AXL: axial length.

3.3. Subgroup Analyses with Different Parameters

In total, there were 37 eyes with ATR usage and 16 eyes with DFCL usage in the moderate myopia population, 12 eyes with ATR usage and 5 eyes with DFCL usage in the moderate astigmatism population, 48 eyes with ATR usage and 22 eyes with DFCL usage in the high-AXL population and 54 eyes with ATR usage and 46 eyes with DFCL usage in the old age population. In the subgroup analysis, the cycloplegic SER progression was insignificant between ATR and DFCL users in all four different subgroups, including the moderate myopia subgroup, moderate astigmatism subgroup, high-AXL subgroup, and the old age subgroup (all $p > 0.05$) (Table 3). Concerning the AXL elongation, the DFCL patients with moderate astigmatism (aOR: 1.893, 95% CI: 1.252–2.557, $p < 0.001$) and high AXL (aOR: 1.994, 95% CI: 1.568–2.817, $p < 0.001$) presented a high risk of AXL elongation compared to the ATR patients under the same conditions, and the trend of AXL elongation demonstrated no difference between the ATR and DFCL users with moderate myopia or old age (both $p < 0.05$) (Table 3).

Table 3. Subgroup analysis for the risk of myopia progression in the DFCL group compared to the ATR group with different characteristics.

Subgroup	aOR #	95%CI	*p* Value
SER			
Moderate myopia	1.008	0.420–1.944	0.778
Moderate astigmatism	0.975	0.126–1.875	0.650
High AXL	1.339	0.638–2.588	0.561
Old age	1.015	0.213–2.487	0.723
AXL			
Moderate myopia	1.064	0.847–1.280	0.540
Moderate astigmatism	1.893	1.252–2.557	<0.001 *
High AXL	1.994	1.568–2.817	<0.001 *
Old age	1.472	0.862–2.514	0.157

aOR: adjusted odds ratio, AXL: axial length, CI: confidence interval, SER: spherical equivalent refraction. * denotes significant difference between groups. # aOR means the DFCL group compared to the ATR group, adjusted for age, sex, pre-treatment BCVA, pre-treatment cycloplegic SE, and pre-treatment AXL.

4. Discussion

Briefly, the current study showed a similar cycloplegic SER progression in the high-concentration ATR and DFCL groups after a follow-up period of one year. Moreover, the speed of AXL elongation was comparable in the participants using DFCLs and the participants using high-concentration ATR. Also, the DFCL users with moderate astigmatism or high AXL tended to develop higher AXL elongation compared to high-concentration ATR users with similar characteristics.

The patients with high-concentration ATR and DFCL applications demonstrated statistically the same cycloplegic SER progression in the current study. In a previous publication, the application of high-concentration 0.1% ATR contributed to a slower SER progression of −0.47 ± 0.91 D compared to −1.06 ± 0.61 D in the control group [16]. On the other hand, the use of DFCLs was also correlated with a 50% decrease in SER compared to the control group using single contact lenses in the previous literature [14]. Nevertheless, previous studies have only compared high-concentration ATR or DFCL users to non-treatment individuals, and the setting of each study was different, which leads to a direct comparison between ATR application and DFCL usage becoming difficult [14,16]. To our knowledge, a preliminary finding may be that the utilization of high-concentration ATR and DFCLs contribute to similar effects on myopia control concerning the rate of SER progression. Except for the similar patient populations between the ATR and DFCL groups in the current study, we adjusted the influence of several confounders for myopic progression, including age, initial refractive power, and initial AXL in the multivariable model [17]. Moreover, the patients using DFCLs and ATR concurrently were excluded from the current study, and thus, the effect of DFCLs on myopic progression was independent. The similar cycloplegic SER progression between the ATR and DFCL groups is contrary to previous publications in which the application of high-concentration ATR was associated with better myopic control than DFCLs [5,14,16]. A possible explanation is that confounders for myopic progression had not been adjusted for in previous studies. On the other hand, high-concentration ATR presented a numerically lower AXL elongation compared to the DFCL population in the current study. AXL is a precise parameter for myopic progression [18], and the results of the current study may indicate similar overall myopic control of ATR and DFCLs. Furthermore, the difference in AXL elongation was 0.15 mm between the ATR group and DFCL group in the current study. Accordingly, the difference in AXL elongation and related myopic progression between high-concentration ATR and DFCL may not be clinically significant.

In the subgroup analysis, the change in cycloplegic SER after the study interval was similar between the high-concentration ATR and DFCL populations in all the specific subgroups. This result is identical to the whole-group analysis between the high-concentration ATR and DFCL groups and indicates that high-concentration ATR and DFCL showed the same effect on cycloplegic SER control in all patients. On the contrary, the individuals with moderate astigmatism and high initial AXL presented a better AXL control with the usage of high-concentration ATR, while the efficiency of AXL control between high-concentration ATR and DFCL was identical in patients with moderate myopia and old age. There was little research reporting this finding. The design of the DFCLs used in the current study did not contain an astigmatism correction function [14,19]. Although low-degree astigmatism can be corrected by spherical contact lenses, according to the experience of orthokeratology contact lenses [20], patients with moderate astigmatism higher than −1.50 D usually require toric orthokeratology contact lenses to obtain a good fit and fair vision [21]. Since the myopic control method was decided by the parents of our patients, some children with moderate astigmatism still applied DFCLs for myopic control. Thus, we speculate that myopic individuals with moderate astigmatism would experience worse visual quality when utilizing DFCLs, which is a risk factor for myopic progression [8]. On the contrary, the individuals who used high-concentration ATR were always equipped with daily spectacles, and their visual quality may be better than that of the DFCL users. The higher AXL elongation of DFCL users with high initial AXL was also observed. Still, the DFCL users showed similar AXL control to high-concentration ATR users regardless of age and myopia degree, and thus, DFCLs may have an advantage in myopic control in those without high AXL and moderate astigmatism because ATR-related complications including photophobia and blurry reading can be avoided [22,23].

With regard to the efficiency of myopic control in our study, a previous publication showed an annual SER progression of −0.87 ± 0.52 D in high-concentration ATR users (0.5 percent) [22]. For the AXL aspect, the range of annual AXL elongation in high-concentration ATR was 0.23 mm to 0.35 mm in a meta-analysis [24]. In the current study, the cycloplegic SER progression and AXL elongation after one year of high-concentration ATR application were −0.31 ± 0.87 D and 0.04 ± 0.39 mm, respectively. Compared to previous studies [5,22,24,25], the effect of ATR-associated myopic control in the current study was acceptable. On the other hand, a previous publication demonstrated SER progression and AXL elongation of −0.51 D and 0.30 mm after a three-year period after DFCL usage [14], and the subsequent experiment of that study presented SER progression and AXL elongation of −0.52 D and 0.23 mm after a six-year interval [26]. The SER progression and AXL elongation were −0.32 ± 0.89 D and 0.19 ± 0.26 mm one year after the application of DFCLs in the current study, which is comparable to preceding studies [14,26]. The comparisons between the current study and previous studies in terms of SER progression and AXL elongation are demonstrated in Table 4. In addition, one study used the combined therapy of low-concentration ATR (0.01 percent) and orthokeratology contact lenses, yielding an annual SER progression and AXL elongation of 0.88 ± 0.31 D and 0.50 ± 0.17 mm [27]. The similar outcome in the DFCL group of the current study may imply that the usage of DFCLs is simpler compared to the combined treatment but has the same efficiency.

Table 4. The changes in myopic progression parameters between the current study and previous publications.

Parameters	Current Study	Previous Studies
SER progression (D)		
ATR	−0.31	−0.87
DFCL	−0.32	−0.51–−0.52
AXL elongation (mm)		
ATR	0.04	0.23–0.35
DFCL	0.19	0.23–0.30

ATR: atropine AXL: axial length, D: diopter, DFCL: dual-focus contact lenses, SER: spherical equivalent refraction.

Concerning the demographic data, the DFCL group demonstrated an older age and higher baseline myopia degree compared to the ATR group in the current study. The possible explanation for this unbalanced demographic data between the two groups could be related to the fact that users of DFCLs must be older [26]. Generally, DFCLs are recommended for children older than 9 years old in Taiwan due to the need to remove DFCLs oneself during daily life. In fact, all contact lenses, including orthokeratology contact lenses, are rarely applied to patients aged younger than 9 years old in Taiwan. As a consequence, the much older age in the DFCL group compared to the ATR group in the current study is reasonable and can reflect the real-world conditions in Taiwan. Similarly, older age was correlated to a higher degree of myopia in a previous study [28], and thus, the older DFCL group should also show higher myopia than the ATR group. Importantly, we adjusted the effects of age and initial SER in the multivariable analysis so that the imbalance in demographic data would not cause significant statistical bias.

There are certain limitations in the current study. Firstly, the retrospective design of the current study diminishes the heterogeneity of our study groups compared to the prospective study, and the differences in age, myopia degree, and AXL of the two groups could cause significant bias. Secondly, the patients in the current study were managed by different ophthalmologists/optometrists in different branches of our clinic. Accordingly, the habits and opinions of each ophthalmologist regarding myopic control tools may influence the parents' choice of myopic control tool, and the different autorefractors in each branch and the different refraction techniques of each optometrist may diminish the integrity of our results. Accordingly, the prescription of DFCLs and the judgment of ATR application may not have a universal standard. In addition, we cannot ensure all the measurement times were within the duration we proposed, which could lead to some bias. Moreover, the follow-up period in the current study was only one year, which may not be adequate compared to some long-term studies [25,26]. Finally, all the participants in the current research were Han Taiwanese, and thus, the external validity of the current study may be reduced. Still, because the genotype and phenotype of Han Taiwanese people are similar to the Chinese people who live in mainland China and several other countries, including America, Singapore, and Canada, the results of the current study can be used as a reference for at least 1.5 billion of the population; thus, the clinical relevance of the current study might not be low.

5. Conclusions

In conclusion, the application of DFCLs showed a similar effect on myopic control concerning cycloplegic SER progression compared to the usage of high-concentration ATR. Furthermore, the suppression of AXL elongation was similar between the DFCL and high-concentration ATR groups in those without moderate astigmatism and higher AXL. Consequently, DFCLs could be recommended to those with low astigmatism and AXL, considering the lower number of side effects. A further large-scale prospective study to survey the effect of combined DFCL and high-concentration ATR usage on myopic control is mandatory.

Author Contributions: Conceptualization, C.-Y.L. and C.-K.C.; methodology, C.-Y.L., S.-F.Y. and Y.-L.C.; software, S.-F.Y.; formal analysis, J.-Y.H.; data curation, I.-B.L.; writing—original draft preparation, C.-Y.L.; writing—review and editing, C.-K.C. and S.-F.Y. All authors have read and agreed to the published version of the manuscript.

Funding: This research received no external funding.

Institutional Review Board Statement: All the procedures performed in the current study adhered to the 1964 Declaration of Helsinki and its later amendments. Additionally, the current study was approved by the National Changhua University of Education (project identification code: NCUEREC-112-071, approved date: 27 September 2023).

Informed Consent Statement: The essentiality of written informed consent was abandoned by the National Changhua University of Education due to the design of the current study.

Data Availability Statement: Data are contained within the article.

Acknowledgments: The authors thank Shu-Hui Chin for table organization and manuscript formatting.

Conflicts of Interest: The authors declare no conflict of interest.

References

1. Huang, J.; Wen, D.; Wang, Q.; McAlinden, C.; Flitcroft, I.; Chen, H.; Saw, S.M.; Chen, H.; Bao, F.; Zhao, Y.; et al. Efficacy Comparison of 16 Interventions for Myopia Control in Children: A Network Meta-analysis. *Ophthalmology* **2016**, *123*, 697–708. [CrossRef] [PubMed]
2. Walline, J.J. Myopia Control: A Review. *Eye Contact Lens* **2016**, *42*, 3–8. [CrossRef]
3. Cooper, J.; Tkatchenko, A.V. A Review of Current Concepts of the Etiology and Treatment of Myopia. *Eye Contact Lens* **2018**, *44*, 231–247. [CrossRef] [PubMed]
4. Morgan, I.G.; Ohno-Matsui, K.; Saw, S.M. Myopia. *Lancet* **2012**, *379*, 1739–1748. [CrossRef] [PubMed]
5. Wu, P.C.; Chuang, M.N.; Choi, J.; Chen, H.; Wu, G.; Ohno-Matsui, K.; Jonas, J.B.; Cheung, C.M.G. Update in myopia and treatment strategy of atropine use in myopia control. *Eye* **2019**, *33*, 3–13. [CrossRef] [PubMed]
6. Remón, L.; Pérez-Merino, P.; Macedo-de-Araújo, R.J.; Amorim-de-Sousa, A.I.; González-Méijome, J.M. Bifocal and Multifocal Contact Lenses for Presbyopia and Myopia Control. *J. Ophthalmol.* **2020**, *2020*, 8067657. [CrossRef] [PubMed]
7. Tran, H.D.M.; Tran, Y.H.; Tran, T.D.; Jong, M.; Coroneo, M.; Sankaridurg, P. A Review of Myopia Control with Atropine. *J. Ocul. Pharmacol. Ther.* **2018**, *34*, 374–379. [CrossRef]
8. Sankaridurg, P. Contact lenses to slow progression of myopia. *Clin. Exp. Optom.* **2017**, *100*, 432–437. [CrossRef]
9. Heng, L.S.; Khoo, C.Y. Can contact lenses control the progression of myopia? *Singap. Med. J.* **1994**, *35*, 367–370.
10. Queirós, A.; Villa-Collar, C.; Gutiérrez, A.R.; Jorge, J.; González-Méijome, J.M. Quality of life of myopic subjects with different methods of visual correction using the NEI RQL-42 questionnaire. *Eye Contact Lens* **2012**, *38*, 116–121. [CrossRef]
11. Bullimore, M.A.; Richdale, K. Myopia Control 2020: Where are we and where are we heading? *Ophthalmic Physiol. Opt.* **2020**, *40*, 254–270. [CrossRef] [PubMed]
12. Cheng, X.; Xu, J.; Chehab, K.; Exford, J.; Brennan, N. Soft Contact Lenses with Positive Spherical Aberration for Myopia Control. *Optom. Vis. Sci.* **2016**, *93*, 353–366. [CrossRef] [PubMed]

13. Gregory, H.R.; Nti, A.N.; Wolffsohn, J.S.; Berntsen, D.A.; Ritchey, E.R. Visual Performance of Center-distance Multifocal Contact Lenses Fit Using a Myopia Control Paradigm. *Optom. Vis. Sci.* **2021**, *98*, 272–279. [CrossRef]
14. Chamberlain, P.; Peixoto-de-Matos, S.C.; Logan, N.S.; Ngo, C.; Jones, D.; Young, G. A 3-year Randomized Clinical Trial of MiSight Lenses for Myopia Control. *Optom. Vis. Sci.* **2019**, *96*, 556–567. [CrossRef] [PubMed]
15. Cabanes-Martí, E.; García-Ayuso, D. Myopia control with dual-focus soft contact lenses during the first year of measures to contain the COVID-19 pandemic. *Ophthalmic Physiol. Opt.* **2022**, *42*, 1227–1231. [CrossRef]
16. Shih, Y.F.; Chen, C.H.; Chou, A.C.; Ho, T.C.; Lin, L.L.; Hung, P.T. Effects of different concentrations of atropine on controlling myopia in myopic children. *J. Ocul. Pharmacol. Ther.* **1999**, *15*, 85–90. [CrossRef]
17. Hyman, L.; Gwiazda, J.; Hussein, M.; Norton, T.T.; Wang, Y.; Marsh-Tootle, W.; Everett, D. Relationship of age, sex, and ethnicity with myopia progression and axial elongation in the correction of myopia evaluation trial. *Arch. Ophthalmol.* **2005**, *123*, 977–987. [CrossRef]
18. Chamberlain, P.; Lazon de la Jara, P.; Arumugam, B.; Bullimore, M.A. Axial length targets for myopia control. *Ophthalmic Physiol. Opt.* **2021**, *41*, 523–531. [CrossRef]
19. Ghorbani-Mojarrad, N.; Cargill, C.; Collard, S.; Terry, L. Patient experience and physiological response to two commercially available daily disposable myopia control contact lenses. *Cont. Lens Anterior Eye* **2022**, *45*, 101426. [CrossRef]
20. Bullimore, M.A.; Johnson, L.A. Overnight orthokeratology. *Cont. Lens Anterior Eye* **2020**, *43*, 322–332. [CrossRef]
21. Chen, C.C.; Cheung, S.W.; Cho, P. Toric orthokeratology for highly astigmatic children. *Optom. Vis. Sci.* **2012**, *89*, 849–855. [CrossRef] [PubMed]
22. Chia, A.; Chua, W.H.; Wen, L.; Fong, A.; Goon, Y.Y.; Tan, D. Atropine for the treatment of childhood myopia: Changes after stopping atropine 0.01%, 0.1% and 0.5%. *Am. J. Ophthalmol.* **2014**, *157*, 451–457.e1. [CrossRef]
23. Woods, J.; Jones, D.; Jones, L.; Jones, S.; Hunt, C.; Chamberlain, P.; McNally, J. Ocular health of children wearing daily disposable contact lenses over a 6-year period. *Cont. Lens Anterior Eye* **2021**, *44*, 101391. [CrossRef] [PubMed]
24. Ha, A.; Kim, S.J.; Shim, S.R.; Kim, Y.K.; Jung, J.H. Efficacy and Safety of 8 Atropine Concentrations for Myopia Control in Children: A Network Meta-Analysis. *Ophthalmology* **2022**, *129*, 322–333. [CrossRef] [PubMed]
25. Chia, A.; Chua, W.H.; Cheung, Y.B.; Wong, W.L.; Lingham, A.; Fong, A.; Tan, D. Atropine for the treatment of childhood myopia: Safety and efficacy of 0.5%, 0.1%, and 0.01% doses (Atropine for the Treatment of Myopia 2). *Ophthalmology* **2012**, *119*, 347–354. [CrossRef]
26. Chamberlain, P.; Bradley, A.; Arumugam, B.; Hammond, D.; McNally, J.; Logan, N.S.; Jones, D.; Ngo, C.; Peixoto-de-Matos, S.C.; Hunt, C.; et al. Long-term Effect of Dual-focus Contact Lenses on Myopia Progression in Children: A 6-year Multicenter Clinical Trial. *Optom. Vis. Sci.* **2022**, *99*, 204–212. [CrossRef]
27. Zhou, H.; Zhao, G.; Li, Y. Adjunctive effects of orthokeratology and atropine 0.01% eye drops on slowing the progression of myopia. *Clin. Exp. Optom.* **2022**, *105*, 520–526. [CrossRef]
28. Morgan, I.G.; French, A.N.; Ashby, R.S.; Guo, X.; Ding, X.; He, M.; Rose, K.A. The epidemics of myopia: Aetiology and prevention. *Prog. Retin. Eye Res.* **2018**, *62*, 134–149. [CrossRef]

life

Article

Evaluation of Reporting Quality of Glaucoma Randomized Controlled Trial Abstracts: Current Status and Future Perspectives

Ana Vucinovic [1], Josipa Bukic [2,*], Doris Rusic [2], Dario Leskur [2], Ana Seselja Perisin [2], Marijana Radic [3], Marko Grahovac [2] and Darko Modun [2]

[1] Department of Ophthalmology, University Hospital Centre Split, Spinciceva 1, 21000 Split, Croatia; avucinovic@kbsplit.hr
[2] Department of Pharmacy, University of Split School of Medicine, Soltanska 2, 21000 Split, Croatia; drusic@mefst.hr (D.R.); dleskur@mefst.hr (D.L.); aperisin@mefst.hr (A.S.P.); marko.grahovac@mefst.hr (M.G.); dmodun@mefst.hr (D.M.)
[3] Department of Neurology, General Hospital Pula, Santoriova 24a, 52100 Pula, Croatia; marijana.radic@obpula.hr
* Correspondence: jbukic@mefst.hr

Abstract: The aim of this study was to explore adherence to the Consolidated Standards of Reporting Trials (CONSORT) reporting standards in abstracts of randomized controlled trials on glaucoma. A cross-sectional observational study was conducted on the aforementioned abstracts, indexed in MEDLINE/PubMed between the years 2017 and 2021. In total, 302 abstracts met the inclusion criteria and were further analyzed. The median score of CONSORT-A items was 8 (interquartile range, 7–10) out of 17 (47.0%). Most analyzed studies were conducted in a single center (80.5%) and the abstracts were predominantly structured (95.0%). Only 20.5% of the abstracts adequately described the trial design, while randomization and funding were described by 6.0% of the abstracts. Higher overall scores were associated with structured abstracts, a multicenter setting, statistically significant results, funding by industry, a higher number of participants, and having been published in journals with impact factors above four ($p < 0.001$, respectively). The results of this study indicate a suboptimal adherence to CONSORT-A reporting standards, especially in particular items such as randomization and funding. Since these factors could contribute to the overall quality of the trials and further translation of trial results into clinical practice, an improvement in glaucoma research reporting transparency is needed.

Keywords: glaucoma; RCT; research; CONSORT

1. Introduction

Glaucoma is a complex multifactorial eye disease that manifests in chronic progressive optic neuropathy. This chronic progressive optic neuropathy could lead to irreversible sight loss, the most devastating consequence of this disease that has tremendous impact on affected patients' quality of life [1]. Studies have shown that in the year 2020, more than 80 million people worldwide were affected by glaucoma, while approximately 10% of all glaucoma cases resulted in bilateral blindness. Interestingly, a study by Shih et al. suggested higher eye-related costs for open-angle glaucoma patients compared with those for ocular hypertension patients. However, the load of glaucoma on healthcare systems could be further evaluated in future studies [2,3]. Most patients suffer from open-angle glaucoma, which has a prevalence of 2.51% from age 40 to 80, and this number is expected to increase to over 112 million by 2040, imposing a major burden on global healthcare [3].

Although glaucoma is not always caused by increased intraocular pressure observed in the patients, according to the literature, increased intraocular pressure is a well-recognized modifiable risk factor of glaucoma [4]. In order to ensure the appropriate treatment of patients with increased intraocular pressure, a correct intraocular pressure measurement is crucial. Currently, it is well-known that there are several modalities to measure intraocular pressure, but Goldmann Applanation Tonometry (which is based on the Imbert–Fick law) is considered to be the gold standard in the assessment of intraocular pressure [5,6]. It should also be noted that intraocular pressure measurement could be influenced by external factors. For instance, the results of a meta-analysis by Albis-Donado et al. suggested there is a higher risk that intraocular pressure measurement could be underestimated when Goldmann Applanation Tonometry is used at higher altitudes. This is particularly the case in patients with glaucoma or those with thinner corneas and a history of corneal refractive surgery. In addition, all IOP measurement modalities, from Goldmann Applanation Tonometry to rebound tonometry, are influenced by other external factors, such as body position, central corneal thickness, corneal astigmatism, altitude, etc. [7,8].

Other important risk factors for glaucoma development described in the scientific literature include older age, not being in the White race group, and a history of glaucoma in one's family [9]. It has also been observed that systemic disease, such as Cushing's disease, and medication use may too predispose individuals to glaucoma. A review by Stein et al. highlighted medicines such as corticosteroids, several medications for depression, medication for epilepsy (topiramat in particular), and anticholinergics as the ones associated with glaucoma occurrence. It should be noted that vision loss caused by glaucoma could be minimized with well-timed recognition of individuals' systemic conditions or medications that increase their risk of glaucoma. It is also very important to refer a high-risk individual for a thorough ophthalmologic examination [10–12]. Lately, a new modifiable glaucoma risk factor has been recognized in the scientific literature. The results of a recently published study by Sun et al., a prospective cohort study which included 409,053 participants from the United Kingdom, revealed that sleep patterns are also associated with glaucoma risk, and individuals who experience insomnia, daytime sleepiness, and snoring have a higher risk of glaucoma development, in comparison with individuals who have healthy sleeping patterns [13].

Glaucoma is often asymptomatic due to the binocular compensation of visual field defects. As a result, patients usually experience the first symptoms only in the advanced stages of the disease when there is significant damage to the visual field [2]. Therefore, making a correct and timely diagnosis and the right choice of therapy for particular patients is essential for sight preservation and improving the quality of life in affected individuals [14]. Diagnostic testing and monitoring for disease progression includes the measurement of intraocular pressure, perimetry, pachymetry, and optical coherence tomography [15]. In addition to the fundoscopic signs of glaucoma—an enlarged optic cup, an increased cup–disc ratio, the loss of the neuroretinal rim, the presence of disc hemorrhages, and parapapillary tissue atrophy—assessing the disease progression can be achieved through a spectral-domain optical coherence tomography evaluation of the optic disc and visual field analysis [16]. The primary objective of the treatment of glaucoma is to reduce the intraocular pressure in order to halt the progression of the disease [17]. The treatment of glaucoma is primarily oriented toward lowering the intraocular pressure with medicaments, lasers, or incisional glaucoma surgery [18]. Unfortunately, none of the currently available treatments can reverse glaucomatous damage to the optic nerve; however, early diagnosis and appropriate treatment can slow down the progression of the disease [19].

Since the global impact of glaucoma is so vast, it is understandable that glaucoma is among the top five most frequently studied eye diseases [20]. The amount of research on glaucoma is growing with new clinical trials bringing potential new advances in this field of medicine [21]. However, clinicians often lack time to thoroughly evaluate each new study on glaucoma as the number of studies is abundant. Therefore, it seems reasonable that abstracts, the only part of published articles freely available to clinicians worldwide, should encompass all crucial data. This inclusivity would aid clinicians in assessing the suitability and usefulness of the found abstract, thereby enabling them to filter and select articles for which they will then seek the full text to read. In order to improve research transparency and to ensure translation of research into clinical practice, reporting guidelines have been introduced. One of them, the CONSORT statement for reporting on randomized trials, was first published in 2010 in order to consolidate the standards of reporting randomized controlled trials [22]. The aforementioned statement is an evidence-based minimum set of recommendations (checklist) for reporting data from randomized controlled trials. Since the introduction of this checklist, many scientific journals have recommended its use for drafting the manuscript in order to ensure the transparent reporting of trials and their easier translation into clinical practice [23,24].

Previous studies evaluated the quality of abstracts (adherence to the CONSORT-A checklist) in several fields of medicine, but to our knowledge, the evaluation of reporting the quality of glaucoma randomized controlled trial abstracts has not yet been conducted. Since it is estimated that the number of glaucoma patients will rise and represent a public health problem, the aim of our study was to assess the adherence of glaucoma randomized controlled trial abstracts to a CONSORT-A checklist.

2. Materials and Methods

We conducted a cross-sectional observational study on abstracts of randomized controlled trials in the field of glaucoma, indexed in MEDLINE/PubMed. Inclusion criteria were the following: randomized controlled study design, studies with a control group, and studies with a comparison of particular intervention with either placebo intervention, active treatment, or no treatment at all. Exclusion criteria were being a cross-sectional, observational, or any other type of study except for randomized controlled trials. Animal studies and studies that did not include glaucoma patients were also excluded from our study.

The study period was from the year 2017 to 2021. The year 2017 was chosen because the guidelines used for our studies were published in 2008, and we assumed that a 10-year period would allow both authors and editors to be familiar with Consolidated Standards of Reporting Trials (CONSORT) guidelines for abstracts [11]. The year 2022 was not included as there was a possibility that some glaucoma articles would still be published during late 2022, and the exclusion of these articles could have an impact on the comparison between each study year.

The search strategy used for article extraction in MEDLINE/PubMed consisted of searching for "*Intraocular Pressure*" [MeSH Terms] OR "*Glaucoma*" [MeSH Terms]) AND ((randomizedcontrolledtrial[Filter]) AND (2017:2021[pdat]). This data extraction method included 426 abstracts. After excluding abstracts that were not conducted on glaucoma patients or human participants, studies that were not designed as randomized controlled trials, and articles for which abstracts were not available, we analyzed 302 abstracts, all abstracts of full-text articles. Diagram flow is presented in Figure 1.

Two authors independently assessed each abstract for the inclusion of CONSORT items. One of the authors is an ophthalmology specialist with previous experience in the conduction of randomized controlled trials, and the second author is an experienced research professional with previously published articles on CONSORT matters. Disagreements between these two authors were resolved through discussion with the third author, the most experienced team member with a background in both randomized controlled trial conduction and CONSORT research.

Data were presented, where applicable, as an overall number and proportion (percent), median and interquartile range (IQR), mean and the standard deviation (SD), or mean and a 95% confidence interval (CI). The Cohen κ coefficient was used to determine interobserver agreement between the authors for individual CONSORT for abstract items. Agreement was considered sufficient for kappa point estimates higher than 0.6. To determine which factors were associated with a higher quality of reporting, a univariate linear regression analysis was conducted. The overall quality score, presented as a percentage of the total score, was a dependent variable. Those factors from the univariate analysis that were significantly associated with a higher quality ($p < 0.05$) were included in the multivariate regression analysis. The statistical analysis was conducted using SPSS (version 16.0, IBM Corporation, Chicago, IL, USA).

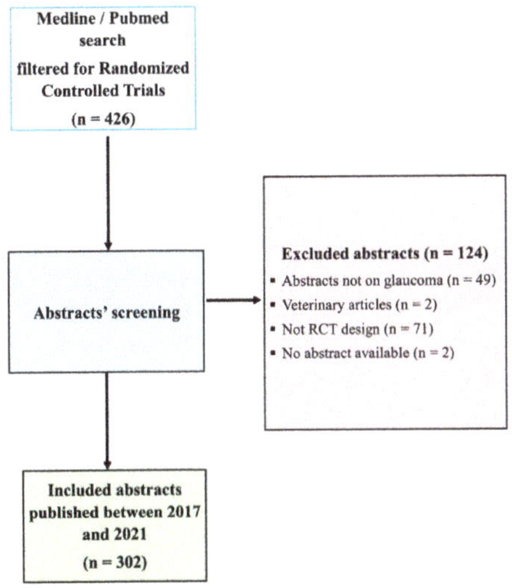

Figure 1. Flow diagram with search strategy and study selection. CONSORT, Consolidated Standards of Reporting Trials.

3. Results

Approximately half of the glaucoma randomized controlled trial abstracts included in this study reported the results of the pharmacological trials (132/302, 43.7%). A similar distribution was noted for the study setting, with 143/302 (47.4%) randomized controlled trials being conducted in a hospital setting, and the number of the participants, with 132/302 (43.7%) randomized controlled trials including more than 100 participants. Most of the studies described in the abstracts were conducted in a single center (243/302, 80.5%), and they had reported results where the main outcome measure was significantly different from the control (194/302, 64.2%). Abstracts were predominantly structured (287/302, 95.0%). On average, abstracts had a median of six authors (IQR 4–8). The mean impact factor of the journals in which they were published was 5.73 (SD = 17.42). A full description of the study characteristics is provided in Table 1.

Table 1. Characteristics of included abstracts.

Characteristics	N	%
Type of intervention		
Non-pharmacological	170	56.3
Pharmacological	132	43.7
Study centers		
Single center	243	80.5
Multicenter	59	19.5
Significance of results		
Non-significant	108	35.8
Significant	194	64.2
Number of participants		
<100	170	56.3
≥100	132	43.7

Table 1. *Cont.*

Characteristics	N	%
Funding		
Non-industry	292	96.7
Industry	10	3.3
Setting		
Non-hospital	159	52.6
Hospital	143	47.4
Abstract structure		
Unstructured abstract	15	5.0
Structured abstract	287	95.0
Quartiles		
Non-ranked	38	12.6
1st	91	30.1
2nd	72	23.8
3rd	79	26.2
4th	22	7.3
	Mean (SD)	**Median (IQR)**
Number of authors	6.54 (3.41)	6.00 (4.00–8.00)
Impact factor	5.73 (17.42)	2.97 (2.02–5.49)

The interobserver agreement in the present study was found to be sufficient as the calculated Cohen κ values for all items were above the recommended threshold value of 0.6, as presented in Table 2.

Table 2. Interobserver agreement for abstract reporting items.

Item	Kappa Point	Kappa > 0.60
Title	0.888	*
Authors	0.953	*
Trial design	0.791	*
Methods		
Participants	0.958	*
Interventions	0.607	*
Objective	0.722	*
Outcome	0.864	*
Randomization	0.607	*
Blinding	0.684	*
Results		
Numbers randomized	0.637	*
Recruitment	0.954	*
Numbers analyzed	0.969	*
Outcome	0.737	*
Harms	0.639	*
Conclusions	0.607	*
Trial registration	0.895	*
Funding	0.830	*

* Kappa > 0.60.

Only 62 (20.5%) of all the included abstracts adequately described the trial design (e.g., parallel, crossover, etc.). A proper title and the corresponding author details were provided by 118 and 136 (39.1% and 45.0%) of the included abstracts, respectively. With regards to the methodology section, interventions and objective items were overwhelmingly well-reported (294/302, 97.4% and 296/302, 98.0%, respectively). On the contrary, randomization and blinding were poorly reported by most abstracts, with only 18 (6.0%) and 56 (18.5%)

sufficiently describing those items. Participant items were properly described in 186 (61.6%) abstracts, while the outcome was reported in 222 (73.5%) abstracts.

Results of the primary outcome measures were adequately described in 236 (78.1%) abstracts. The larger proportion of the included abstracts (224, 74.2%) provided the number of participants randomized in each trial group; however, most abstracts failed to report the number of participants included in the analysis, with only 61 (20.2%) abstracts providing this valuable information. Another poorly reported item was the side effects and adverse events, which were described in only 87 (28.8%) of the included abstracts. Funding statement was provided by only 18 (6.0%) abstracts. Fifty abstracts (16.6%) gave the trial registration information. Adequate conclusions were provided by the vast majority of the abstracts (295, 97.7%). The adherence of each item to the CONSORT for the abstract guideline is provided in Table 3.

Table 3. Quality of the individual CONSORT for abstract items.

Items	N	%
Title	118	39.1
Authors	136	45.0
Trial design	62	20.5
Methods		
Participants	186	61.6
Interventions	294	97.4
Objective	296	98.0
Outcome	222	73.5
Randomization	18	6.0
Blinding	56	18.5
Results		
Numbers randomized	224	74.2
Recruitment	143	47.4
Numbers analyzed	61	20.2
Outcome	236	78.1
Harms	87	28.8
Conclusions	295	97.7
Trial registration	50	16.6
Funding	18	6.0

Only one abstract adequately reported every item and had a maximum score of 17. The median score was 8 (IQR 7–10) out of 17 (47.0%) items. The average overall reporting scores of the included abstracts are described in Table 4.

Table 4. Overall reporting quality score.

	Score	**Score (%)**
Mean	8.28	48.32
SD	2.34	13.61
95% CI	8.02–8.55	46.77–49.86
Median	8.00	47.00
IQR	7.00–10.00	41.00–58.00

The overall quality score for each study characteristic of interest that was included in the regression analysis is presented in Table 5.

Table 5. Overall reporting quality score for each study characteristic.

Characteristics	Mean Score (%)	95% CI
Type of intervention		
Non-pharmacological	46.45	44.44–48.45
Pharmacological	50.72	48.35–53.09
Study centers		
Single center	46.12	44.59–47.66
Multicenter	57.34	53.29–61.39
Significance of results		
Non-significant	44.60	42.00–47.20
Significant	50.38	48.51–52.25
Number of participants		
<100	45.12	43.29–46.95
≥100	52.42	49.95–54.90
Funding		
Non-industry	47.59	46.10–49.07
Industry	69.60	56.94–82.26
Number of authors		
<5	44.63	41.90–47.36
5–7	45.10	42.85–47.35
>7	51.40	48.21–54.59
Collaboration	57.38	52.82–61.93
Setting		
Non-hospital	47.79	45.56–50.01
Hospital	48.90	46.77–51.04
Abstract structure		
Unstructured abstract	34.53	22.54–46.53
Structured abstract	49.04	47.56–50.52
Impact factor		
<2.200	42.69	40.13–45.24
2.201–4	44.51	42.60–46.41
>4	56.60	53.96–59.23
Quartiles		
Non-ranked	39.00	35.21–42.79
1st	55.28	52.60–57.95
2nd	50.06	46.33–53.74
3rd	44.46	42.29–46.62
4th	43.77	39.76–47.79

Table 6 presents the results of the linear regression analysis. Cutoff values of 2.200 and 4.000 for journal impact factors were chosen to create three approximately equal groups. This decision was made to facilitate a balanced categorization of journals based on their impact factors. The goal was to have comparable representation in each group, which enhanced the robustness of the analysis and provided a more nuanced understanding of the data.

Table 6. Linear-regression-derived estimates and 95% CI with the dependent variable defined as the mean overall quality score shown as a percentage.

Characteristics	Univariate Analysis, Estimate 95% CI	Multivariate Analysis, Estimate 95% CI
Type of intervention		
Non-pharmacological	Reference	Reference
Pharmacological	4.273 (1.198–7.347) **	2.406 (−0.170–4.982)
Study centers		
Single center	Reference	Reference
Multicenter	11.216 (7.536–14.895) ***	4.367 (0.822–7.911) *
Significance of results		
Non-significant	Reference	Reference
Significant	5.780 (2.626–8.933) ***	2.946 (0.335–5.557) *
Number of participants		
<100	Reference	Reference
≥100	7.301 (4.300–10.301) ***	2.424 (−0.304–5.152)
Funding		
Non-industry	Reference	Reference
Industry	22.014 (13.756–30.273) ***	12.341 (4.775–19.907) **
Number of authors		
<5	Reference	Reference
5–7	0.466 (−3.347–4.279)	0.686 (−2.597–3.968)
>7	6.770 (2.767–10.772) **	2.358 (−1.152–5.869)
Collaboration	12.742 (7.816–17.669) ***	3.339 (−1.570–8.248)
Setting		
Non-hospital	Reference	
Hospital	1.116 (−1.974–4.206)	
Abstract structure		
Unstructured abstract	Reference	Reference
Structured abstract	14.502 (7.588–21.415) ***	14.784 (8.867–20.700) ***
Impact factor		
<2.200	Reference	Reference
2.201–4	1.820 (−1.617–5.257)	−4.277 (−8.521- (−0.032)) *
>4	13.912 (10.535–17.288) ***	11.327 (4.396–18.259) **
Quartiles		
Non-ranked	Reference	Reference
1st	16.275 (11.533–21.016) ***	−0.701 (−8.894–7.491)
2nd	11.056 (6.133–15.978) ***	8.299 (2.820–13.778) **
3rd	5.456 (0.609–10.302) *	6.943 (1.464–12.423) *
4th	4.773 (−1.804–11.350)	2.820 (−2.933–8.572)

* $p < 0.05$, ** $p < 0.01$, *** $p < 0.001$.

In a univariate model, the higher overall scores were associated with structured abstracts ($p < 0.001$), pharmacological intervention ($p < 0.01$), a multicenter setting ($p < 0.001$), statistically significant results ($p < 0.001$), funding by the industry ($p < 0.001$), a higher number of participants ($p < 0.001$), having been published in journals with impact factors above 4 ($p < 0.001$) and in journals in the first three quartiles, as well as having more authors, namely above seven ($p < 0.01$), and being authored by a collaboration ($p < 0.001$). As no significant association was found with the study setting, it was omitted from the multivariate analysis. A higher overall score remained associated with structured abstracts ($p < 0.001$), a multicenter setting ($p < 0.05$), statistically significant results ($p < 0.05$), industry funding ($p < 0.01$), being published in the second ($p < 0.01$) and third quartile ($p < 0.05$), and having been published in journals with impact factors above four ($p < 0.01$) in the multiple regression model. The overall score was adversely impacted by being published in journals with impact factors between 2.201 and 4.

4. Discussion

This study analyzed 302 abstracts of glaucoma randomized controlled trials and found scarce reporting of CONSORT-A checklist items, as the majority of abstracts included mostly half of all items. It should be noted that only one abstract included all the checklist items. Further, items such as randomization and funding were reported in less than 10% of all abstracts. The results of our study should raise awareness of the current status of the reporting quality in the field of glaucoma. Since this is a rising field, inadequate reporting quality could have an impact on the design of future studies and also on the translation of current conclusions into clinical practice.

The results of our study showed that adverse effects were reported in merely 30% of glaucoma randomized controlled trial abstracts. Since it could be assumed that clinicians did not have time to read through the whole manuscript in search of high-quality information for their patients, the omission of adverse effect data in abstracts could lead to inappropriate intervention in particular patients. In general, due to both time limitations and very often, the non-availability of the full-text articles, most clinicians and scientists perform the preliminary evaluation of the quality and validity of a clinical trial just by screening the abstracts. Therefore, it is of great importance that the abstract is well-written, detailed, and transparent, as this eliminates bias and confounding factors.

The results of our study were in accordance with the results of several previous studies, which reported a low adherence to the CONSORT-A guidelines [25–27]. Song et al. reported that although the reporting quality of psychiatry randomized controlled trial abstracts improved after the publication of the CONSORT-A guidelines, it still remained suboptimal with an overall quality score of just 45% [25]. Janackovic et al. reported that randomized controlled trials published in the seven top anesthesiology journals did not adhere to CONSORT-A guidelines with a median adherence of only 41% [26]. Baulig et al. reported that none of the 136 investigated abstracts on macular degeneration reported all of the CONSORT-A items, and the median number of reported items was seven [27].

A number of authors showed that there was substandard reporting of funding in randomized controlled trial abstracts, also observed in our study, which could be misleading to the reader, as it is well-known that funding by industry could be associated with the positive results of randomized controlled trials [28,29]. Previous research has also demonstrated that inaccurate or omitted funding information could lead to the uncritical incorporation of those results into clinical practice [30]. Fundytus et al. showed that the vast majority of oncology randomized controlled trials are now funded by industry—they are larger, more likely to be positive, and published in higher impact journals than trials without industry support [31]. Furthermore, the results of a study by Wiehn et al. showed that adequate reporting varied considerably across CONSORT items with information on blinding and adverse effects being the least reported [32]. Although the results of several studies have concluded that funding is mostly not included in the abstract of randomized controlled trials, it has been observed that funding is reported in the full text of the randomized controlled trial articles. For instance, a study by Alharbi et al. reported that funding was included in 76.9% of periodontal studies, published in three of the most citable journals in the field. This proportion was more than ten times higher when compared to our results. However, there is a possibility that the majority of journals include additional sections for acknowledgements, conflicts of interest, and funding. Nonetheless, as mentioned before, not all scientific articles are freely available, and readers should be able to distinguish between funded and non-funded research based on the abstract data [33].

Improving the reporting quality of randomized controlled trial abstracts requires concerted efforts and considerations. Firstly, addressing the limitation imposed by word count restrictions on abstract length is crucial. Journals should reconsider these limitations, recognizing that comprehensive reporting may necessitate additional space. Secondly, promoting structured abstracts is paramount, given our findings on their significantly better reporting quality. Journals not endorsing structured abstracts should consider adopting this practice, while those already doing so could refine the designated structure to align more closely with CONSORT-A guidelines. Thirdly, educating authors on the effective utilization of CONSORT-A guidelines for abstract writing is imperative. Workshops and resources should be provided to enhance authors' understanding and application of these guidelines. Additionally, educating peer reviewers to encourage authors to structure their abstracts in accordance with CONSORT-A guidelines is essential for maintaining reporting standards. Furthermore, editors should play a proactive role by insisting on stricter adherence to these guidelines during the review process. Finally, journals should explicitly endorse CONSORT-A guidelines in their submission guidelines for authors, reinforcing the importance of compliance. Stricter enforcement mechanisms should be implemented to ensure that these guidelines become an integral part of the abstract writing process, fostering a culture of comprehensive reporting in the field of glaucoma research.

It is worth mentioning that published glaucoma articles, or their available abstracts, could be used as study materials for both students during their formal education and the general population while initiating public health interventions. For instance, an advanced approach to formal education for medical students was described by Marin et al. The authors provided valuable data on experience with a pilot model of ophthalmology longitudinal integrated clerkships, which improved students' knowledge in this field, but the authors also recognized the need for future studies that would evaluate the relationship between medical curricula and students' interest in ophthalmology. Similarly, a need for accurate information that would allow glaucoma patients to make informed decisions on their condition was recognized in a study by Cohen et al., where authors evaluated patient education materials available online [34,35]. Therefore, in order to ensure that study materials are of high quality, items such as funding, but also harms and outcomes, must be represented in article abstracts.

The limitation of this study was that we used only one database—MEDLINE/PubMed—because of the fact that it is the most used database for medical professionals worldwide and it is a free-access database. The strengths of this study were its reproducibility and selection criterion transparency, as well as a wide timeframe from 2017 to 2022. Finally, we would like to emphasize that the interobserver agreement measured by Cohen's kappa was adequate in all the checklist items.

5. Conclusions

Our study indicated that the publication of the CONSORT-A guidelines has not yet translated into better randomized controlled trial abstract reporting in the field of glaucoma research. Glaucoma is a common and serious condition with an increasing need for high-quality, evidence-based information; however, the reporting quality of randomized controlled trial abstracts concerning glaucoma had not been assessed until this study was conducted. Since items included in the abstracts could assist the evaluation of the quality of the presented trials and the further translation of the trial results into clinical practice, an improvement in glaucoma research reporting transparency is needed. Further efforts on implementing the guidelines are required to enhance the quality of reported data and facilitate the translation of scientific research into clinical practice.

Author Contributions: Conceptualization, A.V., J.B. and D.M.; data curation, D.L. and M.G.; formal analysis, J.B. and M.R.; methodology, A.V., A.S.P., M.R. and M.G.; software, D.R. and D.L.; supervision, D.M.; validation, D.R.; visualization, A.S.P.; writing—original draft, A.V. and J.B.; writing—review and editing, D.R., D.L., A.S.P., M.R., M.G. and D.M. All authors have read and agreed to the published version of the manuscript.

Funding: This research received no external funding.

Institutional Review Board Statement: Not applicable.

Informed Consent Statement: Not applicable.

Data Availability Statement: The data are available upon reasonable request to the corresponding author.

Conflicts of Interest: The authors declare no conflicts of interest.

References

1. Basavarajappa, D.; Galindo-Romero, C.; Gupta, V.; Agudo-Barriuso, M.; Gupta, V.B.; Graham, S.L.; Chitranshi, N. Signalling pathways and cell death mechanisms in glaucoma: Insights into the molecular pathophysiology. *Mol. Aspects Med.* **2023**, *94*, 101216. [CrossRef]
2. Shih, V.; Parekh, M.; Multani, J.K.; McGuiness, C.B.; Chen, C.C.; Campbell, J.H.; Miller-Ellis, E.; Olivier, M.M.G. Clinical and Economic Burden of Glaucoma by Disease Severity: A United States Claims-Based Analysis. *Ophthalmol. Glaucoma* **2021**, *4*, 490–503. [CrossRef] [PubMed]
3. Tham, Y.C.; Li, X.; Wong, T.Y.; Quigley, H.A.; Aung, T.; Cheng, C.Y. Global prevalence of glaucoma and projections of glaucoma burden through 2040: A systematic review and meta-analysis. *Ophthalmology* **2014**, *121*, 2081–2090. [CrossRef]
4. Mahabadi, N.; Foris, L.A.; Tripathy, K. *Open Angle Glaucoma*; StatPearls Publishing: Treasure Island, FL, USA, 2023.
5. De Bernardo, M.; Casaburi, C.; De Pascale, I.; Capasso, L.; Cione, F.; Rosa, N. Comparison between dynamic contour tonometry and Goldmann applanation tonometry correcting equations. *Sci. Rep.* **2022**, *12*, 20190. [CrossRef]
6. Markiewitz, H.H. The so-called Imbert-Fick law. *Arch. Ophthalmol.* **1960**, *64*, 159. [CrossRef] [PubMed]
7. Albis-Donado, O.; Ramirez-Neria, P.; Rios-Acosta, N.; Stalmans, I. The influence of altitude on the differences between Goldmann tonometry and Pascal dynamic contour tonometry: An ecological meta-analysis. *Indian J. Ophthalmol.* **2023**. [CrossRef] [PubMed]
8. De Bernardo, M.; Abbinante, G.; Borrelli, M.; Di Stasi, M.; Cione, F.; Rosa, N. Intraocular Pressure Measurements in Standing, Sitting, and Supine Position: Comparison between Tono-Pen Avia and Icare Pro Tonometers. *J. Clin. Med.* **2022**, *11*, 6234. [CrossRef] [PubMed]
9. Wang, Y.; Dong, X.X.; Hou, X.W.; Pan, C.W. Risk Factors for Primary Angle-closure Glaucoma: A Systematic Review and Meta-Analysis of 45 Studies. *Optom. Vis. Sci.* **2023**, *100*, 606–613. [CrossRef]
10. Stein, J.D.; Khawaja, A.P.; Weizer, J.S. Glaucoma in Adults-Screening, Diagnosis, and Management: A Review. *JAMA* **2021**, *325*, 164–174. [CrossRef]
11. Sun, J.; Li, T.; Zhao, X.; Lu, B.; Chen, J.; Liu, W.; Zhou, M.; Sun, X. Prevalence and Risk Factors of Glaucoma among Chinese People from the China Health and Retirement Longitudinal Study. *J. Glaucoma* **2022**, *31*, 789–795. [CrossRef]
12. Lee, J.H.; Kwon, Y.J.; Lee, H.S.; Han, J.H.; Joung, B.; Kim, S.J. Fatty Liver Is an Independent Risk Factor for Elevated Intraocular Pressure. *Nutrients* **2022**, *14*, 4455. [CrossRef]
13. Sun, C.; Yang, H.; Hu, Y.; Qu, Y.; Hu, Y.; Sun, Y.; Ying, Z.; Song, H. Association of sleep behaviour and pattern with the risk of glaucoma: A prospective cohort study in the UK Biobank. *BMJ Open* **2022**, *12*, e063676. [CrossRef] [PubMed]
14. Dhawan, M.; Hans, T.; Sandhu, P.S.; Midha, N. Evaluation of Vision-related Quality of Life in Patients with Glaucoma: A Hospital-based Study. *J. Curr. Glaucoma Pract.* **2019**, *13*, 9–15. [CrossRef]
15. Aspberg, J.; Heijl, A.; Bengtsson, B. Screening for Open-Angle Glaucoma and Its Effect on Blindness. *Am. J. Ophthalmol.* **2021**, *228*, 106–116. [CrossRef] [PubMed]
16. Singh, R.; Rauscher, F.G.; Li, Y.; Eslami, M.; Kazeminasab, S.; Zebardast, N.; Wang, M.; Elze, T. Normative Percentiles of Retinal Nerve Fiber Layer Thickness and Glaucomatous Visual Field Loss. *Transl. Vis. Sci. Technol.* **2023**, *12*, 13. [CrossRef]
17. Buonfiglio, F.; Pfeiffer, N.; Gericke, A. Immunomodulatory and Antioxidant Drugs in Glaucoma Treatment. *Pharmaceuticals* **2023**, *16*, 1193. [CrossRef]
18. Kang, J.M.; Tanna, A.P. Glaucoma. *Med. Clin. N. Am.* **2021**, *105*, 493–510. [CrossRef] [PubMed]
19. Wagner, I.V.; Stewart, M.W.; Dorairaj, S.K. Updates on the Diagnosis and Management of Glaucoma. *Mayo Clin. Proc. Innov. Qual. Outcomes* **2022**, *6*, 618–635. [CrossRef]
20. Boudry, C.; Denion, E.; Mortemousque, B.; Mouriaux, F. Trends and topics in eye disease research in PubMed from 2010 to 2014. *PeerJ* **2016**, *4*, e1557. [CrossRef]
21. Mohan, N.; Chakrabarti, A.; Nazm, N.; Mehta, R.; Edward, D.P. Newer advances in medical management of glaucoma. *Indian J. Ophthalmol.* **2022**, *70*, 1920–1930. [CrossRef]
22. Speich, B.; Schroter, S.; Briel, M.; Moher, D.; Puebla, I.; Clark, A.; Schlüssel, M.M.; Ravaud, P.; Boutron, I.; Hopewell, S. Impact of a short version of the CONSORT checklist for peer reviewers to improve the reporting of randomised controlled trials published in biomedical journals: Study protocol for a randomised controlled trial. *BMJ Open* **2020**, *10*, e035114. [CrossRef]
23. Imran, M.; Kwakkenbos, L.; McCall, S.J.; McCord, K.A.; Fröbert, O.; Hemkens, L.G.; Zwarenstein, M.; Relton, C.; Rice, D.B.; Langan, S.M.; et al. Methods and results used in the development of a consensus-driven extension to the Consolidated Standards of Reporting Trials (CONSORT) statement for trials conducted using cohorts and routinely collected data (CONSORT-ROUTINE). *BMJ Open* **2021**, *11*, e049093. [CrossRef]
24. Hopewell, S.; Clarke, M.; Moher, D.; Wager, E.; Middleton, P.; Altman, D.G.; Schulz, K.F.; The CONSORT Group. CONSORT for reporting randomized controlled trials in journal and conference abstracts: Explanation and elaboration. *PLoS Med.* **2008**, *5*, e20. [CrossRef]

25. Song, S.Y.; Kim, B.; Kim, I.; Kim, S.; Kwon, M.; Han, C.; Kim, E. Assessing reporting quality of randomized controlled trial abstracts in psychiatry: Adherence to CONSORT for abstracts: A systematic review. *PLoS ONE* **2017**, *12*, e0187807. [CrossRef] [PubMed]
26. Janackovic, K.; Puljak, L. Reporting quality of randomized controlled trial abstracts in the seven highest-ranking anesthesiology journals. *Trials* **2018**, *19*, 591. [CrossRef] [PubMed]
27. Baulig, C.; Krummenauer, F.; Geis, B.; Tulka, S.; Knippschild, S. Reporting quality of randomised controlled trial abstracts on age-related macular degeneration health care: A cross-sectional quantification of the adherence to CONSORT abstract reporting recommendations. *BMJ Open* **2018**, *8*, e021912. [CrossRef] [PubMed]
28. Vrebalov Cindro, P.; Bukic, J.; Pranic, S.; Leskur, D.; Rusic, D.; Seselja Perisin, A.; Bozic, J.; Vukovic, J.; Modun, D. Did an introduction of CONSORT for abstracts guidelines improve reporting quality of randomised controlled trials' abstracts on *Helicobacter pylori* infection? Observational study. *BMJ Open* **2022**, *12*, e054978. [CrossRef]
29. Xie, L.; Qin, W.; Gu, Y.; Pathak, J.; Zeng, S.; Du, M. Quality assessment of randomized controlled trial Abstracts on drug therapy of periodontal disease from the Abstracts published in dental science citation indexed journals in the last ten years. *Med. Oral Patol. Oral Cir. Bucal* **2020**, *25*, e626–e633. [CrossRef]
30. Lundh, A.; Lexchin, J.; Mintzes, B.; Schroll, J.B.; Bero, L. Industry sponsorship and research outcome. *Cochrane Database Syst. Rev.* **2017**, *2*, MR000033. [CrossRef]
31. Fundytus, A.; Wells, J.C.; Sharma, S.; Hopman, W.; Del Paggio, J.; Gyawali, B.; Mukherji, D.; Hammad, N.; Pramesh, C.; Aggarwal, A.; et al. Industry Funding of Oncology Randomised Controlled Trials: Implications for Design, Results and Interpretation. *Clin. Oncol.* **2022**, *34*, 28–35. [CrossRef]
32. Wiehn, J.; Nonte, J.; Prugger, C. Reporting quality for abstracts of randomised trials on child and adolescent depression prevention: A meta-epidemiological study on adherence to CONSORT for abstracts. *BMJ Open* **2022**, *12*, e061873. [CrossRef] [PubMed]
33. Alharbi, F.; Gufran, K.; Ahmed, M.M.; Alsakr, A.; Almutairi, A. Quality of Reporting Randomized Controlled Trials Published in Three of the Most Citable Periodontal Journals from 2018 to 2022. *Healthcare* **2023**, *11*, 3180. [CrossRef] [PubMed]
34. Marin, A.I.; Silva, H.N.D.; Chen, H.; Mehta, N.; Nguyen, L.K.; SooHoo, J.R.; Adams, J.E.; Singh, J.K. A Third-Year Medical School Ophthalmology Curriculum for a Longitudinal Integrated Clerkship Model. *J. Acad. Ophthalmol.* **2022**, *14*, e209–e215. [CrossRef] [PubMed]
35. Cohen, S.A.; Fisher, A.C.; Pershing, S. Analysis of the Readability and Accountability of Online Patient Education Materials Related to Glaucoma Diagnosis and Treatment. *Clin. Ophthalmol.* **2023**, *17*, 779–788. [CrossRef]

life

MDPI

Review

The Role of the Ubiquitin System in Eye Diseases

Sandra Carolina Durán-Cristiano [1,*], Laura de Diego-García [2,*], Alba Martín-Gil [3] and Gonzalo Carracedo [3]

1 Basic Sciences Group, Faculty of Medicine, Universidad CES, Medellín 050021, Colombia
2 Department of Biochemistry and Molecular Biology, Faculty of Optics and Optometry, Universidad Complutense de Madrid, 28037 Madrid, Spain
3 Department of Optometry and Vision, Faculty of Optics and Optometry, Universidad Complutense de Madrid, 28037 Madrid, Spain; amartingil@opt.ucm.es (A.M.-G.); jgcarrac@ucm.es (G.C.)
* Correspondence: sdurancod@gmail.com (S.C.D.-C.); laura.dediego@vet.ucm.es (L.d.D.-G.)

Abstract: The ubiquitin–proteasome system (UPS) is a fundamental process that regulates various biological functions, including immune response, cell cycle, oxidative stress, migration, and cellular proliferation. This system is responsible for the degradation of proteins, while proteasomes play a significant role in mechanisms involved in health and human diseases. The participation of the UPS in immune response is particularly relevant, leading to the involvement of immunoproteasomes. This specialized proteasome is involved in the processing and presentation of antigenic peptides, making it crucial for proper immune function. Moreover, the impact of the UPS is considered essential in understanding several diseases, such as neurodegenerative disorders, infections, and vascular diseases. The dysregulation of the UPS may contribute to the pathogenesis of these conditions, highlighting its importance as a potential therapeutic target. Interestingly, the UPS is also related to ocular structures, playing a role in visual perception and ocular homeostasis. This involvement in the regulation of various ocular processes suggests its potential impact on both anterior and posterior eye pathologies. This review aims to discuss the general considerations of the UPS and provide information about its participation in anterior and posterior eye pathologies. By understanding its role in ocular health and disease, researchers and clinicians may explore novel therapeutic strategies targeting the UPS for the treatment of various eye conditions. In conclusion, the UPS is a crucial player in biological processes, with far-reaching implications in health and disease, including the anterior and posterior segments of the eye. Further research in this field may lead to the development of innovative therapies and a better understanding of the complex mechanisms underlying various eye disorders.

Keywords: proteasome; ubiquitin; ocular surface; retinal diseases; immunoproteasome

1. Introduction

The ubiquitin–proteasome system (UPS) is one of the most specialized and critical systems in mammals, playing a profound role in protein degradation and essential cellular processes such as cell cycle regulation, immune responses, and signaling pathways [1–4]. The UPS operates through two key components: ubiquitination, a post-translational modification that regulates various cellular events, and the proteasome, a multi-subunit complex responsible for recognizing polyubiquitinated proteins and initiating their degradation [5,6].

Due to the participation of the UPS in different biological processes in the cell, this system has been a therapeutic target in many diseases such as multiple myeloma, lung cancer, autoimmunity, peripheral neuropathy, and neurodegenerative disorders [7,8].

Cell death and cellular degeneration may arise from imbalances in cellular systems or biological processes, which are associated with various ocular pathologies that present with distinct clinical manifestations. Among these events, the role of oxidative stress has been considered in recent years [9]. For example, its impact on the levels of reactive oxygen species (ROS) that promote lipid peroxidation and subsequent mitochondrial damage, reflected in pathologies such as glaucoma, macular degeneration, diabetic retinopathy, keratoconus and dry eye, suggests that oxidative stress may be involved in pathophysiology [9] and is, in turn, influenced by the activity of the UPS [10–13].

Recent research has highlighted the significant role of the UPS in a variety of diseases that disrupt cellular homeostasis, particularly in anterior and posterior ocular pathologies. These conditions share common biological mechanisms involving ubiquitin–proteasome activity, which is vital for maintaining cellular proteostasis.

This review aims to provide a comprehensive overview of the UPS and its involvement in specific ocular pathologies. Additionally, we will examine the immunoproteasome and its influence on ocular mechanisms across various physiological processes, thereby enhancing our understanding of diverse ocular diseases.

A systematic literature search was conducted using databases such as PubMed, Scopus, and Google Scholar. Keywords related to ocular diseases, treatments, ubiquitination and proteasome inhibitors were used to identify relevant studies. Articles were initially screened based on titles and abstracts to assess their relevance to the research topic. Full-text articles were then reviewed to ensure they met the inclusion criteria. The following inclusion criteria were applied: (1) studies published in peer-reviewed journals, (2) studies published in English, (3) studies focusing on ocular diseases and the relationship between UPS and eye, and (4) studies conducted to capture the most recent developments in the field. Exclusion criteria included: (1) studies not related to ocular diseases, (2) studies with incomplete data or unclear methodologies, and (3) sources that did not provide primary data (e.g., opinion pieces or editorials).

2. The Ubiquitin–Proteasome System

2.1. *Ubiquitination*

Proteins play a crucial role as regulatory elements in numerous essential biological processes in living beings and, in some cases, it is necessary for certain chemical modifications. These modifications, known as "post-translational modifications" (PTMs), serve to determine the catalytic activity of proteins, as well as modify their function and localization within the cell. These PTMs can involve the addition of functional groups, such as acetyl, phosphate, or methyl groups, to specific amino acid residues within the protein. Alternatively, PTMs can include the removal of certain groups or the formation of disulfide bridges between cysteine residues [14].

By altering the catalytic activity, stability, interactions, or localization of proteins, PTMs play a crucial role in regulating numerous biological processes, such as cell signaling, gene expression, metabolism, and immune response [15]. Dysregulation of PTMs has been implicated in various diseases, including cancer, neurodegenerative disorders, and autoimmune diseases. Understanding the complex interplay of PTMs and their impact on protein function is an active area of research in biology and medicine with potential applications in the development of targeted therapies and biomarkers for disease diagnosis and prognosis [16].

Among the most common PTMs that proteins undergo are palmitoylation, phosphorylation, glycosylation, methylation, and ubiquitination. Ubiquitination is a process that the vast majority of eukaryotic cells present, characterized by the covalent attachment of one or more ubiquitin (Ub) molecules to a target protein, leading to changes in its function, location, structure, or activity [17]. Ub is a small yet essential protein, composed of 76 amino acids, that plays a critical role in regulating various cellular processes. Its high conservation across eukaryotic species underscores its fundamental importance in cellular function. Covalent binding serves as a significant signal for protein degradation, particularly within the context of targeted protein degradation by proteasome.

In 2004, scientists Hershko, Ciechanover, and Rose were awarded the Nobel Prize in Chemistry for their contributions to in vitro proteolysis, where they elucidated the role of Ub in protein degradation [18].

For the ubiquitination process to occur, the activity of several actors is required in a three-step sequential manner: first, a Ub molecule is activated by the activating enzyme or E1 in an ATP-dependent manner; then, a conjugating enzyme or E2 transports the Ub to the substrate protein; and, finally, it culminates in the formation of an isopeptide bond between the terminal α-carboxyl group of Ub and the ε-amino group of a lysine (K) present in the target protein, a function carried out by E3 ligases [10,19] (Figure 1).

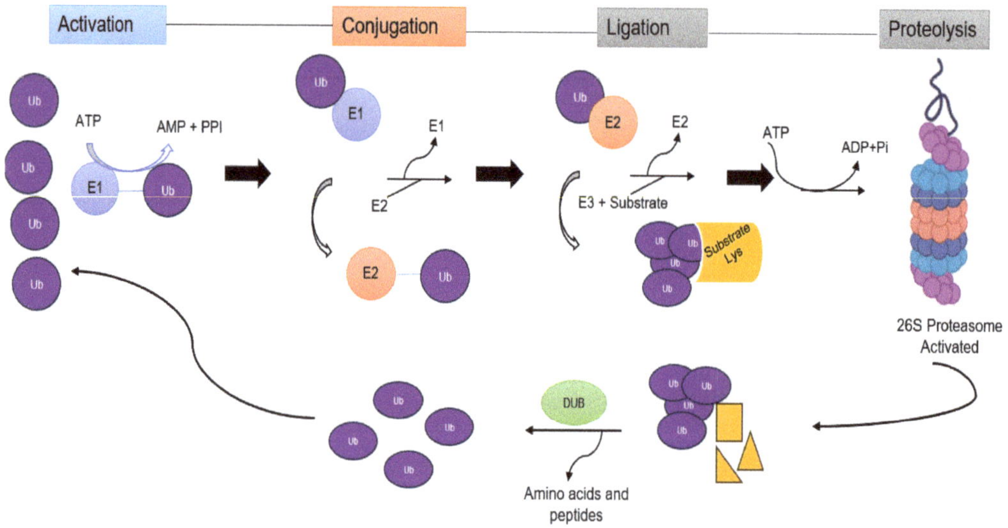

Figure 1. The Ubiquitin–Proteasome System (UPS). Ubiquitination is a post-translational protein modification that occurs in three key steps: activation (E1), where ubiquitin is activated; conjugation, in which ubiquitin is transferred to a ubiquitin-conjugating enzyme (E2); and ligation, where ubiquitin is attached to a substrate protein through the action of an E3 ubiquitin ligase. The polyubiquitinated protein is then recognized by the proteasome and degraded into small peptides. Deubiquitinating enzymes (DUBs) can remove the ubiquitin, allowing it to be recycled for further rounds of ubiquitination.

Certainly, one of the aspects crucial to the diversity and intricacy of ubiquitination is the activity of the E3 ligase enzyme. Once bound and loaded with the substrate, the E3 ligase directs and determines the biological function of the modified protein (substrate). In the human genome, 2 genes have been identified as coding for E1, 40 for E2, and over 600 for E3, which demonstrates the diversity and complexity in the functions of ubiquitination [20]. The E3 ligase are classified into four types according to its structure and function: HECT type, U-box type, RBR type, and RING type [21].

The ubiquitination process, unlike other PTMs, is more complex; it involves the binding of a Ub molecule to the target protein (monoubiquitination), but also the presence of seven lysine residues (K6, K11, K27, K29, K33, K48, and K63) in the Ub enabling the formation of various polyubiquitin chains (polyubiquitination). In this case, the initially inserted Ub acts as the "acceptor or mark" for the insertion of additional Ubs. The type of linkage between the Ub molecules determines the route or destination of the ubiquitinated protein [22]. This diversity makes ubiquitination a complex process influencing multiple cellular and molecular processes [23].

Proteomic analysis has revealed that ubiquitination can occur in both cytosolic proteins located in the membrane and the cell nucleus [23]. In fact, it is well known that ubiquitination regulates a wide range of cellular processes, including cell cycle progression, endocytosis, intracellular trafficking, DNA repair, transcription, signaling and antigen presentation in the immune response, among others [7,24,25]. For instance, Jarome et al. demonstrated that ubiquitination induces changes even in gene expression by modifying histones such as histone H2B, thereby facilitating trimethylation of lysine 4 H3 in genes associated with hippocampal learning [26]. Consequently, Collins P.E. et al. described the importance of ubiquitination in the transcriptional activity of NF-κB (nuclear factor kappa enhancer in the light chain of activated B cells), the principal regulator of the immune response [27].

Just as cells have machinery that provides the insertion of Ub, and this modification triggers a cellular response, there exists a mechanism to remove Ub from proteins, thus reversing the Ub action. This process is referred to as *Deubiquitination* (DUB), and enzymes possessing this capability play a crucial role in the process. In humans, approximately 100 DUBs have been described. Generally, DUBs bind to the isopeptide bond, counteracting the Ub ligase activity and disrupting the regulation by Ub [28]. Consequently, the functions of DUBs include the following: editing Ub chains, recycling Ub molecules during the ubiquitination process, processing Ub precursors and their significant role in regulating proteasomal activity is well-documented [29,30].

2.2. Proteasome

The proteasome is a complex with protease activity that requires energy, predominantly found in eukaryotic cells, and is involved in the cellular machinery that modulates a significant portion of protein degradation. Activation of the proteasome via ubiquitination signaling necessitates polyubiquitination of residue 48, which serves as cue to initiate degradation through the proteasomal pathway [31–33]. In contrast, if the chain is formed through lysine 63, it does not act as a signal for degradation; instead, it is involved in various non-proteolytic functions, including transcription activation, protein kinase activation, DNA repair and replication, and intracellular trafficking [34,35].

Once the substrate has been marked for degradation, the proteasome, in its 26S conformation and with a molecular weight of approximately 2500 kDa, functions as a large multicatalytic protease. It is composed of the following two main complexes: the 20S core complex (the catalytic core) and the 19S regulatory complex [36]. The 20S catalytic complex features two outer α rings and two inner β rings, each comprising seven subunits that provide structural integrity (α1–α7 and β1–β7). The inner β rings exhibit the following distinct catalytic activities: post-glutamyl (β1) activity, which resembles that of caspases and cleaves substrates at acidic residues; trypsin-like (β2) activity, which targets basic residues; and chymotrypsin-like (β5) activity, which cleaves hydrophobic residues [37]. This intricate structure allows the proteasome to efficiently process and degrade ubiquitinated proteins, thereby playing a crucial role in cellular homeostasis.

The 19S complex is located at the end of the 20S center, composed of the following two structures: the base and the lid. The entry to the proteolytic chamber is typically obstructed by the N-terminal ends of the α subunits [38]. The base is the regulatory subunit (19S), which is responsible for binding, deubiquitination, unfolding, and translocating substrates to the catalytic core. It is formed by six subunits with ATPase activity that belong to the AAA family (Rpt1-Rpt6) and three subunits, namely Rpn1 and Rpn2 (scaffolding proteins) and Rpn10 (a ubiquitin receptor), lack ATPase activity. These subunits link the cap and the base of the proteasome complex and play a crucial role in stabilizing it [39]. The ATPase subunits meet the α subunits of the 20s complex [40]. The lid is formed by nine non-ATPase subunits (Rpn3, 5-9, 11, 12, and small adhesive proteins SEM1) [1,41]. Both substrate recognition and unfolding are energy-dependent processes, relying on the ATPase activity of the subunits to provide necessary metabolic energy [42,43].

In addition to the 19S regulatory complex, there are other lesser-known activating complexes, including the 11S complex (also referred to as PA28/PA26/REG) and the PA200 complex [44]. Unlike the 19S complex, both the 11S and PA200 complexes lack ATPase activity and do not unfold proteins. However, they are capable of inducing the opening of the 20S channel, thereby facilitating substrate access [45].

Proteolysis is conducted through different steps that involve the recognition of the substrate, developing translocation and deubiquitination. The substrate protein must have at least four Ubs attached to be recognized. Rpn10 is associated with polyubiquitin while Rpn1-Rpn2 binds to the protein.

Deubiquitinating enzymes separate the Ubs and the subunits with ATPase activity, using the energy of ATP, they produce the unfolding of the protein and make it pass towards the inner chamber of the central particle through conformational changes in the alpha subunits that obstruct the entry [46]. As the protein traverses the chamber, hydrolysis of the peptide bonds takes place, resulting in the release of peptides through the regulatory particle [41]. The proteasome degrades the substrate into fragments, which are subsequently processed into smaller peptides of uniform size. These peptides are then further degraded into free amino acids by the action of endopeptidases or exopeptidases, ultimately leading to their breakdown.

The proteasome is extensively documented to be involved in numerous pathological processes, including cancer, inflammatory conditions, and neurodegenerative diseases [47–49]. Its role in these diseases underscores the importance of the UPS in maintaining cellular homeostasis. Disruptions in proteasomal function can lead to accumulation of damaged or misfolded proteins, contributing to cellular dysfunction and disease progression. In particular, the UPS has been implicated in the pathogenesis of neurodegenerative disorders such as Alzheimer's and Parkinson's disease, where the failure to degrade ubiquitinated proteins results in toxic aggregates that exacerbate neuronal damage [50–53]. Understanding the mechanisms by which the proteasome influences these pathological states is crucial for developing therapeutic strategies aimed at restoring proteostasis and mitigating disease effects.

2.3. *Immunoproteasome*

The immunoproteasome is a specialized variant of the proteasome that plays vital roles in both health and disease. It is instrumental in immune responses through several mechanisms. Notably, it generates peptides for presentation by Major Histocompatibility Complex (MHC) class I molecules, a process essential for activating CD8+ T cells in response to viral infections [54,55]. The immunoproteasome differs from the standard proteasome in its peptide cleavage properties, which enhances its ability to efficiently produce antigenic peptides. Furthermore, it supports the differentiation of pro-inflammatory T helper cell subsets, such as Th1 and Th17, and facilitates the production of pro-inflammatory cytokines, including interferons, TNF-alpha, IL-6, IL-17, and IL-23 [56,57]. These cytokines contribute to the development and persistence of autoimmune diseases. Consequently, targeting and inhibiting the immunoproteasome presents a promising therapeutic strategy for managing autoimmune conditions and influencing viral infections [58].

Hematopoietic origin cells or cells stimulated with pro-inflammatory agents leads to the replacement the constitutive catalytic subunits of the proteasome (β1, β2, β5) with the inducible catalytic subunits of Low-Molecular-Weight Peptides LMP2 (β1i) and LMP7 (β5i), or with the Multi-Catalytic Endopeptidase Complex-Like MECL-1 (β2i) during proteasomal neosynthesis, forming what is known as the immunoproteasome [59,60]. Under inflammatory conditions, the 19S regulatory subunit is also substituted by the 11S subunit (also called PA28), which consists of two subunits, PA28α and PA28β. This complex is significantly smaller [61] and its involvement has been studied in various neurodevelopmental disorders, including epilepsy [62].

Furthermore, the immunoproteasome is implicated in a range of diseases. For example, its dysfunction has been associated with cardiovascular and pulmonary conditions, including chronic obstructive pulmonary disease [63–65]. For instance, the immunoproteasome is continuously expressed in alveolar macrophages and is quickly activated in respiratory cells during viral infections, highlighting its role in antiviral immunity in the lungs [66–68]. Additionally, the immunoproteasome is involved in the degradation of oxidatively damaged proteins, particularly under conditions of stress and disease [57,69]. Given these roles, it is plausible to consider its involvement in ocular pathologies, where dysregulation of the immunoproteasome has been linked to diseases characterized by protein aggregation.

In summary, the immunoproteasome is essential for antigen presentation, immune regulation, and protein homeostasis. Its dysregulation has been associated with various diseases, making it a potential therapeutic target and biomarker for disease prediction and progression.

3. Role of the UPS in Eye

Advancements in biology have significantly enhanced our understanding of the pathophysiological events underlying ocular diseases, including the critical roles played by specific metabolic pathways and signaling cascades. These discoveries have provided deeper insights into the mechanisms driving various ocular conditions, thus paving the way for more targeted interventions in diagnosis and treatment [70]. A notable example is the potential involvement of the UPS, whose association with protein accumulation may play a pivotal role in the pathogenesis of ocular diseases. In fact, recent studies suggest that UPS plays a key role in retinal development, photoreceptor survival, and neuroinflammation (REF). These functions are crucial in eye diseases such as glaucoma and ocular surface disorders, where inflammation and cell death are prominent.

Currently, for the management of various anterior segment ocular pathologies, pharmacological and surgical treatments are available to minimize the risk of vision loss, although their effectiveness is limited in some cases [71]. However, the development of novel therapies that can intervene at the early stages of biological processes, such as inflammation, oxidative stress, or apoptosis, holds the potential for more effective treatment prior to the manifestation of clinical signs and symptoms. One example of this is the use of proteasome inhibitors, which have been proposed as a therapeutic option in diseases like cancer. Additionally, the dysregulation of enzymatic activity in the ubiquitination process could be a key factor in the treatment of various ocular pathologies.

In Drosophila Melanogaster, ocular development requires ubiquitination to activate retinal morphogenesis and photoreceptor cells viability [72]. Furthermore, neuroinflammation plays a crucial role in glaucoma, as inflammatory mediators influence cellular responses in the retina, ultimately leading to cell loss via apoptosis. Moreover, the regulation of ubiquitination activity is vital in various ocular surface diseases, as it is maintains cellular homeostasis and influence disease progression [73,74]. However, the role of the

UPS in ocular pathologies is not so widely studied, considering that the multiple roles of the UPS include regulation of inflammation, so it could be thought that some biological phenomena involved in pathologies of both the anterior segment and the posterior segment of the eye could be explained by the Ubiquitin–Proteasome pathway (Figure 2).

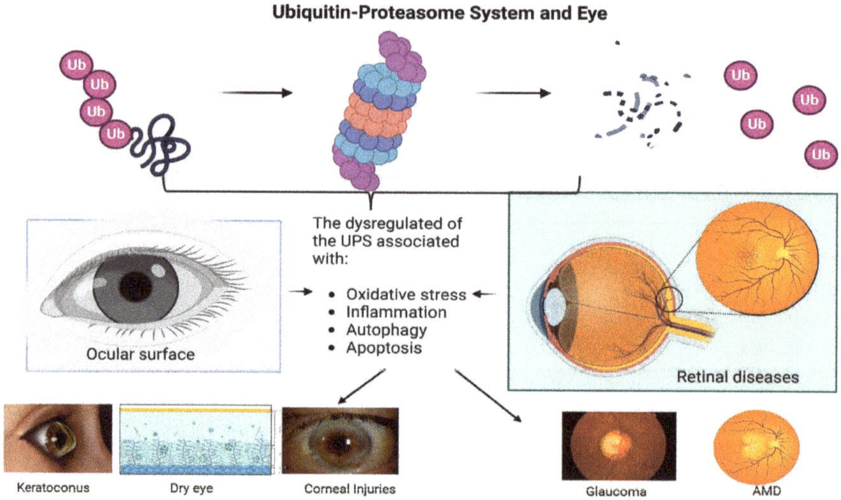

Figure 2. The UPS regulates key biological processes such as inflammation, oxidative stress, and cell death. Its dysfunction could be involved in anterior segment ocular diseases, such as dry eye and keratoconus, which are associated with chronic inflammation and abnormal protein degradation. In the posterior segment, the UPS may influence conditions such as glaucoma and age-related macular degeneration (AMD), where impaired protein degradation and stress response contribute to disease progression.

In this section, we discuss the role of the UPS in both anterior segment pathologies (such as dry eye and keratoconus) and posterior segment pathologies (including macular degeneration and glaucoma), highlighting its clinical relevance in the diagnosis and treatment of these conditions.

3.1. Anterior Segment of the Eye

3.1.1. Dry Eye

Dry eye disease (DED) is a multifactorial disease that results in the loss of homeostasis of the Lacrimal Functional Unit (LFU), causing ocular symptoms and signs that, in some cases, result in visual impairment and loss of quality of life [75]. In recent decades, significant contributions from molecular and cellular biologist has allowed us to understand and establish the various events involved in the pathogenesis of the disease. Such is the case for inflammation, where once various transcription factors such as NF-κB are activated, they modulate the gene expression of cytokines such as IL-6, IL-22, and tumor necrosis factor (TNFα) and this leads to an inflammatory process [76] that modifies tear film, corneal, and conjunctival stability.

Key biological events in dry eye disease include hyperosmolarity, instability of the tear film, loss of homeostasis, inflammation, and neurosensory abnormalities [77]. These events are closely related to changes in tear quality, which in turn disrupt the LFU. This dysregulation may be associated with alterations in the proteins on the ocular surface, which can accumulate and induce apoptosis in conjunctival, epithelial cells, and Meibomian glands. Therefore, dysfunction in the UPS could lead to a loss of protein balance, potentially inducing remodeling of the ocular surface.

Accordingly, experimental studies suggest that inflammation plays a role in the diagnosis and treatment of dry eye. Thus, Kuklinski E.J. et al., demonstrated in vitro that dendrite cells (DC) are activated, and these initially mediate the activation of the innate and adaptive immune response on the ocular surface in a dry eye model [78]. However, it is necessary to recognize that antigen presentation by DC can be carried out by MHC class I and II. Although a large participation in DED is associated with the activity of MHC class II and its mechanism which modulates the activation of Th1 lymphocytes, and thus the secretion of pro-inflammatory cytokines such as TNF, IL-2, IL-17. In the case of recognition by MHC class I, once DCs are activated, they induce the production of A and B proteins related to MHC class I, which activate NK cells, and these produce IFN-γ, which leads to conjunctival and corneal epithelial activation, causing activation of Th1 cells. Interestingly, recognition by MHC class I requires proteasomal and immunoproteasome activity [59].

Recently, Xie M. et al. (2022) demonstrated, in C57BL/6 mice with dry eye and stimulated with acacetin, a natural flavone, a reduction in the activity of the NLRP3 inflammasome, and, thus, a decrease in corneal staining and an increase in the number of goblet cells in the conjunctiva. Interestingly, acacetin inactivated the NLRP3 signal through its ubiquitination, where glycoprotein 78 (gp78), known as E3 ligase, suppressed the activation of NLRP3 and attenuated the inflammatory response, suggesting a promising therapeutic target, where ubiquitination activity is involved [79].

Inflammation plays a key role in the immunopathology of dry eye, with emerging therapies focusing on suppressing this response. A critical factor in ocular surface inflammation is nuclear factor kappa B (NF-κB) [80], which promotes the secretion of pro-inflammatory cytokines [81]. The activation of NF-κB depends on the UPS, which labels IκB with Ub for degradation. Once IκB is degraded, NF-κB translocates to the nucleus and activates inflammatory gene transcription. Consequently, studies suggest that proteasome inhibitors could help reduce inflammatory mediators in diseases where inflammation is a central factor [27,82].

On the other hand, IL-17 has been studied as a therapeutic target promoter in dry eye. Alam J. (2022) established elevated levels of both IL-17 and IL-23 in corneal and conjunctival tissues in an animal model with receptor-deficient nuclear RXRα. In transcriptomic analyses, they found that ubiquitination was involved within the pathways related to IL-17 signaling [83]. This aspect is consistent with what was published by Rong Z. et al. (2007), who found that TRAF mediates the ubiquitination of IL-17R induced by IL-17F, and that its E3 ligase activity was necessary for said signaling [84], the role of residue 48 in polyubiquitination is considered crucial in determining the specific type of dry eye condition that involves the Th17 phenotype [85].

Dry eye is associated with other ocular disorders. During the process of aging and cellular senescence, ocular structures undergo important changes, especially those of the ocular surface. Nättinen J. et al. (2019) examined the effects of aging on the tear proteome, finding a relationship between age and several tear proteins related to cell death and inflammatory response, and several proteins of the ubiquitination complex [86].

In addition, ocular manifestations of limbal stem cell deficiency (LSCD) include dry eye. In an LSCD model, an increase in inflammatory cells and the activity of immunoproteasome formation with a decrease in constitutive proteasome formation was found [87,88]. Furthermore, the immunoproteasome has been implicated in the pathophysiology of dry eye disease, particularly in conditions such as Sjögren's syndrome [89]. For example, the dysregulation of immune responses, including those mediated by the immunoproteasome, can lead to the destruction of lacrimal glands and reduced tear production, further aggravating dry eye symptoms [90]. The above suggests that it may lead to rapid immunoproteasome response and reduce constitutive proteasome activity, a change in the proteasome population after the immune response.

In studies of chronic inflammation, constitutive proteasome activity has been shown to decrease and immunoproteasome activity to increase. Therefore, in chronic stages of dry eye, it is possible that the activity of the constitutive proteasome may be affected, leading to the non-degradation of proteins via the proteasome, and, therefore, this leads to the accumulation of proteins, which subsequently contributes to oxidative stress, activation of autophagy, and subsequent cell death [91–93]. Thus, given its involvement in inflammation and immune regulation, the immunoproteasome is being explored as a potential therapeutic target for dry eye treatment, especially in autoimmune contexts, and as focusing on inhibitors of the immunoproteasome may help mitigate the inflammatory responses associated with dry eye conditions.

3.1.2. Keratoconus

Keratoconus (KC) is a degenerative disease of the cornea characterized by cone-like steepening and irregular stromal thinning, which distorts vision. In recent years, attention has been focused on the role of inflammation as a regulator of the disease's development and progression [94]. Understanding the pathophysiology of KC, from a molecular perspective, allows us to recognize the clinical significance of biological events such as inflammation, oxidative stress, alterations in the extracellular matrix, and the activation of apoptosis [95].

For many decades, inflammation was thought to be irrelevant in KC. However, experimental studies have demonstrated its influence on specific signals that contribute to cellular stress, alterations in the extracellular matrix, and the activation of apoptotic pathways, ultimately leading to damage in keratocytes and fibroblasts at the corneal level [96]. Nonetheless, the role of the UPS in protein regulation and stability at the corneal level remains underexplored.

The corneal epithelium has the capacity to express K3/K12 keratins and maintains regular functions related to the renewal process in the face of an injury [88]. For this, it is necessary to modulate the amount of keratin present in affected tissue and ensure that it does not accumulate and is not added at undesirable times. In addition, the constitutive proteasome plays a crucial role in protein degradation, as highlighted by Chan J.K.L. et al. (2018), who emphasized the importance of keratin 6a (K6a) and its post-translational modification by Ub. This modification influences proteasomal processing to produce antimicrobial peptides derived from keratin, which contribute to the innate immune response in the corneal epithelium, particularly in cytoskeletal remodeling in UPS-mediated infections [97]. This underscores the system's role in generating antigenic fragments during immune responses.

Bardag-Gorce et al. characterized the proteasome in corneal epithelial cells [87] and later investigated its effects in an animal model following corneal injury. They found that the epithelial keratins K3 and K13 are polyubiquitinated for proteasomal degradation. However, corneal injury leads to impaired proteasome activity, resulting in keratin aggregation and subsequent UPS activation [88]. This suggests that proteasome activity is crucial for the formation and removal of corneal keratin aggresomes, with potential therapeutic implications for ocular surface injuries such as Limbal Stem Cell Deficiency (LSCD) and other conditions that promote corneal opacity, including keratoconus.

In addition, Ferrington D.A. et al. (2013) proposed that the immunoproteasome is key in corneal healing. Following the induction of inflammatory cytokine secretion, the constitutive proteasome becomes unstable, and the immunoproteasome is rapidly activated.

This activation enables the production of peptides that are ultimately bound to MHC class I molecules [98].

On the other hand, Lomako J. et al. (2010), highlighted the importance of the proteasome in regulating MUC4, a membrane mucin involved in eye protection. They demonstrated that TGF-β induces the degradation of MUC4 in the basal and intermediate layers of the cornea, and that this effect is reversed by proteasome inhibitors (MG132), leading to an increased expression of MUC4 on corneal tissue [99]. This suggests that proteasome inhibitors could be a promising therapeutic approach for treating corneal injuries and stabilizing mucin in cases of ocular surface damage. Additionally, recent omics-based studies of corneal tissue have revealed that the UPS pathway plays a role in keratoconus (KC), with its upregulation potentially contributing to KC progression [100,101]. Thus, targeting the UPS may offer a novel therapeutic strategy for the treatment of KC.

Indeed, several studies in transcriptomics and proteomics affirm that hypothesis. Shinde V. et al. (2019), evaluated corneas of healthy individuals and those with keratoconus using mass spectrometry, detecting a total of 3132 proteins, of which 627 were overregulated in ectatic corneas. Interestingly, within these proteins, some E3 ligases (CUL2, CUL3 and CUL4B), SUMO3 and UBA6 [100] were involved in the proteasomal pathway, among them some E3 ligases (CUL2, CUL3 and CUL4B), which could in the future be used as new therapeutic targets.

Cellular proteases, particularly those such as metalloproteinases (MMP), play a critical role in the degradation compression of the extracellular matrix and corneal thinning [102]. Several factors regulate the activity of these enzymes, with vascular endothelial growth factor (VEGF) being a prominent example, as it is expressed in both corneal epithelial and endothelial cells. Once activated, VEGF stimulates the expression of MMP-2 and MMP-9 in the cornea, leading to inflammation, scarring, and loss of corneal transparency.

Consequently, antiangiogenic factors can modulate the activity of VEGF; thrombospondin-1 (TSP-1) serves as a notable example. Bardag-Gorce F. et al. demonstrated, in cultures of epithelial cells within a neovascularization model, that TSP-1 levels decreased. However, when the proteasome was inhibited, TSP-1 levels increased, while VEGF decreased [103]. This finding is clinically relevant for the development of corneal neovascularization with proteasome inhibitors, potentially reducing visual loss.

The immunoproteasome is abundantly expressed in the corneal epithelium and plays a crucial role in maintaining corneal integrity and function. The immunoproteasome has been implicated in the pathogenesis of keratoconus, though its exact role is still being investigated. For example, immunoproteasome deficiency leads to increased apoptosis in corneal epithelial cells and delayed wound healing in mouse models [87,98].

Recently, its function has been involved in regulating inflammation, with findings suggesting a significant role in mediating oxidative stress responses [104] may be relevant in keratoconus pathogenesis. Further studies are essential to elucidate the specific mechanisms through which the immunoproteasome and protein accumulation resulting from proteasome dysfunction may contribute to corneal thinning and the structural changes characteristic of keratoconus. Such research could provide valuable insights into potential therapeutic strategies for addressing these pathological alterations.

In ocular surface diseases, including dry eye and keratoconus, effective management is crucial for enhancing visual quality. However, current treatments often fall short of expectations, primarily focusing on alleviating symptoms while neglecting underlying factors such as oxidative stress, inflammation, and protein accumulation, which significantly contribute to the pathophysiology of these diseases. Therefore, future research should investigate the role of the UPS in disease biology, as a comprehensive understanding of its function could provide insights into more effective therapeutic strategies that target the root causes of these conditions.

3.2. Posterior Segment of the Eye

3.2.1. Age-Related Macular Degeneration

Age-related macular degeneration (AMD) is one of the causes of global blindness [105]. Within its etiopathogenesis, there are various factors, including mutagenesis in some candidate genes, epigenetic factors, and lifestyle factors [106–109]. Biological events are related to protein degradation or PTMs that some proteins may undergo that maintain retinal homeostasis from visual development to retinal neurodegeneration processes [110].

The immunoproteasome plays a significant role in retinal function and health, particularly in the context of visual transmission [111,112]. For instance, immunoproteasomes are present in high concentrations in the photoreceptors and synaptic regions of the retina, suggesting their importance in visual transmission. Studies using immunoproteasome knockout (KO) mice have demonstrated that a deficiency in immunoproteasome subunits leads to defects in bipolar cell responses, resulting in a decrease in the amplitude of electroretinography (ERG) b-waves by approximately 25% [111]. This highlights their relevance in retinal physiology and physiopathology processes.

On the other hand, the immunoproteasome has been shown to provide cytoprotective effects in the retina under conditions of oxidative stress and injury [12]. For instance, retinal pigment epithelial cells lacking immunoproteasome components exhibited increased susceptibility to peroxide-induced cell death, indicating that the immunoproteasome plays a protective role against oxidative damage and its possible implication in age-related macular degeneration.

Considering that the retina has a high metabolic rate, rapid and efficient activities are required for the modification of proteins and, where appropriate, to lead them to degradation. However, as age advances and adds to other factors, such as UV exposure, poor diet, and cigarette intake [113], these degradation processes and modifications in proteins can alter in a more accelerated manner. Therefore, the accumulation of proteins in the macular area and its relationship with cellular senescence and aging can be explained by autophagy and UPS activity [114,115].

In an animal model, it has been demonstrated that inhibiting the activity of the proteasome results in the accumulation of oxidized proteins, including lipofuscin; this is a key component in the formation of the dominated "drusen" [3]. Therefore, there is an implication of proteasome activity. The proteasome not only focuses on protein degradation, but also how relevant processes, such as oxidative stress, cell signaling, inflammation, and key elements in the physiopathogenesis of AMD, can be regulated through the ubiquitination–proteasome pathway.

Consequently, Lee H. et al. reported that, in aqueous humor samples of individuals with AMD, analyzed by proteomics, a significant increase in proteins related to proteasome activity could be seen, including the regulatory subunit Rpn2 [116]. In addition, Qin et al., proposed that inhibiting the proteasome pharmacologically in RPE cells induced deregulation of the NF-κB pathway, which finally led to the differential expression of pro-inflammatory and proapoptotic genes, aspects that agree with what was reported by Fernandez A.F. et al. and Qin T. et al., who suggested that UPS has a role both in inflammation, and oxidative stress in AMD [117,118]. The above shows that the activity of the UPS influences many events in the retinal tissue and that this could be a critical element in the search for therapeutic interventions for AMD [114,119], considering its multiple roles in both retinal development and neurodegeneration.

3.2.2. Glaucoma

Glaucoma is defined as a neurodegenerative disease that includes a variety of biological events including glutamate excitotoxicity, mitochondrial dysfunction, cholinergic deregulation, etc., which lead to loss of retinal ganglion cells (RGCs), clinically converted by the loss of the nerve fiber layer of the retina, in some cases with an increase in intraocular pressure (IOP) and, with these, changes in functions such as contrast sensitivity and visual field [73].

Recent studies reveal molecular mechanisms that include protein misfolding, protein aggregation, and the role of UPS activity in regulating protein degradation processes. An event that has been highlighted in the pathophysiology of neurodegenerative diseases.

Indeed, several studies support that glaucoma should not only be considered an eye disease, but it can also become a risk factor for Alzheimer's disease [120,121]. In fact, the pathophysiological mechanisms of glaucoma converge with Alzheimer's when comparing characteristics such as cholinergic deficiency, glutamate excitotoxicity, and neuroinflammation [73]. For instance, Korac J et al. (2013) demonstrated the role of ubiquitination in the formation of misfolded proteins in different neurodegenerative diseases such as Alzheimer's, Parkinson's, and amyotrophic lateral sclerosis (ALS) [122].

Optineurin (OPTN) is a protein that interacts with a series of events, including cell morphogenesis, vesicular trafficking, transcriptional regulation, and autophagy, and has been a genetic marker in normal tension glaucoma and primary open-angle glaucoma (POAG) [123,124]. Under physiological conditions, OPTN interacts with LC3 to degrade its substrates through autophagy [125]. Thus, when analyzing the protein structure, it can be seen that it contains a ubiquitin-binding domain, and studies such as that of Shen WC have shown that mutations in the region related to Ub recognition in the OPTN gene interfere with the process of autophagy, and, thus, OPTN colocalizes with misfolded proteins [126].

Conversely, Kageyama et al. indicated that chemical inhibition of the proteasome leads to a reduction in proteasome activity and an increase in the level of polyubiquitinated proteins, ultimately resulting in retinal degeneration and the death of photoreceptors and retinal ganglion cells [127]. Similar findings were reported by Hayat B et al. in patients with pseudoexfoliation glaucoma, who exhibited increased expression of ER-stress markers and decreased proteasome activity [128]. This imbalance in proteasome function underscores its clinical significance and highlights the UPS as a promising therapeutic target in retinal diseases such as glaucoma.

From another point of view, inflammation has been considered a possible etiology for the release of inflammatory mediators from trabecular meshwork (TM) cells [73,129]. Indeed, studies of tear proteomes and aqueous humor samples from glaucoma patients demonstrate a pro-inflammatory profile, supporting the role of inflammation in glaucoma [130]. Keller K.E. and Wirtz M.K. described that the *ASB10* gene is associated with the development of glaucoma and, interestingly, *ASB10* is regulated by pro-inflammatory cytokines that, in turn, contain the suppressor of cytokine signaling (SOCS) gene family that contains ubiquitination domains and could recruit complexes of Ub ligase for subsequent degradation by the proteasome [131].

In studies of POAG individuals with elevated IOP levels, differential expression of *ASB10* has been identified; it has a role in regulating aqueous humor outflow and maintaining IOP homeostasis [132]. Although direct involvement of the immunoproteasome in glaucoma pathology has not been thoroughly investigated, its established role in other neurodegenerative conditions and its significance in regulating inflammation position it as a promising candidate for further study.

Consequently, Keller K.E. et al. (2013) demonstrated that TM cells express ASB10 and contain motifs facilitated by two proteins: Cullin5 and elonginBC. This study suggests that

ASB10 may function as a Ub ligand, promoting the degradation of specific proteins in TM cells. This mechanism is crucial for understanding of the regulation of cellular homeostasis and provides insights into glaucoma pathogenesis, where the accumulation of misfolded or excess proteins can lead to cellular dysfunction and impaired tissue function. [133].

The immunoproteasome has emerged as a potential therapeutic target in various neurodegenerative diseases, including Alzheimer's disease and cardiovascular diseases [49,63]. In Alzheimer's disease, increased immunoproteasome activity has been observed in reactive glial cells surrounding amyloid plaques, suggesting its involvement in disease pathogenesis [134]. Tezel et al. have proposed that proteasome activity could serve as a biomarker in human glaucoma models [135]. The immunoproteasome offers valuable insights into disease progression and holds promise as a therapeutic target. Its involvement in neurodegenerative diseases, along with its potential as a biomarker and treatment target, warrants further investigation, particularly in glaucoma. Exploring the immunoproteasome's role in glaucoma pathophysiology could pave the way for novel treatment strategies targeting this proteasome subtype.

Age-related retinal degeneration represents a significant public health concern, given the increasing number of individuals in older age groups. Understanding the biological events occurring within the retina is crucial, as it could lead to early detection of changes primarily associated with protein accumulation and dysfunction in key biological systems, such as the UPS. This knowledge may pave the way for more effective diagnostic and therapeutic strategies aimed at mitigating the impact of retinal degeneration in aging populations.

4. Treatments Targeting the Proteasome in Ocular Pathologies

The proteasome has garnered significant attention as a potential therapeutic target in various diseases [136]. Recent advances in understanding the role of proteasomal dysfunction in the pathogenesis of multiple conditions have led to the exploration of novel drug development strategies focused on modulating proteasomal activity [137].

In the context of ocular diseases, where protein homeostasis is crucial for maintaining cellular integrity, proteasome-targeted therapies hold great promise. Diseases like keratoconus, dry eye, glaucoma, and age-related macular degeneration (AMD) have been linked to impaired protein degradation, leading to the accumulation of misfolded or dysfunctional proteins [138]. These accumulated proteins can trigger cellular stress, inflammation, and tissue damage, which ultimately contribute to disease progression. Therefore, restoring proper proteasomal function could be a pivotal strategy in preventing or even reversing disease processes.

The development of small molecules or biologics that either enhance or inhibit proteasomal activity offers a promising avenue for therapeutic intervention. Proteasome activators could help with improving protein degradation, especially in diseases characterized by the accumulation of damaged proteins [137]. Conversely, proteasome inhibitors could be utilized to selectively degrade or to induce cell death in cancer cells where excessive protein degradation may be beneficial [139,140].

Targeting the proteasome holds promise for developing more specific and effective therapies, potentially improving patient outcomes and transforming the management of ocular diseases. Further investigation into the precise mechanisms underlying proteasomal regulation and the optimal modulation of its activity will be crucial to fully unlock the therapeutic potential of this approach. Currently, proteasome inhibitors are being explored in the contexts of cancer, autoimmunity, and viral infections, and this strategy could potentially be adapted as a novel therapeutic approach for ocular diseases (Table 1).

Table 1. Treatments targeting the proteasome in ocular pathologies.

Treatment	Mechanism of Action	Ocular Pathologies	Outcome/Effect	Refs.
Bortezomib	Inhibits the 26S proteasome, preventing protein degradation	Wet AMD, diabetic retinopathy	Reduces inflammation, prevents retinal cell death, and exerts a neuroprotective effect.	[141,142]
Carfilzomib	Inhibits the proteasome by binding to its catalytic subunits	Glaucoma, retinal degeneration	Reduces oxidative stress, and prevents retinal damage.	[143]
Lactacystin	Inhibits proteasomal activity by binding to the proteasome catalytic site	AMD	May modulate inflammatory pathways, retinal aging, and cell survival.	[127,144]
MG132	A potent, reversible proteasome inhibitor	Corneal injury, keratoconjunctivitis sicca.	Reduces cellular apoptosis, and promotes tissue repair.	[145,146]
		Glaucoma	MG132 could enhance the efficiency of transduction by a FIV vector expressing green fluorescent protein (GFP) in immortalized human trabecular meshwork cells.	[147]
Epoxomicin	Selectively inhibits the 20S proteasome, blocking protein degradation	AMD, Glaucoma	Suppresses pro-inflammatory signaling, mitigates retinal cell death, and promotes anti-inflammatory activity.	[148,149]
Ubistatin	Inhibits the ubiquitin-proteasome pathway	Retinal pathology	Enhances retinal neuron survival and may promote neurite growth and synaptogenesis.	[150]

All findings presented in this table are based on studies of proteasome inhibitors. FIV: feline immunodeficiency virus. AMD: Age-related macular degeneration. GFP: green fluorescent protein.

5. Conclusions and Future Perspectives

The eye is a target organ for many biological events, including oxidative stress, inflammation, and processes that are required by the UPS to maintain ocular homeostasis. However, due to various exogenous and endogenous factors, this balance can be lost, generating an accumulation of protein components that can trigger responses that favor the appearance of diseases such as dry eye, glaucoma, AMD, and others, which is why, in the last decade, a significant number of publications have focused their attention on understanding what happens with "cellular proteostasis" and how, from the loss of proteostasis, pathways can appear that lead to the development of the disease [8,151,152].

This highlights the critical role of the UPS in regulating the activity and maintenance of numerous proteins, either through ubiquitination signals or by directing them for degradation via proteasomal pathways. The involvement of the UPS in ocular health provides valuable insights not only into the pathophysiology of ocular diseases but also in identifying potential biomarkers associated with UPS dysfunction. For example, retinal degenerative diseases are frequently marked by the accumulation of misfolded proteins and protein aggregation, which are key pathological features [153]. These insights open the door to exploring pharmacological interventions targeting proteasome in the treatment of eye diseases.

Although numerous studies are included in this review concerning the role of the UPS, several limitations exist regarding the therapeutic approaches to the ocular pathologies described. While the UPS is indeed involved in protein accumulation and recycling, further research is essential to determine whether specific E3 ligases are associated with protein buildup in ocular tissues, and to explore whether the proteasome and immunoproteasome could serve as viable therapeutic targets.

Additionally, the UPS plays a crucial role in the removal of damaged or misfolded proteins, and its dysfunction can lead to the accumulation of toxic proteins, resulting in inflammation, cell death, and further vision impairment. Investigating the molecular mechanisms underlying UPS failure in retinal cells could provide valuable insights into potential strategies for targeting this system to slow or prevent disease progression.

Currently, within pharmacological interventions for many diseases such as cancer, autoimmune and neurodegenerative disease, have been described as either activating or inhibiting the activity of the proteasome [137,154–156]. Therefore, considering the implications of UPS activity on various ocular structures, one can think of future and novel therapeutic approaches to various ocular disorders.

In fact, medications based on proteasome inhibitors have already been patented for the treatment of dry eye [157], which shows that they can be a therapeutic line to explore for many diseases of both the anterior and posterior segments of the eye.

In comparison to other conditions, such as neurodegenerative disorders, autoimmune conditions, infectious diseases, and cancer, the investigation of the role of the UPS in ophthalmology remains in its early stages. Nonetheless, this progress has been facilitated by a deeper understanding of the biological events associated with ocular diseases, supported by insights from omics approaches, in vitro assays, and other methods. These efforts have enabled the identification of disrupted metabolic pathways and have clarified the relationship between the UPS and additional biological pathways that maintain cellular homeostasis. Consequently, there remains significant scope for further research and development in this area for application in the field of ophthalmology.

Author Contributions: Conceptualization, S.C.D.-C.; writing—original draft preparation, S.C.D.-C., L.d.D.-G., A.M.-G. and G.C.; writing—review and editing, S.C.D.-C. and L.d.D.-G. All authors have read and agreed to the published version of the manuscript.

Funding: This research was funded by the Programa de Atracción de Talento de la Comunidad de Madrid, grant number 2020-T2/BMD-20180.

Institutional Review Board Statement: Not applicable.

Informed Consent Statement: Not applicable.

Data Availability Statement: Data are contained within the article.

Conflicts of Interest: The authors declare no conflicts of interest.

References

1. Bard, J.A.M.; Goodall, E.A.; Greene, E.R.; Jonsson, E.; Dong, K.C.; Martin, A. Structure and Function of the 26S Proteasome. *Annu. Rev. Biochem.* **2018**, *87*, 697–724. [CrossRef] [PubMed]
2. Liu, W.J.; Ye, L.; Huang, W.F.; Guo, L.J.; Xu, Z.G.; Wu, H.L.; Yang, C.; Liu, H.F. p62 links the autophagy pathway and the ubiqutin-proteasome system upon ubiquitinated protein degradation. *Cell. Mol. Biol. Lett.* **2016**, *21*, 29. [CrossRef]
3. Shang, F.; Taylor, A. Roles for the ubiquitin-proteasome pathway in protein quality control and signaling in the retina: Implications in the pathogenesis of age-related macular degeneration. *Mol. Aspects Med.* **2012**, *33*, 446–466. [CrossRef]
4. Wang, Y.; Li, S.; Wang, W. The ubiquitin-proteasome system in the tumor immune microenvironment: A key force in combination therapy. *Front. Immunol.* **2024**, *15*, 1436174. [CrossRef]
5. Peth, A.; Besche, H.C.; Goldberg, A.L. Ubiquitinated proteins activate the proteasome by binding to Usp14/Ubp6, which causes 20S gate opening. *Mol. Cell* **2009**, *36*, 794–804. [CrossRef]
6. Liao, Y.; Zhang, W.; Liu, Y.; Zhu, C.; Zou, Z. The role of ubiquitination in health and disease. *MedComm* **2024**, *5*, e736. [CrossRef]

7. Stekel, Z.; Sheng, Y.; Zhang, W. The Multifaceted Role of the Ubiquitin Proteasome System in Pathogenesis and Diseases. *Biomolecules* **2022**, *12*, 925. [CrossRef]
8. Höhn, A.; Tramutola, A.; Cascella, R. Proteostasis Failure in Neurodegenerative Diseases: Focus on Oxidative Stress. *Oxid. Med. Cell. Longev.* **2020**, *2020*, 5497046. [CrossRef]
9. Dammak, A.; Pastrana, C.; Martin-Gil, A.; Carpena-Torres, C.; Peral Cerda, A.; Simovart, M.; Alarma, P.; Huete-Toral, F.; Carracedo, G. Oxidative Stress in the Anterior Ocular Diseases: Diagnostic and Treatment. *Biomedicines* **2023**, *11*, 292. [CrossRef]
10. Shang, F.; Taylor, A. Ubiquitin-proteasome pathway and cellular responses to oxidative stress. *Free Radic. Biol. Med.* **2011**, *51*, 5–16. [CrossRef]
11. Pandino, I.; Giammaria, S.; Zingale, G.A.; Roberti, G.; Michelessi, M.; Coletta, M.; Manni, G.; Agnifili, L.; Vercellin, A.V.; Harris, A.; et al. Ubiquitin proteasome system and glaucoma: A survey of genetics and molecular biology studies supporting a link with pathogenic and therapeutic relevance. *Mol. Aspects Med.* **2023**, *94*, 101226. [CrossRef]
12. Plafker, S.M. Oxidative stress and the ubiquitin proteolytic system in age-related macular degeneration. *Adv. Exp. Med. Biol.* **2010**, *664*, 447–456. [CrossRef]
13. Hurley, D.J.; Normile, C.; Irnaten, M.; O'Brien, C. The Intertwined Roles of Oxidative Stress and Endoplasmic Reticulum Stress in Glaucoma. *Antioxidants* **2022**, *11*, 886. [CrossRef] [PubMed]
14. Chen, L.; Kashina, A. Post-translational Modifications of the Protein Termini. *Front. Cell Dev. Biol.* **2021**, *9*, 719590. [CrossRef] [PubMed]
15. Landini, A.; Trbojević-Akmačić, I.; Navarro, P.; Tsepilov, Y.A.; Sharapov, S.Z.; Vučković, F.; Polašek, O.; Hayward, C.; Petrović, T.; Vilaj, M.; et al. Genetic regulation of post-translational modification of two distinct proteins. *Nat. Commun.* **2022**, *13*, 1586. [CrossRef] [PubMed]
16. Zhong, Q.; Xiao, X.; Qiu, Y.; Xu, Z.; Chen, C.; Chong, B.; Zhao, X.; Hai, S.; Li, S.; An, Z.; et al. Protein posttranslational modifications in health and diseases: Functions, regulatory mechanisms, and therapeutic implications. *Med. Comm* **2023**, *4*, e261. [CrossRef]
17. Glickman, M.H.; Ciechanover, A. The ubiquitin-proteasome proteolytic pathway: Destruction for the sake of construction. *Physiol. Rev.* **2002**, *82*, 373–428. [CrossRef]
18. Kresge, N.; Simoni, R.D.; Hill, R.L. The Discovery of Ubiquitin-mediated Proteolysis by Aaron Ciechanover, Avram Hershko, and Irwin Rose. *J. Biol. Chem.* **2006**, *281*, e32–e36. [CrossRef]
19. Metzger, M.B.; Hristova, V.A.; Weissman, A.M. HECT and RING finger families of E3 ubiquitin ligases at a glance. *J. Cell Sci.* **2012**, *125*, 531–537. [CrossRef]
20. Toma-Fukai, S.; Shimizu, T. Structural Diversity of Ubiquitin E3 Ligase. *Molecules* **2021**, *26*, 6682. [CrossRef]
21. Yang, Q.; Zhao, J.; Chen, D.; Wang, Y. E3 ubiquitin ligases: Styles, structures and functions. *Mol. Biomed.* **2021**, *2*, 23. [CrossRef]
22. Dougherty, S.E.; Maduka, A.O.; Inada, T.; Silva, G.M. Expanding Role of Ubiquitin in Translational Control. *Int. J. Mol. Sci.* **2020**, *21*, 1151. [CrossRef] [PubMed]
23. Callis, J. The ubiquitination machinery of the ubiquitin system. *Arab. B.* **2014**, *12*, e0174. [CrossRef]
24. Groothuis, T.A.M.; Dantuma, N.P.; Neefjes, J.; Salomons, F.A. Ubiquitin crosstalk connecting cellular processes. *Cell Div.* **2006**, *1*, 21. [CrossRef]
25. Damgaard, R.B. The ubiquitin system: From cell signalling to disease biology and new therapeutic opportunities. *Cell Death Differ.* **2021**, *28*, 423–426. [CrossRef]
26. Jarome, T.J.; Perez, G.A.; Webb, W.M.; Hatch, K.M.; Navabpour, S.; Musaus, M.; Farrell, K.; Hauser, R.M.; McFadden, T.; Martin, K.; et al. Ubiquitination of Histone H2B by Proteasome Subunit RPT6 Controls Histone Methylation Chromatin Dynamics During Memory Formation. *Biol. Psychiatry* **2021**, *89*, 1176–1187. [CrossRef] [PubMed]
27. Collins, P.E.; Mitxitorena, I.; Carmody, R.J. The Ubiquitination of NF-κB Subunits in the Control of Transcription. *Cells* **2016**, *5*, 23. [CrossRef]
28. Wang, W.; Cai, X.; Chen, X.-L. Recent Progress of Deubiquitinating Enzymes in Human and Plant Pathogenic Fungi. *Biomolecules* **2022**, *12*, 1424. [CrossRef] [PubMed]
29. Snyder, N.A.; Silva, G.M. Deubiquitinating enzymes (DUBs): Regulation, homeostasis, and oxidative stress response. *J. Biol. Chem.* **2021**, *297*, 101077. [CrossRef]
30. Eletr, Z.M.; Wilkinson, K.D. Regulation of proteolysis by human deubiquitinating enzymes. *Biochim. Biophys. Acta* **2014**, *1843*, 114–128. [CrossRef]
31. Hershko, A.; Ciechanover, A. The ubiquitin system. *Annu. Rev. Biochem.* **1998**, *67*, 425–479. [CrossRef] [PubMed]
32. Blount, J.R.; Johnson, S.L.; Todi, S. V Unanchored Ubiquitin Chains, Revisited. *Front. Cell Dev. Biol.* **2020**, *8*, 582361. [CrossRef]
33. Thibaudeau, T.A.; Smith, D.M. A Practical Review of Proteasome Pharmacology. *Pharmacol. Rev.* **2019**, *71*, 170–197. [CrossRef] [PubMed]
34. Tracz, M.; Bialek, W. Beyond K48 and K63: Non-canonical protein ubiquitination. *Cell. Mol. Biol. Lett.* **2021**, *26*, 1. [CrossRef] [PubMed]

35. Hochrainer, K.; Lipp, J. Ubiquitylation within signaling pathways in- and outside of inflammation. *Thromb. Haemost.* **2007**, *97*, 370–377.
36. DeMartino, G.N.; Slaughter, C.A. The proteasome, a novel protease regulated by multiple mechanisms. *J. Biol. Chem.* **1999**, *274*, 22123–22126. [CrossRef]
37. Saha, A.; Oanca, G.; Mondal, D.; Warshel, A. Exploring the Proteolysis Mechanism of the Proteasomes. *J. Phys. Chem. B* **2020**, *124*, 5626–5635. [CrossRef]
38. Groll, M.; Bajorek, M.; Köhler, A.; Moroder, L.; Rubin, D.M.; Huber, R.; Glickman, M.H.; Finley, D. A gated channel into the proteasome core particle. *Nat. Struct. Biol.* **2000**, *7*, 1062–1067. [CrossRef]
39. Lander, G.C.; Estrin, E.; Matyskiela, M.E.; Bashore, C.; Nogales, E.; Martin, A. Complete subunit architecture of the proteasome regulatory particle. *Nature* **2012**, *482*, 186–191. [CrossRef]
40. Lee, S.-H.; Moon, J.-H.; Yoon, S.K.; Yoon, J.-B. Stable incorporation of ATPase subunits into 19 S regulatory particle of human proteasome requires nucleotide binding and C-terminal tails. *J. Biol. Chem.* **2012**, *287*, 9269–9279. [CrossRef]
41. Budenholzer, L.; Cheng, C.L.; Li, Y.; Hochstrasser, M. Proteasome Structure and Assembly. *J. Mol. Biol.* **2017**, *429*, 3500–3524. [CrossRef] [PubMed]
42. Murata, S.; Yashiroda, H.; Tanaka, K. Molecular mechanisms of proteasome assembly. *Nat. Rev. Mol. Cell Biol.* **2009**, *10*, 104–115. [CrossRef] [PubMed]
43. Wen, X.; Klionsky, D.J. The proteasome subunit RPN10 functions as a specific receptor for degradation of the 26S proteasome by macroautophagy in Arabidopsis. *Autophagy* **2016**, *12*, 905–906. [CrossRef]
44. Rechsteiner, M.; Hill, C.P. Mobilizing the proteolytic machine: Cell biological roles of proteasome activators and inhibitors. *Trends Cell Biol.* **2005**, *15*, 27–33. [CrossRef] [PubMed]
45. Cheng, Y. Toward an atomic model of the 26S proteasome. *Curr. Opin. Struct. Biol.* **2009**, *19*, 203–208. [CrossRef]
46. Goldberg, A.L.; Kim, H.T.; Lee, D.; Collins, G.A. Mechanisms That Activate 26S Proteasomes and Enhance Protein Degradation. *Biomolecules* **2021**, *11*, 779. [CrossRef]
47. Chen, B.; Zhu, H.; Yang, B.; Cao, J. The dichotomous role of immunoproteasome in cancer: Friend or foe? *Acta Pharm. Sin. B* **2023**, *13*, 1976–1989. [CrossRef]
48. Imbesi, C.; Ettari, R.; Irrera, N.; Zappalà, M.; Pallio, G.; Bitto, A.; Mannino, F. Blunting Neuroinflammation by Targeting the Immunoproteasome with Novel Amide Derivatives. *Int. J. Mol. Sci.* **2023**, *24*, 732. [CrossRef]
49. Lee, M.J.; Bhattarai, D.; Jang, H.; Baek, A.; Yeo, I.J.; Lee, S.; Miller, Z.; Lee, S.; Hong, J.T.; Kim, D.-E.; et al. Macrocyclic Immunoproteasome Inhibitors as a Potential Therapy for Alzheimer's Disease. *J. Med. Chem.* **2021**, *64*, 10934–10950. [CrossRef]
50. Wagner, L.K.; Gilling, K.E.; Schormann, E.; Kloetzel, P.M.; Heppner, F.L.; Krüger, E.; Prokop, S. Immunoproteasome deficiency alters microglial cytokine response and improves cognitive deficits in Alzheimer's disease-like APPPS1 mice. *Acta Neuropathol. Commun.* **2017**, *5*, 52. [CrossRef]
51. Nguyen, H.D.; Kim, Y.E.; Nhat Nguyen, L.T.; Kwak, I.H.; Lee, Y.K.; Kim, Y.J.; Hai Nguyen, T.T.; Pham, H.N.; Ma, H.-I. Upregulation of immunoproteasome PSMB8 is associated with Parkinson's disease. *Parkinsonism Relat. Disord.* **2023**, *114*, 105797. [CrossRef] [PubMed]
52. Madsen, D.A.; Schmidt, S.I.; Blaabjerg, M.; Meyer, M. Interaction between Parkin and α-Synuclein in PARK2-Mediated Parkinson's Disease. *Cells* **2021**, *10*, 283. [CrossRef] [PubMed]
53. Moon, S.P.; Balana, A.T.; Galesic, A.; Rakshit, A.; Pratt, M.R. Ubiquitination Can Change the Structure of the α-Synuclein Amyloid Fiber in a Site Selective Fashion. *J. Org. Chem.* **2020**, *85*, 1548–1555. [CrossRef] [PubMed]
54. Kasahara, M. Role of immunoproteasomes and thymoproteasomes in health and disease. *Pathol. Int.* **2021**, *71*, 371–382. [CrossRef]
55. McCarthy, M.K.; Weinberg, J.B. The immunoproteasome and viral infection: A complex regulator of inflammation. *Front. Microbiol.* **2015**, *6*, 21. [CrossRef]
56. Abi Habib, J.; Lesenfants, J.; Vigneron, N.; Van den Eynde, B.J. Functional Differences between Proteasome Subtypes. *Cells* **2022**, *11*, 421. [CrossRef]
57. Basler, M.; Groettrup, M. On the Role of the Immunoproteasome in Protein Homeostasis. *Cells* **2021**, *10*, 3216. [CrossRef]
58. Basler, M.; Mundt, S.; Bitzer, A.; Schmidt, C.; Groettrup, M. The immunoproteasome: A novel drug target for autoimmune diseases. *Clin. Exp. Rheumatol.* **2015**, *33* (Suppl S92), S74–S79.
59. Sijts, E.J.A.M.; Kloetzel, P.M. The role of the proteasome in the generation of MHC class I ligands and immune responses. *Cell. Mol. Life Sci.* **2011**, *68*, 1491–1502. [CrossRef]
60. Vagapova, E.; Burov, A.; Spasskaya, D.; Lebedev, T.; Astakhova, T.; Spirin, P.; Prassolov, V.; Karpov, V.; Morozov, A. Immunoproteasome Activity and Content Determine Hematopoietic Cell Sensitivity to ONX-0914 and to the Infection of Cells with Lentiviruses. *Cells* **2021**, *10*, 1185. [CrossRef]
61. Kisselev, A.F.; Goldberg, A.L. Proteasome inhibitors: From research tools to drug candidates. *Chem. Biol.* **2001**, *8*, 739–758. [CrossRef] [PubMed]

62. Leister, H.; Krause, F.F.; Gil, B.; Prus, R.; Prus, I.; Hellhund-Zingel, A.; Mitra, M.; Da Rosa Gerbatin, R.; Delanty, N.; Beausang, A.; et al. Immunoproteasome deficiency results in age-dependent development of epilepsy. *Brain Commun.* **2024**, *6*, fcae017. [CrossRef]
63. Schaftenaar, F.H.; van Dam, A.D.; de Bruin, G.; Depuydt, M.A.C.; de Mol, J.; Amersfoort, J.; Douna, H.; Meijer, M.; Kröner, M.J.; van Santbrink, P.J.; et al. Immunoproteasomal Inhibition With ONX-0914 Attenuates Atherosclerosis and Reduces White Adipose Tissue Mass and Metabolic Syndrome in Mice. *Arterioscler. Thromb. Vasc. Biol.* **2024**, *44*, 1346–1364. [CrossRef]
64. Keller, I.E.; Vosyka, O.; Takenaka, S.; Kloß, A.; Dahlmann, B.; Willems, L.I.; Verdoes, M.; Overkleeft, H.S.; Marcos, E.; Adnot, S.; et al. Regulation of Immunoproteasome Function in the Lung. *Sci. Rep.* **2015**, *5*, 10230. [CrossRef]
65. Arya, R.; Kedar, V.; Hwang, J.R.; McDonough, H.; Li, H.-H.; Taylor, J.; Patterson, C. Muscle ring finger protein-1 inhibits PKC{epsilon} activation and prevents cardiomyocyte hypertrophy. *J. Cell Biol.* **2004**, *167*, 1147–1159. [CrossRef] [PubMed]
66. Kammerl, I.E.; Hardy, S.; Flexeder, C.; Urmann, A.; Peierl, J.; Wang, Y.; Vosyka, O.; Frankenberger, M.; Milger, K.; Behr, J.; et al. Activation of immune cell proteasomes in peripheral blood of smokers and COPD patients: Implications for therapy. *Eur. Respir. J.* **2022**, *59*, 2101798. [CrossRef]
67. Lin, Y.-C.; Jeng, K.-S.; Lai, M.M.C. CNOT4-Mediated Ubiquitination of Influenza A Virus Nucleoprotein Promotes Viral RNA Replication. *MBio* **2017**, *8*, e00597-17. [CrossRef]
68. Liao, T.-L.; Wu, C.-Y.; Su, W.-C.; Jeng, K.-S.; Lai, M.M.C. Ubiquitination and deubiquitination of NP protein regulates influenza A virus RNA replication. *EMBO J.* **2010**, *29*, 3879–3890. [CrossRef] [PubMed]
69. Pickering, A.M.; Davies, K.J.A. Degradation of damaged proteins: The main function of the 20S proteasome. *Prog. Mol. Biol. Transl. Sci.* **2012**, *109*, 227–248. [CrossRef]
70. Rosenbaum, J.T.; Sibley, C.H.; Choi, D.; Harrington, C.A.; Planck, S.R. Molecular diagnosis: Implications for ophthalmology. *Prog. Retin. Eye Res.* **2016**, *50*, 25–33. [CrossRef]
71. Ong, F.S.; Kuo, J.Z.; Wu, W.-C.; Cheng, C.-Y.; Blackwell, W.-L.B.; Taylor, B.L.; Grody, W.W.; Rotter, J.I.; Lai, C.-C.; Wong, T.Y. Personalized Medicine in Ophthalmology: From Pharmacogenetic Biomarkers to Therapeutic and Dosage Optimization. *J. Pers. Med.* **2013**, *3*, 40–69. [CrossRef] [PubMed]
72. Piedade, W.P.; Famulski, J.K. E3 ubiquitin ligase-mediated regulation of vertebrate ocular development; new insights into the function of SIAH enzymes. *Biochem. Soc. Trans.* **2021**, *49*, 327–340. [CrossRef] [PubMed]
73. Durán-Cristiano, S.C. Glaucoma: Biological mechanism and its Clinical Translation. *Curr. Mol. Med.* **2022**. [CrossRef]
74. Zhang, J.; Li, W.; Xiong, Z.; Zhu, J.; Ren, X.; Wang, S.; Kuang, H.; Lin, X.; Mora, A.; Li, X. PDGF-D-induced immunoproteasome activation and cell-cell interactions. *Comput. Struct. Biotechnol. J.* **2023**, *21*, 2405–2418. [CrossRef] [PubMed]
75. Li, M.; Gong, L.; Chapin, W.J.; Zhu, M. Assessment of Vision-Related Quality of Life in Dry Eye Patients. *Invest. Ophthalmol. Vis. Sci.* **2012**, *53*, 5722–5727. [CrossRef]
76. Ganesalingam, K.; Ismail, S.; Sherwin, T.; Craig, J.P. Molecular evidence for the role of inflammation in dry eye disease. *Clin. Exp. Optom.* **2019**, *102*, 446–454. [CrossRef]
77. Bron, A.J.; de Paiva, C.S.; Chauhan, S.K.; Bonini, S.; Gabison, E.E.; Jain, S.; Knop, E.; Markoulli, M.; Ogawa, Y.; Perez, V.; et al. TFOS DEWS II pathophysiology report. *Ocul. Surf.* **2017**, *15*, 438–510. [CrossRef]
78. Kuklinski, E.J.; Yu, Y.; Ying, G.-S.; Asbell, P.A. Association of Ocular Surface Immune Cells with Dry Eye Signs and Symptoms in the Dry Eye Assessment and Management (DREAM) Study. *Invest. Ophthalmol. Vis. Sci.* **2023**, *64*, 7. [CrossRef]
79. Xie, M.; Wang, H.; Peng, J.; Qing, D.; Zhang, X.; Guo, D.; Meng, P.; Luo, Z.; Wang, X.; Peng, Q. Acacetin protects against depression-associated dry eye disease by regulating ubiquitination of NLRP3 through gp78 signal. *Front. Pharmacol.* **2022**, *13*, 984475. [CrossRef]
80. Chen, Z.J. Ubiquitin signalling in the NF-kappaB pathway. *Nat. Cell Biol.* **2005**, *7*, 758–765. [CrossRef]
81. Kravtsova-Ivantsiv, Y.; Ciechanover, A. The ubiquitin-proteasome system and activation of NF-κB: Involvement of the ubiquitin ligase KPC1 in p105 processing and tumor suppression. *Mol. Cell. Oncol.* **2015**, *2*, e1054552. [CrossRef] [PubMed]
82. Yamamoto, Y.; Gaynor, R.B. Therapeutic potential of inhibition of the NF-κB pathway in the treatment of inflammation and cancer. *J. Clin. Invest.* **2001**, *107*, 135–142. [CrossRef]
83. Alam, J.; Yazdanpanah, G.; Ratnapriya, R.; Borcherding, N.; de Paiva, C.S.; Li, D.; Guimaraes de Souza, R.; Yu, Z.; Pflugfelder, S.C. IL-17 Producing Lymphocytes Cause Dry Eye and Corneal Disease with Aging in RXRα Mutant Mouse. *Front. Med.* **2022**, *9*, 849990. [CrossRef]
84. Rong, Z.; Cheng, L.; Ren, Y.; Li, Z.; Li, Y.; Li, X.; Li, H.; Fu, X.-Y.; Chang, Z. Interleukin-17F signaling requires ubiquitination of interleukin-17 receptor via TRAF6. *Cell. Signal.* **2007**, *19*, 1514–1520. [CrossRef] [PubMed]
85. Lin, X.; Rui, K.; Deng, J.; Tian, J.; Wang, X.; Wang, S.; Ko, K.-H.; Jiao, Z.; Chan, V.S.-F.; Lau, C.S.; et al. Th17 cells play a critical role in the development of experimental Sjögren's syndrome. *Ann. Rheum. Dis.* **2015**, *74*, 1302–1310. [CrossRef]
86. Nättinen, J.; Jylhä, A.; Aapola, U.; Mäkinen, P.; Beuerman, R.; Pietilä, J.; Vaajanen, A.; Uusitalo, H. Age-associated changes in human tear proteome. *Clin. Proteomics* **2019**, *16*, 11. [CrossRef] [PubMed]

87. Bardag-Gorce, F.; Hoft, R.; Meepe, I.; Garcia, J.; Tiger, K.; Wood, A.; Laporte, A.; Pan, D.; Makalinao, A.; Niihara, R.; et al. Proteasomes in corneal epithelial cells and cultured autologous oral mucosal epithelial cell sheet (CAOMECS) graft used for the ocular surface regeneration. *Ocul. Surf.* **2017**, *15*, 749–758. [CrossRef]
88. Bardag-Gorce, F.; Makalinao, A.; Meepe, I.; Hoft, R.H.; Cortez, D.; Oliva, J.; Laporte, A.; Stark, J.; Gorce, A.; Di Lorenzo, M.; et al. Corneal keratin aggresome (CKAGG) formation and clearance by proteasome activation. *Heliyon* **2018**, *4*, e01012. [CrossRef]
89. Kamounah, S.; Sembler-Møller, M.L.; Nielsen, C.H.; Pedersen, A.M.L. Sjögren's syndrome: Novel insights from proteomics and miRNA expression analysis. *Front. Immunol.* **2023**, *14*, 1183195. [CrossRef]
90. de Paiva, C.S.; Trujillo-Vargas, C.M.; Schaefer, L.; Yu, Z.; Britton, R.A.; Pflugfelder, S.C. Differentially Expressed Gene Pathways in the Conjunctiva of Sjögren Syndrome Keratoconjunctivitis Sicca. *Front. Immunol.* **2021**, *12*, 702755. [CrossRef]
91. Li, Y.; Li, S.; Wu, H. Ubiquitination-Proteasome System (UPS) and Autophagy Two Main Protein Degradation Machineries in Response to Cell Stress. *Cells* **2022**, *11*, 851. [CrossRef] [PubMed]
92. Liang, Q.; Guo, R.; Tsao, J.-R.; He, Y.; Wang, C.; Jiang, J.; Zhang, D.; Chen, T.; Yue, T.; Hu, K. Salidroside alleviates oxidative stress in dry eye disease by activating autophagy through AMPK-Sirt1 pathway. *Int. Immunopharmacol.* **2023**, *121*, 110397. [CrossRef] [PubMed]
93. Jeyabalan, N.; Pillai, A.M.; Khamar, P.; Shetty, R.; Mohan, R.R.; Ghosh, A. Autophagy in dry eye disease: Therapeutic implications of autophagy modulators on the ocular surface. *Indian. J. Ophthalmol.* **2023**, *71*, 1285–1291. [CrossRef] [PubMed]
94. Nichani, P.A.H.; Solomon, B.; Trinh, T.; Mimouni, M.; Rootman, D.; Singal, N.; Chan, C.C. Investigating the role of inflammation in keratoconus: A retrospective analysis of 551 eyes. *Eur. J. Ophthalmol.* **2023**, *33*, 35–43. [CrossRef]
95. Santodomingo-Rubido, J.; Carracedo, G.; Suzaki, A.; Villa-Collar, C.; Vincent, S.J.; Wolffsohn, J.S. Keratoconus: An updated review. *Cont. Lens Anterior Eye* **2022**, *45*, 101559. [CrossRef]
96. Lalgudi, V.G.; Shetty, R.; Nischal, K.K.; Ziai, S.; Koaik, M.; Sethu, S. Biochemical and molecular alterations and potential clinical applications of biomarkers in keratoconus. *Saudi J. Ophthalmol. Off. J. Saudi Ophthalmol. Soc.* **2022**, *36*, 7–16. [CrossRef]
97. Chan, J.K.L.; Yuen, D.; Too, P.H.-M.; Sun, Y.; Willard, B.; Man, D.; Tam, C. Keratin 6a reorganization for ubiquitin-proteasomal processing is a direct antimicrobial response. *J. Cell Biol.* **2018**, *217*, 731–744. [CrossRef]
98. Ferrington, D.A.; Roehrich, H.; Chang, A.A.; Huang, C.W.; Maldonado, M.; Bratten, W.; Rageh, A.A.; Heuss, N.D.; Gregerson, D.S.; Nelson, E.F.; et al. Corneal wound healing is compromised by immunoproteasome deficiency. *PLoS ONE* **2013**, *8*, e54347. [CrossRef]
99. Lomako, J.; Lomako, W.M.; Carothers Carraway, C.A.; Carraway, K.L. Regulation of the membrane mucin Muc4 in corneal epithelial cells by proteosomal degradation and TGF-beta. *J. Cell. Physiol.* **2010**, *223*, 209–214. [CrossRef]
100. Shinde, V.; Hu, N.; Renuse, S.; Mahale, A.; Pandey, A.; Eberhart, C.; Stone, D.; Al-Swailem, S.A.; Maktabi, A.; Chakravarti, S. Mapping Keratoconus Molecular Substrates by Multiplexed High-Resolution Proteomics of Unpooled Corneas. *OMICS* **2019**, *23*, 583–597. [CrossRef]
101. Ouyang, S.; Ma, J.; Sun, Q.; Li, J.; Chen, Y.; Luo, L. Comprehensive Bioinformatics Analysis to Reveal Key RNA Targets and Hub Competitive Endogenous RNA Network of Keratoconus. *Front. Genet.* **2022**, *13*, 896780. [CrossRef]
102. Balasubramanian, S.A.; Pye, D.C.; Willcox, M.D.P. Are proteinases the reason for keratoconus? *Curr. Eye Res.* **2010**, *35*, 185–191. [CrossRef] [PubMed]
103. Bardag-Gorce, F.; Hoffman, C.; Meepe, I.; Ferrini, M.; Hoft, R.H.; Oliva, J.; Niihara, Y. Thrombospondin-1 induction and VEGF reduction by proteasome inhibition. *Heliyon* **2023**, *9*, e13397. [CrossRef]
104. Johnston-Carey, H.K.; Pomatto, L.C.D.; Davies, K.J.A. The Immunoproteasome in oxidative stress, aging, and disease. *Crit. Rev. Biochem. Mol. Biol.* **2015**, *51*, 268–281. [CrossRef] [PubMed]
105. Chaudhuri, M.; Hassan, Y.; Bakka Vemana, P.P.S.; Bellary Pattanashetty, M.S.; Abdin, Z.U.; Siddiqui, H.F. Age-Related Macular Degeneration: An Exponentially Emerging Imminent Threat of Visual Impairment and Irreversible Blindness. *Cureus* **2023**, *15*, e39624. [CrossRef]
106. Tuo, J.; Bojanowski, C.M.; Chan, C.-C. Genetic factors of age-related macular degeneration. *Prog. Retin. Eye Res.* **2004**, *23*, 229–249. [CrossRef]
107. Ferreira, V.P.; Herbert, A.P.; Cortés, C.; McKee, K.A.; Blaum, B.S.; Esswein, S.T.; Uhrín, D.; Barlow, P.N.; Pangburn, M.K.; Kavanagh, D. The binding of factor H to a complex of physiological polyanions and C3b on cells is impaired in atypical hemolytic uremic syndrome. *J. Immunol.* **2009**, *182*, 7009–7018. [CrossRef]
108. Gemenetzi, M.; Lotery, A.J. Epigenetics in age-related macular degeneration: New discoveries and future perspectives. *Cell. Mol. Life Sci.* **2020**, *77*, 807–818. [CrossRef] [PubMed]
109. de Koning-Backus, A.P.M.; Kiefte-de Jong, J.C.; van Rooij, J.G.J.; Team, A.-L.; Uitterlinden, A.G.; Voortman, T.G.; Meester-Smoor, M.A.; Klaver, C.C.W. Lifestyle Intervention Randomized Controlled Trial for Age-Related Macular Degeneration (AMD-Life): Study Design. *Nutrients* **2023**, *15*, 602. [CrossRef]
110. Garcia-Garcia, J.; Usategui-Martin, R.; Sanabria, M.R.; Fernandez-Perez, E.; Telleria, J.J.; Coco-Martin, R.M. Pathophysiology of Age-Related Macular Degeneration: Implications for Treatment. *Ophthalmic Res.* **2022**, *65*, 615–636. [CrossRef]

111. Hussong, S.A.; Roehrich, H.; Kapphahn, R.J.; Maldonado, M.; Pardue, M.T.; Ferrington, D.A. A novel role for the immunoproteasome in retinal function. *Invest. Ophthalmol. Vis. Sci.* **2011**, *52*, 714–723. [CrossRef] [PubMed]
112. Wang, S.; Li, J.; Bai, J.; Li, J.-M.; Che, Y.-L.; Lin, Q.-Y.; Zhang, Y.-L.; Li, H.-H. The immunoproteasome subunit LMP10 mediates angiotensin II-induced retinopathy in mice. *Redox Biol.* **2018**, *16*, 129–138. [CrossRef] [PubMed]
113. Heesterbeek, T.J.; Lorés-Motta, L.; Hoyng, C.B.; Lechanteur, Y.T.E.; den Hollander, A.I. Risk factors for progression of age-related macular degeneration. *Ophthalmic Physiol. Opt. J. Br. Coll. Ophthalmic Opt.* **2020**, *40*, 140–170. [CrossRef]
114. Blasiak, J.; Pawlowska, E.; Szczepanska, J.; Kaarniranta, K. Interplay between Autophagy and the Ubiquitin-Proteasome System and Its Role in the Pathogenesis of Age-Related Macular Degeneration. *Int. J. Mol. Sci.* **2019**, *20*, 210. [CrossRef] [PubMed]
115. Campello, L.; Esteve-Rudd, J.; Cuenca, N.; Martín-Nieto, J. The ubiquitin-proteasome system in retinal health and disease. *Mol. Neurobiol.* **2013**, *47*, 790–810. [CrossRef] [PubMed]
116. Lee, H.; Choi, A.J.; Kang, G.-Y.; Park, H.S.; Kim, H.C.; Lim, H.J.; Chung, H. Increased 26S proteasome non-ATPase regulatory subunit 1 in the aqueous humor of patients with age-related macular degeneration. *BMB Rep.* **2014**, *47*, 292–297. [CrossRef]
117. Fernandes, A.F.; Zhou, J.; Zhang, X.; Bian, Q.; Sparrow, J.; Taylor, A.; Pereira, P.; Shang, F. Oxidative inactivation of the proteasome in retinal pigment epithelial cells. A potential link between oxidative stress and up-regulation of interleukin-8. *J. Biol. Chem.* **2008**, *283*, 20745–20753. [CrossRef]
118. Qin, T.; Gao, S. Inhibition of Proteasome Activity Upregulates IL-6 Expression in RPE Cells through the Activation of P38 MAPKs. *J. Ophthalmol.* **2018**, *2018*, 5392432. [CrossRef]
119. Wei, J.; Chen, X.; Xiong, Y.; Gao, Y. Advances in Ubiquitination and Proteostasis in Retinal Degeneration. *Front. Biosci. (Landmark Ed.* **2024**, *29*, 260. [CrossRef]
120. Firmani, G.; Salducci, M.; Testa, F.; Covelli, G.P.; Sagnelli, P.; Lambiase, A. Ocular Biomarkers in Alzheimer's Disease: Insights into Early Detection Through Eye-Based Diagnostics—A Literature Review. *Clin. Ter.* **2024**, *175*, 352–361. [CrossRef]
121. Wang, X.; Chen, W.; Zhao, W.; Miao, M. Risk of glaucoma to subsequent dementia or cognitive impairment: A systematic review and meta-analysis. *Aging Clin. Exp. Res.* **2024**, *36*, 172. [CrossRef]
122. Korac, J.; Schaeffer, V.; Kovacevic, I.; Clement, A.M.; Jungblut, B.; Behl, C.; Terzic, J.; Dikic, I. Ubiquitin-independent function of optineurin in autophagic clearance of protein aggregates. *J. Cell Sci.* **2013**, *126*, 580–592. [CrossRef] [PubMed]
123. Ying, H.; Yue, B.Y.J.T. Cellular and molecular biology of optineurin. *Int. Rev. Cell Mol. Biol.* **2012**, *294*, 223–258. [CrossRef] [PubMed]
124. Sayyad, Z.; Kaveti, S.; Bhattacharjee, D.; Vedagiri, D.; Jain, N.; Swarup, G. A glaucoma-associated OPTN polymorphism, M98K sensitizes retinal cells to endoplasmic reticulum stress and tumour necrosis factor α. *FEBS J.* **2023**, *290*, 3110–3127. [CrossRef] [PubMed]
125. Qiu, Y.; Wang, J.; Li, H.; Yang, B.; Wang, J.; He, Q.; Weng, Q. Emerging views of OPTN (optineurin) function in the autophagic process associated with disease. *Autophagy* **2022**, *18*, 73–85. [CrossRef]
126. Li, F.; Xu, D.; Wang, Y.; Zhou, Z.; Liu, J.; Hu, S.; Gong, Y.; Yuan, J.; Pan, L. Structural insights into the ubiquitin recognition by OPTN (optineurin) and its regulation by TBK1-mediated phosphorylation. *Autophagy* **2018**, *14*, 66–79. [CrossRef]
127. Kageyama, M.; Ota, T.; Sasaoka, M.; Katsuta, O.; Shinomiya, K. Chemical proteasome inhibition as a novel animal model of inner retinal degeneration in rats. *PLoS ONE* **2019**, *14*, e0217945. [CrossRef]
128. Hayat, B.; Padhy, B.; Mohanty, P.P.; Alone, D.P. Altered unfolded protein response and proteasome impairment in pseudoexfoliation pathogenesis. *Exp. Eye Res.* **2019**, *181*, 197–207. [CrossRef]
129. Baudouin, C.; Kolko, M.; Melik-Parsadaniantz, S.; Messmer, E.M. Inflammation in Glaucoma: From the back to the front of the eye, and beyond. *Prog. Retin. Eye Res.* **2021**, *83*, 100916. [CrossRef]
130. Gupta, D.; Wen, J.C.; Huebner, J.L.; Stinnett, S.; Kraus, V.B.; Tseng, H.C.; Walsh, M. Cytokine biomarkers in tear film for primary open-angle glaucoma. *Clin. Ophthalmol.* **2017**, *11*, 411–416. [CrossRef]
131. Keller, K.E.; Wirtz, M.K. Working your SOCS off: The role of ASB10 and protein degradation pathways in glaucoma. *Exp. Eye Res.* **2017**, *158*, 154–160. [CrossRef] [PubMed]
132. Pasutto, F.; Keller, K.E.; Weisschuh, N.; Sticht, H.; Samples, J.R.; Yang, Y.-F.; Zenkel, M.; Schlötzer-Schrehardt, U.; Mardin, C.Y.; Frezzotti, P.; et al. Variants in ASB10 are associated with open-angle glaucoma. *Hum. Mol. Genet.* **2012**, *21*, 1336–1349. [CrossRef] [PubMed]
133. Keller, K.E.; Yang, Y.-F.; Sun, Y.Y.; Sykes, R.; Acott, T.S.; Wirtz, M.K. Ankyrin repeat and suppressor of cytokine signaling box containing protein-10 is associated with ubiquitin-mediated degradation pathways in trabecular meshwork cells. *Mol. Vis.* **2013**, *19*, 1639–1655. [PubMed]
134. Orre, M.; Kamphuis, W.; Dooves, S.; Kooijman, L.; Chan, E.T.; Kirk, C.J.; Dimayuga Smith, V.; Koot, S.; Mamber, C.; Jansen, A.H.; et al. Reactive glia show increased immunoproteasome activity in Alzheimer's disease. *Brain* **2013**, *136*, 1415–1431. [CrossRef]
135. Tezel, G.; Thornton, I.L.; Tong, M.G.; Luo, C.; Yang, X.; Cai, J.; Powell, D.W.; Soltau, J.B.; Liebmann, J.M.; Ritch, R. Immunoproteomic analysis of potential serum biomarker candidates in human glaucoma. *Investig. Ophthalmol. Vis. Sci.* **2012**, *53*, 8222–8231. [CrossRef]

136. Osei-Amponsa, V.; Walters, K.J. Proteasome substrate receptors and their therapeutic potential. *Trends Biochem. Sci.* **2022**, *47*, 950–964. [CrossRef]
137. Njomen, E.; Tepe, J.J. Proteasome Activation as a New Therapeutic Approach to Target Proteotoxic Disorders. *J. Med. Chem.* **2019**, *62*, 6469–6481. [CrossRef]
138. Weinberg, J.; Gaur, M.; Swaroop, A.; Taylor, A. Proteostasis in aging-associated ocular disease. *Mol. Aspects Med.* **2022**, *88*, 101157. [CrossRef]
139. Frankland-Searby, S.; Bhaumik, S.R. The 26S proteasome complex: An attractive target for cancer therapy. *Biochim. Biophys. Acta* **2012**, *1825*, 64–76. [CrossRef]
140. Seyoum Tola, F. The Role of Ubiquitin-Proteasome System in the Pathogenesis of Severe Acute Respiratory Syndrome Coronavirus-2 Disease. *Int. J. Inflam.* **2023**, *2023*, 6698069. [CrossRef]
141. Liu, Y.; Feng, M.; Cai, J.; Li, S.; Dai, X.; Shan, G.; Wu, S. Repurposing bortezomib for choroidal neovascularization treatment via antagonizing VEGF-A and PDGF-D mediated signaling. *Exp. Eye Res.* **2021**, *204*, 108446. [CrossRef] [PubMed]
142. Chen, F.-T.; Yang, C.-M.; Yang, C.-H. The protective effects of the proteasome inhibitor bortezomib (velcade) on ischemia-reperfusion injury in the rat retina. *PLoS ONE* **2013**, *8*, e64262. [CrossRef]
143. Forghani, P.; Rashid, A.; Sun, F.; Liu, R.; Li, D.; Lee, M.R.; Hwang, H.; Maxwell, J.T.; Mandawat, A.; Wu, R.; et al. Carfilzomib Treatment Causes Molecular and Functional Alterations of Human Induced Pluripotent Stem Cell-Derived Cardiomyocytes. *J. Am. Heart Assoc.* **2021**, *10*, e022247. [CrossRef] [PubMed]
144. Rockwell, C.E.; Qureshi, N. Differential effects of lactacystin on cytokine production in activated Jurkat cells and murine splenocytes. *Cytokine* **2010**, *51*, 12–17. [CrossRef] [PubMed]
145. Hou, A.; Mohamed Ali, S.; Png, E.; Hunziker, W.; Tong, L. Transglutaminase-2 is critical for corneal epithelial barrier function via positive regulation of Claudin-1. *Ocul. Surf.* **2023**, *28*, 155–164. [CrossRef]
146. Benischke, A.-S.; Vasanth, S.; Miyai, T.; Katikireddy, K.R.; White, T.; Chen, Y.; Halilovic, A.; Price, M.; Price, F.J.; Liton, P.B.; et al. Activation of mitophagy leads to decline in Mfn2 and loss of mitochondrial mass in Fuchs endothelial corneal dystrophy. *Sci. Rep.* **2017**, *7*, 6656. [CrossRef]
147. Aktas, Z.; Rao, H.; Slauson, S.R.; Gabelt, B.T.; Larsen, I.V.; Sheridan, R.T.C.; Herrnberger, L.; Tamm, E.R.; Kaufman, P.L.; Brandt, C.R. Proteasome Inhibition Increases the Efficiency of Lentiviral Vector-Mediated Transduction of Trabecular Meshwork. *Invest. Ophthalmol. Vis. Sci.* **2018**, *59*, 298–310. [CrossRef]
148. Sridevi Gurubaran, I.; Hytti, M.; Kaarniranta, K.; Kauppinen, A. Epoxomicin, a Selective Proteasome Inhibitor, Activates AIM2 Inflammasome in Human Retinal Pigment Epithelium Cells. *Antioxidants* **2022**, *11*, 1288. [CrossRef]
149. Salazar-Chaparro, A.F.; Halder, S.; Trader, D.J. Synthesis and Application of a Clickable Epoxomicin-Based Probe for Proteasome Activity Analysis. *Curr. Protoc.* **2022**, *2*, e490. [CrossRef]
150. Nakasone, M.A.; Lewis, T.A.; Walker, O.; Thakur, A.; Mansour, W.; Castañeda, C.A.; Goeckeler-Fried, J.L.; Parlati, F.; Chou, T.-F.; Hayat, O.; et al. Structural Basis for the Inhibitory Effects of Ubistatins in the Ubiquitin-Proteasome Pathway. *Structure* **2017**, *25*, 1839–1855.e11. [CrossRef]
151. Klaips, C.L.; Jayaraj, G.G.; Hartl, F.U. Pathways of cellular proteostasis in aging and disease. *J. Cell Biol.* **2018**, *217*, 51–63. [CrossRef] [PubMed]
152. Sabath, N.; Levy-Adam, F.; Younis, A.; Rozales, K.; Meller, A.; Hadar, S.; Soueid-Baumgarten, S.; Shalgi, R. Cellular proteostasis decline in human senescence. *Proc. Natl. Acad. Sci. USA* **2020**, *117*, 31902–31913. [CrossRef] [PubMed]
153. Bales, K.L.; Gross, A.K. Aberrant protein trafficking in retinal degenerations: The initial phase of retinal remodeling. *Exp. Eye Res.* **2016**, *150*, 71–80. [CrossRef] [PubMed]
154. Verbrugge, S.E.; Scheper, R.J.; Lems, W.F.; de Gruijl, T.D.; Jansen, G. Proteasome inhibitors as experimental therapeutics of autoimmune diseases. *Arthritis Res. Ther.* **2015**, *17*, 17. [CrossRef]
155. Cao, Y.; Zhu, H.; He, R.; Kong, L.; Shao, J.; Zhuang, R.; Xi, J.; Zhang, J. Proteasome, a Promising Therapeutic Target for Multiple Diseases Beyond Cancer. *Drug Des. Devel. Ther.* **2020**, *14*, 4327–4342. [CrossRef]
156. Davidson, K.; Pickering, A.M. The proteasome: A key modulator of nervous system function, brain aging, and neurodegenerative disease. *Front. cell Dev. Biol.* **2023**, *11*, 1124907. [CrossRef]
157. Klimko, P.G.; Hellberg, M.R. Use of Proteasome Inhibitors to Treat Dry Eye Disorders; National Center for Biotechnology Information. PubChem Patent Summary for US-7112588-B2; Patent Application No. US7112588B2, 26 September 2006.

life

MDPI

Review

Review of Guideline Recommendations for Optimal Anti-VEGF Therapy in Age-Related Macular Degeneration

Andreea Dana Moraru [1,2], Ciprian Danielescu [1,2,*,†], Raluca Eugenia Iorga [1,2,*], Radu Lucian Moraru [3], Mihail Zemba [4,†] and Daniel Constantin Branisteanu [1,5]

1 Department of Ophthalmology, 'Grigore T. Popa' University of Medicine and Pharmacy, 700115 Iași, Romania; oftalmoconsultiasi@yahoo.ro (A.D.M.); daniel.branisteanu@umfiasi.ro (D.C.B.)
2 Department of Ophthalmology, 'N. Oblu' Clinical Hospital, 700309 Iași, Romania
3 'Transmed Expert' Medical Center, 700011 Iași, Romania
4 Department of Ophthalmology, 'Dr. Carol Davila' Central Military Emergency University Hospital, 010825 Bucharest, Romania
5 Department of Ophthalmology, Railway Clinical Hospital, 700506 Iași, Romania
* Correspondence: ciprianmd@yahoo.com (C.D.); ralucadanulescu@yahoo.com (R.E.I.)
† These authors contributed equally to this work.

Abstract: Neovascular age-related macular degeneration is a progressive, blinding macular disease that has become a burden both in healthcare systems and the global economy. The vascular endothelial growth factor (VEGF) is the main agent involved in the pathogenic process of the disease. The main goal of the age-related macular degeneration treatment is to maintain and improve visual acuity by injecting intravitreal anti-VEGF agents in either a reactive or proactive manner. Subretinal and intraretinal fluids are the main biomarkers that should be considered when managing the frequency of the therapy. This review discusses both functional and morphological treatment criteria according to current recommendations as opposed to real-life situations encountered during day-to-day clinical practice and highlights situations in which the benefits of continuing therapy are arguable in terms of improving patients' quality of life. Optimizing the treatment regimen represents an important aim of current clinical ophthalmological practice, as age-related macular degeneration patients usually have a long follow-up period.

Keywords: age-related macular degeneration; anti-VEGF therapy; treat and extend; intraretinal fluid; subretinal fluid

1. Introduction

Neovascular age-related macular degeneration (nAMD), or macular neovascularization as it is currently known (MNV) is a progressive, chronic, blinding retinal disease affecting 8.7% of the world population [1]. One meta-analysis taking into account the European population reported a prevalence of early or late AMD of 0.08% in the group of 50- to 55- year-old participants, which increased with age to a percent of 20.1% in the group of participants over 90 years old [2]. It is estimated that 10% of patients diagnosed with the non-exudative form of age-related macular degeneration eventually develop the exudative form [3]. Visual impairment caused by MNV has become a burden to both the global economy and the overly crowded healthcare system.

The main pathological event in MNV is the formation of a choroidal neovascular membrane (CNV) that penetrates the Bruch membrane, leading to exudation in the subretinal space, retinal edema, hemorrhage, pigment epithelial detachment, and subretinal fibrous scars. Clinical and experimental data have demonstrated that vascular endothelial growth factor (VEGF) is the main agent involved in inflammatory and angiogenetic process [4,5].

VEGF is a neurovascular trophic factor important for the function of both endothelial cells and neurons. VEGF activity is important for sustaining nervous tissue, the cardiovascular system, and the renal system. The eye also intervenes in the development and normal function of the retinal vasculature [6]. VEGF plays an important role in the expression of nitric oxide by endothelial cells; thus, inhibition of VEGF causes dysfunction of the vascular endothelium and may lead to thromboembolic events, systemic hypertension, and renal impairment [7].

Understanding of the physiopathological mechanism has facilitated the emergence of new therapeutic methods. Thus, over the last two decades, several anti-VEGF agents have been studied and approved as first-line treatments for nAMD. Current therapeutic protocols are under continuous evaluation in order to improve the results obtained in real--life treatment of patients with nAMD.

The current review aims to bring into discussion the therapeutic protocols of the available anti-VEGF agents, the main biomarkers useful in guiding the therapy, the risk factors associated with the treatment, and some future directions that may influence clinical practice in the following years.

2. Therapeutic Protocols and Available Drugs

There are currently several drugs that can be used to treat neovascular age-related macular degeneration.

Bevacizumab was the first drug used, off-label, in nAMD therapy. It was administered by intravitreal injection and showed major improvements in visual function and retinal morphology of nAMD patients [8,9].

Ranibizumab is a recombinant humanized immunoglobulin (Ig) G monoclonal antibody fragment that binds to VEGF A, thus inhibiting its effects. It is smaller than a full-size antibody and penetrates the retina with ease, but it is cleared from the vitreous quickly, with a half-life of only 9 days [10]. Its efficacy in maintaining vision was demonstrated in two double-blind studies, ANCHOR and MARINA, over the course of two years. The ANCHOR study also demonstrated that ranibizumab is superior to photodynamic therapy for the treatment of classic neovascular membranes [11].

Aflibercept is a widely used VEGF Trap-Eye, which is a chimeric protein containing the second binding domain of the VEGFR-1 receptor and the third domain of the VEGFR-2 receptor. It has high affinity for all isomers of VEGF A, VEGF B, and placental growth factor. The VIEW 1 and VIEW 2 studies demonstrated its non-inferiority for visual function maintenance compared to ranibizumab [12,13].

Two other drugs were recently approved for the treatment of macular neovascularization: Brolucizumab and faricimab. Brolucizumab is a humanized monoclonal single-chain variable fragment; thus, it is the smallest functional unit of an antibody that binds and inhibits VEGF A at a ratio of 2:1 [14]. Two studies, HAWK and HARRIER, demonstrated its non-inferiority to aflibercept in maintaining visual acuity and its superiority in reducing intraretinal and subretinal fluid as compared to the same drug [15].

Faricimab is a bispecific antibody that binds to both VEGF A and Angiopoietin 2. Its efficacy was demonstrated in two comparative studies, TENAYA and LUCERNE, which showed similar visual function gains between the group treated with aflibercept and those receiving faricimab. The results were maintained throughout the second year of treatment, with the possibility of extending the dosing interval for faricimab to 8, 12, or 16 weeks, depending on the functional and anatomic results [16].

The main goal of MNV treatment is to maintain and improve visual acuity by injecting anti-VEGF agents such as aflibercept, brolucizumab, ranibizumab, and bevacizumab in the vitreous cavity. The treatment can be administered in either a reactive or proactive manner but should be individualized in order to obtain optimal results.

The reactive approach, or pro re nata (PRN), means that injections are administered only when the disease shows signs of activity, such as intraretinal or subretinal fluid. This type of approach reduces the number of injections to which the patient has to be submitted but, requires very rigorous monitoring in order to capture the moment in which a dormant CNV resumes activity. Although patients do not follow a monthly injection regimen, they need to follow a monthly examination schedule, which enables the ophthalmologist to determine if retreatment criteria are met based on clinical, OCT (optical coherence tomography), and angiographic assessment. Recent literature data has shown that PRN usually leads to suboptimal results due to delayed or low-frequency dosing [17,18].

Treat-and-extend (T and E) is a proactive type of therapeutic management for MNV. In T and E, the patient has to follow a regular schedule of injections, starting with an implementation phase, in which the injections are administered monthly, and continuing with a maintenance phase, when the interval between injections is lengthened gradually until the morpho-functional aspect of the disease becomes stable. The advantage of this type of therapeutic approach is that it minimizes the risk of undertreatment or overtreatment of delayed administration and reduces the number of hospital visits compared with a monthly regimen of injections, which does not consider whether the disease shows signs of activity.

Currently, the treatment recommendations for intravitreal anti-VEGF treatment are to perform a loading dose, consisting of three-monthly doses, followed by another injection at eight weeks intervals [17]. If, at this point, the disease becomes stable based on morpho-functional criteria (visual acuity and OCT aspect), the period of time to the 5th injection can be extended by 2 to 4 weeks, to a maximum of 12 weeks. Similarly, the interval to the next injection can be extended to a maximum of 16 weeks if the disease is stable and there are no signs of disease progression. The interval of time should be maintained if changes in visual acuity and OCT morphology occur when a longer period of time between injections is being implemented. However, if visual acuity worsens due to loss of more than 5 ETDRS letters and OCT shows signs of disease activity consisting of subretinal and intraretinal fluid and macular hemorrhages, then the interval between injections should be reduced by 2 to 4 weeks until disease inactivity is achieved (Figure 1).

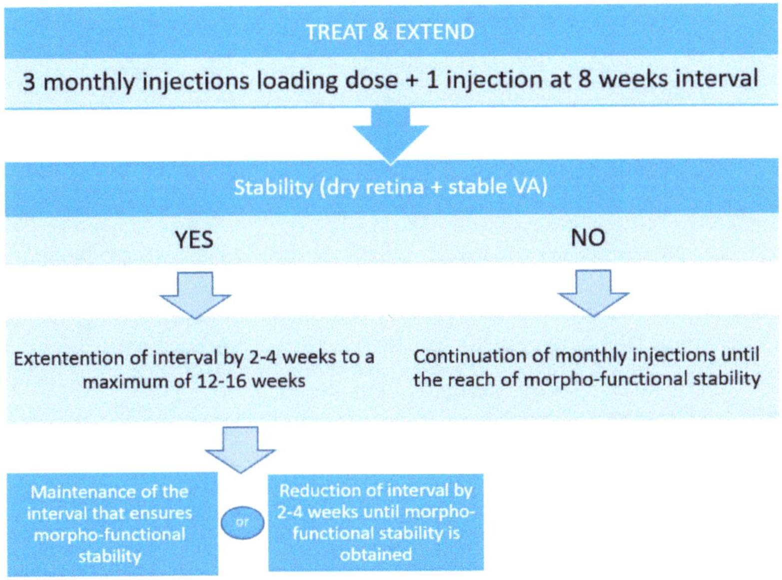

Figure 1. Treat-and-extend algorithm for intravitreal injections in neovascular AMD. Morpho-functional stability is defined as the loss of no more than five ETDRS letters in visual acuity and no fluid or no new fluid on OCT.

Newer studies have shown that an increase in the administered anti-VEGF dosage could lead to relaxation of the therapeutic protocol, with the possibility that after the loading phase, the interval between two intravitreal injections might be lengthened to 8 to 12 weeks. Over the same period, high-dose aflibercept produced better anatomical results, with a greater number of eyes free of macular fluid and no compromises regarding the safety of administration, as compared to standard-dose aflibercept. Despite the better morphological results, the difference between the final visual acuity was not statistically significant between the groups treated with aflibercept 2 mg and 8 mg [19,20].

3. Biomarkers of Treatment Response

Subretinal and intraretinal fluids are the main biomarkers that should be taken into account when managing the T and E regimen. (Table 1) Visual acuity should also be considered in the analysis, but it is not a specific biomarker for disease activity like the morphological changes seen on OCT, as it can be influenced by several other factors, such as cataract progression.

Table 1. Correlation between OCT biomarkers and their influence on visual prognosis.

Biomarkers	OCT Aspect	Influence on Visual Prognosis
Intraretinal fluid (IFR)	Increased retinal thickness, Fluid cysts above the outer plexiform layer	Signs of disease activity Negative prognostic on VA May determine cystic degeneration of the retina
Subretinal fluid (SRF)	Fluid between the RPE and the neurosensory retina	Indicates the need to continue therapy A small and stable quantity may be tolerated without increasing but also without reducing the number of intravitreal injections
Sub- retinal pigment epithelium (RPE) fluid	Pigmentary epithelium detachment (PED)	Less impact on visual acuity
Foveal receptor integrity	Disruption of the ellipsoid zone and the external limiting membrane band	Negative impact on visual acuity (especially on baseline VA)
Hyperreflective dots	Small retinal conglomerates with a reflectivity higher than the RPE, located in all the layers, mostly around the cystoid spaces	Negative prognostic value Correlation with recurrences
Subretinal hyperreflective material	Large retinal conglomerates located between the RPE and the neurosensory retina	Negative impact on visual acuity regardless of its disposition and associated with a lower increase of the visual function after treatment
Vitreomacular interface alterations		
Adhesion	Strong adhesions between the posterior hyaloid and the retina due to the development of the neovascular membrane	Less responsive to anti-VEGF therapy
Traction	Important traction of the retina exerted by the posterior hyaloid may cause alteration of the inner and outer retinal layers	Less responsive to anti-VEGF therapy Benefit from the surgical removal of the traction
Alterations in choroidal morphology		
Sub-RPE hyperreflective columns	Sign of broken RPE Blood, fluid, and neovessels enter the subretinal space	Negative prognostic value
Prechoroidal clefts	Spindle-shaped hyporeflective cavities located between the choroid and the fibrous component of a multilayered PED	Less impact on visual acuity Possible protective effect on the outer retinal layers

Table 1. *Cont.*

Biomarkers	OCT Aspect	Influence on Visual Prognosis
Choroidal caverns	Hyporeflective sub-RPE structures	No prognostic value on VA
Subfoveal choroidal thickness	Assessed by SS-OCT High variability	No prognostic value on VA
Choroidal vascular index	The choroidal vascular lumen area reported to the choroidal stromal area	No prognostic value on VA Correlates choroidal hypoxia
Outer retinal tubulations	Non-specific lesions in which photoreceptors rearrange in a circular manner Hyperreflective borders surrounding a hyporeflective space located in the outer nuclear layer Located at the border between an atrophic lesion and normal retinal tissue, with the RPE absent or altered	Negative prognostic value

Table 1 summarizes the main biomarkers previously discussed, their morphological aspect on OCT, and the influence each of them has on visual rehabilitation and functional prognosis during therapy. The persistence of intraretinal fluid (IFR), disruption of foveal receptor integrity, presence of hyperreflective dots, subretinal hyperreflective material or sub-RPE hyperreflective columns, and appearance of outer retinal tubulations are highly suggestive of a poor functional prognosis.

Subretinal fluid (SRF) should be treated until the disease becomes stable and the subretinal space is dry. Sometimes, despite correct and frequent treatment, a small quantity of SRF persists. Recent studies have shown that a small and stable quantity of SRF can be safely tolerated by patients without the need to increase the number of injections. The exact volume of SRF considered tolerable should be determined by the supervising physician. The stability of SRF levels and absence of new morphological changes are key factors in the management of these cases. Both the CATT and FLUID studies showed no significant difference in visual acuity at 1 year follow-up between patients with and without a small amount of SRF. The FLUID study demonstrated that visual acuity at 1 year was similar in those who followed a T and E dosing protocol aimed at eradicating all SRF and those who received fewer injections and tolerated a fluid volume of less than 200 µm [21,22].

A retrospective analysis after 1 year of treatment with aflibercept showed that the gain in visual acuity was similar in patients with inactive and active disease, defined by the presence of SRF, intraretinal cysts, and intraretinal fluid and that after the loading dose, the macular status could predict the results obtained at 1 year interval [23].

The occurrence of pigment epithelial detachment, hemorrhage, and modifications of the choroidal neovascular membrane, together with the persistence or addition of new SRF, are signs of retreatment necessity.

Currently, there is no consensus regarding the extent to which residual SRF can be considered tolerable. Recently, an artificial intelligence-assisted analysis of patients enrolled in the FLUID study stated that an SRF-tolerant treat-and-extend regimen was associated with worse functional prognosis. Extended intervals between injections, despite the presence of residual SRF, were associated with higher volumes of SRF in the central 6 mm area of the macula [24].

Intraretinal fluid (IRF) represents a sign of disease activity, and it is associated with a lower visual acuity than SRF, both at baseline and after treatment. CATT study showed that at both 1 and 5 years of treatment, the gain in visual acuity was reduced in patients with IRF compared with those without IRF [10]. IRF present at baseline correlates with disease activity and is a sign of poor prognosis even in treatment-naïve patients [25].

IRF can cause morphological alterations in the retina due to the loss of photoreceptors. The presence of IRF for a long time may determine cystic degeneration of the retina over areas of atrophy and fibrosis [26]. This is why many eyes do not improve significantly in visual acuity despite following a strict protocol of treatment.

Two recent studies used artificial intelligence technology to analyze OCT data and correlate the quantity and disposition of the SRF and IRF with the functional benefit obtained after anti-VEGF therapy [27,28].

Schmidt-Erfurth et al. demonstrated in these studies that the presence of IRF is the most important biomarker for predicting visual acuity regression, while the influence of SRF is much weaker. The presence of SRF in the juxtafoveal area also depends on volume, but not in the central foveal region, which is associated with a decrease in visual acuity. The IRF has a reverse association, as its presence in the central fovea and, to a lesser extent, in the juxtafoveal area is associated with poorer visual function [27].

IRF should not be confused with outer retinal tubulation. **Outer retinal tubulation** is a retinal feature associated with degeneration, in which the photoreceptors are rearranged in a circular pattern associated with degenerative diseases of the retinal tissue, including age-related macular degeneration, dystrophies, etc. [29].

This lesion is non-specific and needs to be differentiated from an IRF for proper management. On optical coherence tomography (OCT) images, outer retinal tubulation can be distinguished from an intraretinal cyst by its hyperreflective borders surrounding a hyporeflective space located in the outer nuclear layer [30].

This aspect is due to the loss of the adhesion of the photoreceptors, which fold inward with the outer limiting membrane. The tubular structure protects the photoreceptors from injuries as they are located in the lumen. The structure is located at the border between an atrophic lesion and normal retinal tissue, where the retinal pigment epithelium is absent or altered [31].

The outer retinal tubulation is non-responsive and does not require anti-VEGF treatment, which is a factor of reserved visual prognosis [32].

Sub–retinal pigmentary epithelium (sub-RPE) fluid, usually described on OCT as pigmentary epithelium detachment (PED), seems to have a less important impact on the visual function prognosis. In the VIEW and HARBOR studies, the patients who were diagnosed with PED had a higher visual acuity at baseline than those without, but the association was weaker during the follow-up period. At 2 years follow-up, the eyes with better visual acuity at baseline maintained superior visual function compared to the rest [33]. The presence of foveal PED was associated with better visual acuity at 5 years in the CATT study, as sub-RPE fluid may have a trophic effect on the retina [34].

However, eyes that presented with complete resolution of PED at 24 months had a higher risk of developing macular atrophy [35].

The integrity of the **foveal receptor layer** is another biomarker with important implications for visual prognosis. The disruption of the ellipsoid zone and the external limiting membrane band negatively affects the outcome of anti-VEGF therapy [36–38].

However, the correlation between the integrity of these layers and the visual acuity appears to be stronger at baseline assessment than after VEGF therapy [39].

Hyperreflective dots are retinal lesions scattered throughout all layers, but with a preferred disposition around the cystoid spaces, with a higher reflectivity than the RPE. They are thought to be formed by lipid-filled microglia and migrated RPE cells [40].

The presence of hyperreflective dots has negative prognostic value. These lesions are associated with lower visual acuity at baseline and their persistence inside the retinal layers is correlated with worse visual function after treatment [41].

Subretinal hyperreflective material, located between the RPE and the neurosensory retina, is thought to consist of fibrin, blood, fluid, scar, or macular neovascularization and is associated with a lower visual acuity, regardless of its disposition and with less improvement in visual function after treatment [42]. Its composition can change over time. If the subretinal hypereflective material has a neovascular component, which can be identified by OCT angiography, then the response to anti-VEGF therapy is usually weak [43]. One study suggested that if reflectivity decreases after treatment, the visual prognosis could be better [44].

Recently, a higher incidence of **vitreomacular interface alterations**, in particular, vitreomacular adhesions and vitreomacular traction, has been described [45]. This correlation seems to be caused by the development of the neovascular membrane with its exudative and fibrotic phases, making the adhesions between the posterior hyaloid and the retina stronger [46]. These eyes tend to respond poorly to anti-VEGF therapy and require a greater number of intravitreal injections [47].

Vitreomacular traction may cause alteration of the inner and outer retinal layers and lead to chronic inflammation, which may accelerate the progression of MNV [48]. Eyes with vitreomacular traction might benefit from surgical removal of traction by reducing the number of intravitreal injections needed to stabilize the neovascular membrane [49].

Some **alterations in choroidal morphology** may also be biomarkers that influence the outcomes of intravitreal anti-VEGF therapy. These include sub-RPE hyperreflective columns, prechoroidal clefts, choroidal caverns, subfoveal choroidal thickness, and the choroidal vascular index [50].

Sub-RPE hyperreflective columns are a sign of broken RPE, which may open the path for blood, fluid, and neovessels to enter the subretinal space [51].

Prechoroidal clefts appear in eyes with chronic fibrovascular and multilayered PED as hyporeflective cavities between the choroid and the fibrous component of the PED. They usually have a spindle shape and are surrounded by hyperreflective lamella with contractile properties. The exudation and contraction of the sub-RPE neovascular membrane cause delamination of the RPE—Bruch's membrane complex and of the choroid. These eyes maintain good visual acuity because the lesion is located under the RPE and responds to anti-VEGF therapy [52]. Another explanation for the preservation of relatively good visual function is the possible nutritional effect of the sub-RPE complex on the outer retinal layers, thus protecting the retina from geographic atrophy [53]. Due to its morphology, the prechoroidal cleft is associated with a lower risk of developing RPE tears.

In AMD, the choroidal caverns may be associated with neovascular membranes or geographic atrophy. They appear as hyporeflective sub-RPE structures visible on en-face and cress-sectional OCT. They are thought to be either non-perfused ghost vessels at the site of a previous neovascular membrane or lipid-rich Friedman globules, and do not require treatment [54,55].

The influence of subfoveal choroidal thickness and choroidal volume on visual prognosis and treatment outcomes is still under debate. Choroidal thickness can be assessed by swept-source OCT, and it is influenced by circadian rhythm, injected anti-VEGF drug volume, and systemic pressure [56].

However, choroidal hypoperfusion is considered a risk factor for the development of AMD. Several studies have reported a reduction in the choroidal vascular index in relation to the progression of AMD lesions toward neovascular membranes [57].

The choroidal vascular index is defined as the area of the choroidal vascular lumen within the area of the choroidal stroma. A reduction in this index correlates with choroidal hypoxia [58].

4. Signs of Choroidal Neovascular Membrane Reactivation

Despite a good response to therapy and achievement of disease stability, a significant number of cases reactivate over a variable period of time. After following the T and E protocol, the risk of reactivation was higher when the interval between injections was longer. One-fifth of the patients that were treated at 16 weeks intervals suffered from recurrence of symptoms [59].

New signs of CNV activity include recurrence or increased amount of SRF and/or IRF, subretinal hemorrhage, new CNV, or pigmentary epithelium detachment that was not present in previous examinations. These cases need to be treated immediately either by reducing the interval between injections by 2–4 weeks or by beginning a new loading phase with 3 monthly injections, depending on the gravity of lesions observed on OCT. Switching between anti-VEGF agents may also be an option [17].

5. Non-Responsive Cases

Non-responsiveness to treatment is usually associated with subretinal fibrosis present in the final stage of the disease or the development of atrophic changes in the retinal pigmentary epithelium (RPE) and the photoreceptor layer.

The reduced therapeutic effect from the outset may be due to a diagnostic error, most likely due to confusion between CNV and polypoidal choroidal vasculopathy or retinal angiomatous proliferation. The involvement of VEGF in the pathogenesis of polypoidal choroidal vasculopathy is less important than in MNV; thus, the response to anti-VEGF therapy is limited. Encouraging morpho-functional results have been obtained with aflibercept treatment [60].

Retinal angiomatous proliferation is considered a type 3 neovascularization with a suboptimal response to anti-VEGF therapy [61].

The pathogenesis of retinal angiomatous proliferation is both ischemic and inflammatory, with multiple growth factors involved in the development of lesions, accounting for the limited response to intravitreal treatment.

Studies based on genetic testing have concluded that there are some genetic variants of MNV that are less responsive to anti-VEGF therapy and more prone to frequent recurrences [62]. Future treatment guidelines might have to take into account an individualized treatment regimen based on genetic variants.

There is a subgroup of patients who show either minimal or no response to therapy from the outset. Morphological assessment of these eyes shows persistence of intraretinal, subretinal, or sub-RPE fluid and sometimes additional hemorrhages. The unresponsiveness of these eyes is due to chronic alterations in the retinal tissue, RPE, and fibrosis. This may also be due to an exudative syndrome other than MNV.

Chronic central serous chorioretinopathy may present with subretinal and sub-RPE fluid and chronic cystoid degeneration of the retinal tissue that is similar to MNV. Polypoidal choroidal vasculopathy (PCV) is part of the neovascular proliferation spectrum, but it has different characteristics from MNV and is usually less responsive to anti-VEGF injections. This pathological entity is part of the pachychoroid spectrum of diseases, which has been shown to respond poorly to intravitreal therapy [63]. Nevertheless, several studies (EVEREST, LAPTOP, PLANET, EPIC) have shown that both functional and morphological results are better when PCV is treated with intravitreal anti-VEGF therapy, either as monotherapy or in combination with photodynamic therapy [64–67].

Neovascular membranes that develop as a result of an inflammatory disease tend to be less responsive to anti-VEGF agents because the VEGF pathway is not the only pathway responsible for the pathogenic process. The use of steroids and immunosuppressive agents may be beneficial in these cases [68].

The development of drug tolerance is another cause of poor treatment response. The inflammatory cells that are located in the neovascular membrane respond to anti-VEGF therapy by upregulating the number of VEGF receptors and the production of VEGF. At the same time, the immune system's response to the drug, and the secretion of neutralizing antibodies, accelerates the clearance of the injected substance from the eye. Both the ANCHOR and MARINA studies described an increase in immunoreactivity to anti-VEGF after the first year of monthly administration of the drug [69,70].

In theory, an increase in the dosage or frequency of administration may overcome poor response to therapy. Several studies, including the HARBOR trial, demonstrated that a higher dose of anti-VEGF does not lead to a better morpho-functional result in all patients [71–73].

The HARBOR study compared outcomes following the administration of either a standard 0.5 mg dose of ranibizumab or a 2 mg dose of the same drug. This study found no statistically significant differences between the two groups in terms of anatomical and functional outcomes in treatment-naïve patients. Two other studies, LAST and SAVE, demonstrated a minor improvement in visual acuity and morphological results at 6 months when treatment-resistant patients were switched from a 0.5 mg dose to a 2 mg dose of ranibizumab [74,75].

Increasing the frequency of administration may also improve morpho-functional outcomes. This is due to the higher levels of anti-VEGF achieved by increasing the frequency of administration compared to increasing the dose. The maximum reduction in the neovascular membrane size was achieved 12 to 18 days after treatment [76].

While twice-monthly dosing may improve immediate morphological outcomes, it may also open the door to more aggressive disease regression with the development of more SRF and IRF and decreased patient compliance [77].

Tachyphylaxis to anti-VEGF agents was considered a possible cause of the lack or insufficient response to therapy despite following a strict protocol. Tachyphylaxis is quantified by assessing the improvement in central retinal thickness and was defined in a recent study as no reduction or worsening of this parameter after at least two monthly injections [78].

Hara et al. observed that tachyphylaxis to anti-VEGF agents was more likely to occur in eyes with neovascular lesions under the RPE than in eyes with occult CNV and polypoidal choroidal vasculopathy but not in eyes with intraretinal edema [78].

One possible approach to tachyphylaxis is to switch anti-VEGF agents to take advantage of the superior binding affinity or pharmacokinetics of another drug [79–81].

Since the introduction of aflibercept, many studies have analyzed outcomes after replacing ranibizumab or bevacizumab with aflibercept [82,83].

Most of these studies reported an improvement in macular morphology but less benefit in visual acuity [84,85].

In some cases, anti-VEGF treatment not only does not bring the expected morpho-functional improvement, but is also accompanied by worsening visual acuity and a higher quantity of subretinal fluid. This is due to the development of an RPE tear, most likely a result of CNV membrane contraction after anti-VEGF therapy. The incidence of RPE tears is approximately one-fifth of cases treated with anti-VEGF agents, which is higher than the number of tears associated with the natural evolution of a CNV membrane [86]. Several risk factors for the development of an RPE tear have been identified, such as a large pigmentary epithelium detachment, both in height and basal diameter, recent, multilobular or fibrovascular pigmentary epithelium detachment, and smaller size of the CNV membrane by comparison to the detachment size [87]. The imminent development of an RPE tear may be indicated by the appearance of wrinkling of the RPE surface visible on OCT examination or radial lines visible on the infrared image. The presence of these signs may be an indication of treatment postponement. After tear development, fluid leakage may be greater due to the absence of the RPE, but the CNV progresses toward fibrosis and, thus, reduction of exudation. Stopping treatment does not appear to offer any benefit, especially if the disease is showing signs of activity. Patients with small tears may experience a small increase in visual acuity if treatment is continued, and patients with large tears may benefit from continued treatment by achieving stabilization and preventing further visual loss [88]. Therapy should be individualized by careful monitoring of these cases. The visual prognosis for these eyes is usually poor, especially if the RPE tear involves the fovea or is associated with subretinal scars or hemorrhage [89].

Another possibility for disease evolution is the sudden onset of massive hemorrhaging under the retina or the RPE. This is most often associated with the rupture of the fragile neo-vessels. Some risk factors include anticoagulant therapy, blood dyscrasias, trauma, Valsalva maneuvers, and more than three months interval between anti-VEGF agent administration [90].

Small hemorrhages may benefit from more frequent anti-VEGF therapy. However, large hemorrhages can be treated by surgical removal of blood but have poor functional prognosis.

The lack of response to anti-VEGF treatment, consisting of persistent exudation after 6 months of monthly treatment, is considered by one expert group to be refractory or treatment-resistant MNV [91]. The same study group classified cases that presented with either recurrence of SRF, IRF, or a new subretinal hemorrhage, despite an initial favorable response to treatment, such as recurrent MNV. Seventy% of patients fall into this category, as they present with a recurrence of symptoms between the first and second years of therapy [92]. Many cases with recurrence of disease tend to have a good response to retreatment, while others develop refractory MNV.

6. Anti-VEGF Therapy Ocular Side Effects

The main event associated with long-term anti-VEGF therapy is geographic atrophy. A five-year follow-up of more than 1000 MNV patients treated with intravitreal injections reported an incidence of 12–17% at one and two years and almost 40% after five years of therapy in eyes that were not previously diagnosed with geographic atrophy [93].

The same conclusion is supported by the HARBOR, SEVEN-UP, and IVAN studies [94–96].

The follow-up period for the SEVEN-UP study was eight years of ranibizumab treatment and reported a 98% incidence of geographic atrophy detected by fundus auto-fluorescence.

Some experimental studies conducted on rat and primate eyes have shown that intravitreal anti-VEGF treatment generates geographic atrophy as a result of the reduced fenestration of the choriocapillaris during treatment [97].

A few risk factors associated with the development of macular atrophy have been identified: lower baseline visual acuity, reticular pseudodrusen, depigmentation, a lower number of anti-VEGF injections, and retinal angiomatous proliferation [98].

In contrast, the presence of SRF alone, without IRF, seems to be a protective factor against the development of macular atrophy [99,100].

A common event associated with intravitreal anti-VEGF therapy is ocular hypertension. In most cases, the increase in ocular pressure is transient and is related to the volume of drug injected. Approximately 10% of patients who follow intravitreal anti-VEGF treatment for a long period develop chronic ocular hypertension. The risk factors include pre-diagnosed glaucoma, a large number of injections, and a high frequency of intravitreal administration [101].

The pathogenic mechanism is reported to be a decrease in the aqueous humor outflow facility due to the inflammatory effects of anti-VEGF agents on the trabecular meshwork and its direct obstruction by drug particles [102].

The less common adverse effects of intravitreal anti-VEGF therapy include exacerbation of macular ischemia, retinal vascular occlusions, anterior optic neuropathy, and tractional retinal detachment [103].

The OCTOPUS and SWIFT studies analyzed the incidence of ocular inflammatory events associated with brolucizumab treatment in naive patients and in patients previously treated with ranibizumab. Brolucizumab therapy was associated with a higher risk of ocular inflammation than other agents, estimated at 10.5% of the treated patients, of which 3.4% presented with either retinal vasculitis or vascular occlusion, besides vitritis [104]. A few other studies have examined the relationship between brolucizumab therapy and ocular inflammation, suggesting that, in some patients, the anti-VEGF agent triggers an autoimmune response. Although the inflammatory response is mild in most eyes, some have experienced significant vision loss [105–108].

7. When to Stop Treatment

Disease stability is the main criterion for stopping treatment. Recent studies have concluded that it is safe to discontinue the T and E protocol when morpho-functional stability is achieved after two or three intravitreal injections administered at 12-to-16-week intervals [109,110].

The disease should then be monitored three to four times per year, and both visual function and macular morphology should be assessed using OCT, angiography, or OCT angiography. Recurrence should be treated with a monthly regimen followed by an extension of the interval of administration. The success rate of anti-VEGF therapy is greatly influenced by the prevention of recurrences, and such a proactive approach to treatment allows better control of the disease, reduces the likelihood of treatment delays, and helps anticipate and plan the next steps in treatment [111].

8. Future Directions in Neovascular AMD

Several studies have used artificial intelligence (AI) to analyze the morphological features of neovascular AMD. Thus, it is possible to predict the evolutionary trend of the disease, risk of exudation, need for therapy, number of intravitreal injections required to achieve stability of the neovascular membrane, visual outcomes obtained with therapy, better choice of treatment, and risk of conversion to geographic atrophy [112–117].

Thus, new biomarkers are likely to emerge, and the future of intravitreal therapy is likely to be greatly aided by AI, which can only be seen as an improvement in case management and reduction in the socioeconomic burden of this disease.

9. Conclusions

As the number of patients affected by neovascular age-related macular degeneration continues to increase, so does the demand for intravitreal anti-VEGF therapy, which, if properly administered, can put significant strain on the ophthalmic healthcare system. A large number of patients benefit from this treatment, which improves the stability of visual acuity. Strict adherence to the chosen protocol of administration ensures a high success rate in most cases, as long as the selection of cases is based on a thorough follow-up of the main biomarkers that guide therapy. Discriminating cases that benefit from therapy from those that should discontinue it could make a great difference in the quality of medical care offered to patients.

Author Contributions: All authors contributed equally to the design of the study and participated in the preparation and reviewing of the manuscript. C.D., R.L.M., M.Z. and D.C.B. contributed to the literature research and analysis and critical interpretation of the data. A.D.M., R.E.I. and D.C.B. conceived the review and revised the manuscript. All authors have read and agreed to the published version of the manuscript.

Funding: This research received no external funding.

Data Availability Statement: The datasets used and/or analyzed during the current study are available from the corresponding author upon reasonable request.

Conflicts of Interest: The authors declare no conflict of interest.

References

1. Wong, W.L.; Su, X.; Li, X.; Cheung, C.M.; Klein, R.; Cheng, C.Y.; Wong, T.Y. Global prevalence of age-related macular degeneration and disease burden projection for 2020 and 2040: A systematic review and meta-analysis. *Lancet Glob. Health* **2014**, *2*, e106–e116. [CrossRef]
2. Rudnicka, A.R.; Jarrar, Z.; Wormald, R.; Cook, D.G.; Fletcher, A.; Owen, C.G. Age and gender variations in age-related macular degeneration prevalence in populations of European ancestry: A meta-analysis. *Ophthalmology* **2012**, *119*, 571–580. [CrossRef]
3. Hobbs, S.D.; Pierce, K. *Wet Age-Related Macular Degeneration (Wet AMD)*; StatPearls: St Petersburg, Russia, 2022.
4. Spilsbury, K.; Garrett, K.L.; Shen, W.Y.; Constable, I.J.; Rakoczy, P.E. Over-expression of vascular endothelial growth factor (VEGF) in the retinal pigment epithelium leads to the development of choroidal neovascularization. *Am. J. Pathol.* **2000**, *157*, 135–144. [CrossRef]
5. Wong, T.Y.; Liew, G.; Mitchell, P. Clinical update: New treatments for age-related macular degeneration. *Lancet* **2007**, *370*, 204–206. [CrossRef]
6. Usui, Y.; Westenskow, P.D.; Kurihara, T.; Aguilar, E.; Sakimoto, S.; Paris, L.P.; Wittgrove, C.; Feitelberg, D.; Friedlander, M.S.; Moreno, S.K.; et al. Neurovascular crosstalk between interneurons and capillaries is required for vision. *J. Clin. Investig.* **2015**, *125*, 2335–2346. [CrossRef]
7. Zhao, T.; Wang, X.; Xu, T.; Xu, X.; Liu, Z. Bevacizumab significantly increases the risks of hypertension and proteinuria in cancer patients: A systematic review and comprehensive meta-analysis. *Oncotarget* **2017**, *8*, 51492–51506. [CrossRef]
8. Spaide, R.F.; Laud, K.; Fine, H.F.; Klancnik, J.M., Jr.; Meyerle, C.B.; Yannuzzi, L.A.; Sorenson, J.; Slakter, J.; Fisher, Y.L.; Cooney, M.J. Intravitreal bevacizumab treatment of choroidal neovascularization secondary to age-related macular degeneration. *Retina* **2006**, *26*, 383–390. [CrossRef]

9. Rosenfeld, P.J.; Moshfeghi, A.A.; Puliafito, C.A. Optical coherence tomography findings after an intravitreal injection of bevacizumab (avastin) for neovascular age-related macular degeneration. *Ophthalmic Surg. Lasers Imaging* **2005**, *36*, 331–335. [CrossRef]
10. Lucentis—Ranibizumab Injection, Solution. DailyMed. Available online: https://dailymed.nlm.nih.gov/dailymed/lookup.cfm?setid=de4e66cc-ca05-4dc9-8262-e00e9b41c36d (accessed on 27 June 2024).
11. Brown, D.M.; Michels, M.; Kaiser, P.K.; Heier, J.S.; Sy, J.P.; Ianchulev, T.; ANCHOR Study Group. Ranibizumab versus verteporfin photodynamic therapy for neovascular age-related macular degeneration: Two-year results of the ANCHOR study. *Ophthalmology* **2009**, *116*, 57–65. [CrossRef]
12. Nguyen, Q.D.; Heier, J.; Brown, D.; Ho, A.; Kaiser, P.; Vitti, R. Randomized, double-masked, active-controlled phase 3 trial of the efficacy and safety of intravitreal VEGF trap-eye in wet AMD: One-year results of the View-1 study. *Investig. Ophthalmol. Vis. Sci.* **2011**, *52*, 3073.
13. Schmidt-Erfurth, U.; Chong, V.; Kirchof, B.; Korobelnik, J.F.; Papp, A.; Anderesi, M.; Groetzbach, G.; Sommerauer, B.; Sandbrink, R.; Ogura, Y. Primary results of an international phase III study using intravitreal VEGF trap-eye compared to ranibizumab in patients with wet AMD (VIEW 2). *Investig. Ophthalmol. Vis. Sci.* **2011**, *52*, 1650.
14. Tadayoni, R.; Sararols, L.; Weissgerber, G.; Verma, R.; Clemens, A.; Holz, F.G. Brolucizumab: A Newly Developed Anti-VEGF Molecule for the Treatment of Neovascular Age-Related Macular Degeneration. *Ophthalmologica* **2021**, *244*, 93–101. [CrossRef]
15. Dugel, P.U.; Koh, A.; Ogura, Y.; Jaffe, G.J.; Schmidt-Erfurth, U.; Brown, D.M.; Gomes, A.V.; Warburton, J.; Weichselberger, A.; Holz, F.G.; et al. HAWK and HARRIER: Phase 3, Multicenter, Randomized, Double-Masked Trials of Brolucizumab for Neovascular Age-Related Macular Degeneration. *Ophthalmology* **2020**, *127*, 72–84. [CrossRef]
16. Khanani, A.M.; Kotecha, A.; Chang, A.; Chen, S.J.; Chen, Y.; Guymer, R.; Heier, J.S.; Holz, F.G.; Iida, T.; Ives, J.A.; et al. TENAYA and LUCERNE Investigators. TENAYA and LUCERNE: Two-Year Results from the Phase 3 Neovascular Age-Related Macular Degeneration Trials of Faricimab with Treat-and-Extend Dosing in Year 2. *Ophthalmology* **2024**, *131*, 914–926. [CrossRef]
17. Ross, A.H.; Downey, L.; Devonport, H.; Gale, R.P.; Kotagiri, A.; Mahmood, S.; Mehta, H.; Narendran, N.; Patel, P.J.; Parmar, N.; et al. Recommendations by a UK expert panel on an aflibercept treat-and-extend pathway for the treatment of neovascular age-related macular degeneration. *Eye* **2020**, *34*, 1825–1834. [CrossRef]
18. Mantel, I. Optimizing the anti-VEGF treatment strategy for neovascular age-related macular degeneration: From clinical trials to real-life requirements. *Transl. Vis. Sci. Technol.* **2015**, *4*, 6. [CrossRef]
19. Bayer. *Study to Gather Information on Safety and Use of High Dose Aflibercept Injection into the Eye in Patients with an Age Related Eye Disorder that Causes Blurred Vision or a Blind Spot Due to Abnormal Blood Vessels that Leak Fluid into the Light Sensitive Lining Inside the Eye (PULSAR)*; Bayer: Leverkusen, Germany, 2019; Clinicaltrials.gov Identifier: NCT04423718.
20. Wykoff, C.C.; Brown, D.M.; Reed, K.; Berliner, A.J.; Gerstenblith, A.T.; Breazna, A.; Abraham, P.; Fein, J.G.; Chu, K.W.; Clark, W.L.; et al. Effect of High-Dose Intravitreal Aflibercept, 8 mg, in Patients With Neovascular Age-Related Macular Degeneration: The Phase 2 CANDELA Randomized Clinical Trial. *JAMA Ophthalmol.* **2023**, *141*, 834–842. [CrossRef]
21. CATT Research Group; Martin, D.F.; Maguire, M.G.; Ying, G.S.; Grunwald, J.E.; Fine, S.L.; Jaffe, G.J. Ranibizumab and bevacizumab for neovascular age-related macular degeneration. *N. Engl. J. Med.* **2011**, *364*, 1897–1908.
22. Guymer, R.H.; Markey, C.M.; McAllister, I.L.; Gillies, M.C.; Hunyor, A.P.; Arnold, J.J.; FLUID Investigators. Tolerating subretinal fluid in neovascular age-related macular degeneration treated with ranibizumab using a treat-and-extend regimen: FLUID study 24-month results. *Ophthalmology* **2019**, *126*, 723–734. [CrossRef]
23. Almuhtaseb, H.; Kanavati, S.; Rufai, S.; Lotery, A.J. One-year real-world outcomes in patients receiving fixed-dosing aflibercept for neovascular age-related macular degeneration. *Eye* **2017**, *31*, 878–883. [CrossRef]
24. Grechenig, C.; Reiter, G.S.; Riedl, S.; Arnold, J.; Guymer, R.; Gerendas, B.S.; Bogunović, H.; Schmidt-Erfurth, U. Impact of Residual Subretinal Fluid Volumes on Treatment Outcomes in a Subretinal Fluid-Tolerant Treat-and-Extend Regimen. *Retina* **2021**, *41*, 2221–2228. [CrossRef]
25. Waldstein, S.M.; Philip, A.M.; Leitner, R.; Simader, C.; Langs, G.; Gerendas, B.S.; Schmidt-Erfurth, U. Correlation of 3-dimensionally quantified intraretinal and subretinal fluid with visual acuity in neovascular age-related macular degeneration. *JAMA Ophthalmol.* **2016**, *134*, 182–190. [CrossRef]
26. Miotto, S.; Zemella, N.; Gusson, E.; Panozzo, G.; Saviano, S.; Scarpa, G.; Boschi, G.; Piermarocchi, S. Morphologic Criteria of Lesion Activity in Neovascular Age-Related Macular Degeneration: A Consensus Article. *J. Ocul. Pharmacol. Ther.* **2018**, *34*, 298–308. [CrossRef]
27. Schmidt-Erfurth, U.; Vogl, W.D.; Jampol, L.M.; Bogunović, H. Application of automated quantification of fluid volumes to anti-VEGF therapy of neovascular age-related macular degeneration. *Ophthalmology* **2020**, *127*, 1211–1219. [CrossRef]
28. Reiter, G.S.; Grechenig, C.; Vogl, W.D.; Guymer, R.H.; Arnold, J.J.; Bogunovic, H.; Schmidt-Erfurth, U. Analysis of fluid volume and its impact on visual acuity in the fluid study as quantified with deep learning. *Retina* **2021**, *41*, 1318–1328. [CrossRef]
29. Jung, J.J.; Freund, K.B. Long-term follow-up of outer retinal tubulation documented by eye-tracked and en face spectral-domain optical coherence tomography. *Arch. Ophthalmol.* **2012**, *130*, 1618–1619. [CrossRef]
30. Zweifel, S.A.; Engelbert, M.; Laud, K.; Margolis, R.; Spaide, R.F.; Freund, K.B. Outer retinal tubulation: A novel optical coherence tomography finding. *Arch. Ophthalmol.* **2009**, *127*, 1596–1602. [CrossRef]
31. Litts, K.M.; Messinger, J.D.; Dellatorre, K.; Yannuzzi, L.A.; Freund, K.B.; Curcio, C.A. Clinicopathological correlation of outer retinal tubulation in age-related macular degeneration. *JAMA Ophthalmol.* **2015**, *133*, 609–612. [CrossRef]

32. Kovacs, A.; Kiss, T.; Rarosi, F.; Somfai, G.M.; Facsko, A.; Degi, R. The effect of ranibizumab and aflibercept treatment on the prevalence of outer retinal tubulation and its influence on retreatment in neovascular age-related macular degeneration. *BMC Ophthalmol.* **2018**, *18*, 298. [CrossRef]
33. Schmidt-Erfurth, U.; Waldstein, S.M.; Deak, G.G.; Kundi, M.; Simader, C. Pigment epithelial detachment followed by retinal cystoid degeneration leads to vision loss in treatment of neovascular age-related macular degeneration. *Ophthalmology* **2015**, *122*, 822–832. [CrossRef]
34. Jaffe, G.J.; Ying, G.S.; Toth, C.A.; Daniel, E.; Grunwald, J.E.; Martin, D.F.; Maguire, M.G. Macular morphology and visual acuity in year five of the comparison of age-related macular degeneration treatments trials. *Ophthalmology* **2019**, *126*, 252–260. [CrossRef] [PubMed]
35. Sarraf, D.; London, N.J.S.; Khurana, R.N.; Dugel, P.U.; Gune, S.; Hill, L.; Tuomi, L. Ranibizumab treatment for pigment epithelial detachment secondary to neovascular age-related macular degeneration: Post hoc analysis of the HARBOR study. *Ophthalmology* **2016**, *123*, 2213–2224. [CrossRef] [PubMed]
36. Riedl, S.; Cooney, L.; Grechenig, C.; Sadeghipour, A.; Pablik, E.; Seaman, J.W., 3rd; Waldstein, S.M.; Schmidt-Erfurth, U. Topographic analysis of photoreceptor loss correlated with disease morphology in neovascular age-related macular degeneration. *Retina* **2020**, *40*, 2148–2157. [CrossRef] [PubMed]
37. Woronkowicz, M.; Lightman, S.; Tomkins-Netzer, O. The prognostic value of total macular external limiting membrane and ellipsoid zone damage for clinical outcome in treatment-resistant neovascular age-related macular degeneration. *Graefe's Arch. Clin. Exp. Ophthalmol.* **2020**, *258*, 2373–2378. [CrossRef]
38. Shin, H.J.; Chung, H.; Kim, H.C. Association between foveal microstructure and visual outcome in age-related macular degeneration. *Retina* **2011**, *31*, 1627–1636. [CrossRef]
39. Coscas, F.; Coscas, G.; Lupidi, M.; Dirani, A.; Srour, M.; Semoun, O.; Français, C.; Souied, E.H. Restoration of outer retinal layers after aflibercept therapy in exudative AMD: Prognostic value. *Investig. Opthalmol. Vis. Sci.* **2015**, *56*, 4129–4134. [CrossRef]
40. Curcio, C.A.; Zanzottera, E.C.; Ach, T.; Balaratnasingam, C.; Freund, K.B. Activated retinal pigment epithelium, an optical coherence tomography biomarker for progression in age-related macular degeneration. *Investig. Ophthalmol. Vis. Sci.* **2017**, *58*, BIO211–BIO226.
41. Coscas, G.; De Benedetto, U.; Coscas, F.; Li Calzi, C.I.; Vismara, S.; Roudot-Thoraval, F.; Bandello, F.; Souied, E. Hyperreflective dots: A new spectral-domain optical coherence tomography entity for follow-up and prognosis in exudative age-related macular degeneration. *Ophthalmologica* **2013**, *229*, 32–37. [CrossRef]
42. Willoughby, A.S.; Ying, G.S.; Toth, C.A.; Maguire, M.G.; Burns, R.E.; Grunwald, J.E.; Daniel, E.; Jaffe, G.J. Subretinal hyperreflective material in the comparison of age-related macular degeneration treatments trials. *Ophthalmology* **2015**, *122*, 1846.e5–1853.e5. [CrossRef]
43. Kawashima, Y.; Hata, M.; Oishi, A.; Ooto, S.; Yamashiro, K.; Tamura, H.; Miyata, M.; Uji, A.; Ueda-Arakawa, N.; Tsujikawa, A. Association of vascular versus avascular subretinal hyperreflective material with aflibercept response in age-related macular degeneration. *Am. J. Ophthalmol.* **2017**, *181*, 61–70. [CrossRef]
44. Kumar, J.B.; Stinnett, S.; Han, J.I.L.; Jaffe, G.J. Correlation of subretinal hyperreflective material morphology and visual acuity in neovascular age-related macular degeneration. *Retina* **2020**, *40*, 845–856. [CrossRef] [PubMed]
45. Ashraf, M.; Souka, A.; Adelman, R.A. Association between the vitreomacular interface and optical coherence tomography characteristics in wet age-related macular degeneration. *Retina* **2017**, *37*, 1738–1745. [CrossRef] [PubMed]
46. Kanadani, T.C.M.; Dos Reis Veloso, C.E.; Dorairaj, S.; Nehemy, M.B. Influence of vitreomacular adhesion on anti-vascular endothelial growth factor treatment for neovascular age-related macular degeneration. *Ophthalmic Res.* **2017**, *58*, 18–26. [CrossRef] [PubMed]
47. Lee, S.J.; Koh, H.J. Effects of vitreomacular adhesion on anti-vascular endothelial growth factor treatment for exudative age-related macular degeneration. *Ophthalmology* **2011**, *118*, 101–110. [CrossRef] [PubMed]
48. Xie, P.; Zheng, X.; Yu, Y.; Ye, X.; Hu, Z.; Yuan, D.; Liu, Q. Vitreomacular adhesion or vitreomacular traction may affect antivascular endothelium growth factor treatment for neovascular age-related macular degeneration. *Br. J. Ophthalmol.* **2017**, *101*, 1003–1010. [CrossRef]
49. Kimura, S.; Morizane, Y.; Toshima, S.; Hosogi, M.; Kumase, F.; Hosokawa, M.; Shiode, Y.; Fujiwara, A.; Shiraga, F. Efficacy of vitrectomy and inner limiting membrane peeling in age-related macular degeneration resistant to anti-vascular endothelial growth factor therapy, with vitreomacular traction or epiretinal membrane. *Graefe's Arch. Clin. Exp. Ophthalmol.* **2016**, *254*, 1731–1736. [CrossRef]
50. Metrangolo, C.; Donati, S.; Mazzola, M.; Fontanel, L.; Messina, W.; D'alterio, G.; Rubino, M.; Radice, P.; Premi, E.; Azzolini, C. OCT Biomarkers in Neovascular Age-Related Macular Degeneration: A Narrative Review. *J. Ophthalmol.* **2021**, *2021*, 9994098. [CrossRef]
51. Padnick-Silver, L.; Weinberg, A.B.; Lafranco, F.P.; Macsai, M.S. Pilot study for the detection of early exudative age-related macular degeneration with optical coherence tomography. *Retina* **2012**, *32*, 1045–1056. [CrossRef]
52. Kim, J.M.; Kang, S.W.; Son, D.Y.; Bae, K. Risk factors and clinical significance of prechoroidal cleft in neovascular age-related macular degeneration. *Retina* **2017**, *37*, 2047–2055. [CrossRef]

53. Dolz-Marco, R.; Glover, J.P.; Gal-Or, O.; Litts, K.M.; Messinger, J.D.; Zhang, Y.; Cozzi, M.; Pellegrini, M.; Freund, K.B.; Staurenghi, G.; et al. Choroidal and sub-retinal pigment epithelium caverns: Multimodal imaging and correspondence with friedman lipid globules. *Ophthalmology* **2018**, *125*, 1287–1301. [CrossRef]
54. Querques, G.; Costanzo, E.; Miere, A.; Capuano, V.; Souied, E.H. Choroidal caverns: A novel optical coherence tomography finding in geographic atrophy. *Investig. Opthalmol. Vis. Sci.* **2016**, *57*, 2578–2582. [CrossRef] [PubMed]
55. Friedman, E.; Smith, T.R. Clinical and pathological study of choroidal lipid globules. *Arch. Ophthalmol.* **1966**, *75*, 334–336. [CrossRef] [PubMed]
56. Singh, S.R.; Vupparaboina, K.K.; Goud, A.; Dansingani, K.K.; Chhablani, J. Choroidal imaging biomarkers. *Surv. Ophthalmol.* **2019**, *64*, 312–333. [CrossRef]
57. Gupta, P.; Ting, D.S.W.; Thakku, S.G.; Wong, T.Y.; Cheng, C.Y.; Wong, E.; Mathur, R.; Wong, D.; Yeo, I.; Gemmy Cheung, C.M. Detailed characterization of choroidal morphologic and vascular features in age-related macular degeneration and polypoidal choroidal vasculopathy. *Retina* **2017**, *37*, 2269–2280. [CrossRef] [PubMed]
58. Agrawal, R.; Gupta, P.; Tan, K.A.; Cheung, C.M.G.; Wong, T.Y.; Cheng, C.Y. Choroidal vascularity index as a measure of vascular status of the choroid: Measurements in healthy eyes from a population-based study. *Sci. Rep.* **2016**, *6*, 21090. [CrossRef]
59. Essex, R.W.; Nguyen, V.; Walton, R.; Arnold, J.J.; McAllister, I.L.; Guymer, R.H.; Morlet, N.; Young, S.; Barthelmes, D.; Gillies, M.C. Treatment patterns and visual outcomes during the maintenance phase of treat-and-extend therapy for age-related macular degeneration. *Ophthalmology* **2016**, *123*, 2393–2400. [CrossRef]
60. Yamamoto, A.; Okada, A.A.; Kano, M.; Koizumi, H.; Saito, M.; Maruko, I.; Sekiryu, T.; Iida, T. One-Year results of intravitreal aflibercept for polypoidal choroidal vasculopathy. *Ophthalmology* **2015**, *122*, 1866–1872. [CrossRef]
61. Hemeida, T.S.; Keane, P.A.; Dustin, L.; Sadda, S.R.; Fawzi, A.A. Long-term visual and anatomical outcomes following anti-VEGF monotherapy for retinal angiomatous proliferation. *Br. J. Ophthalmol.* **2010**, *94*, 701–705. [CrossRef]
62. Abedi, F.; Wickremasinghe, S.; Richardson, A.J.; Islam, A.F.; Guymer, R.H.; Baird, P.N. Genetic influences on the outcome of anti-vascular endothelial growth factor treatment in neovascular age-related macular degeneration. *Ophthalmology* **2013**, *120*, 1641–1648. [CrossRef]
63. Kimk, H.; Lee, S.C.; Kwon, K.Y.; Lee, J.H.; Koh, H.J.; Byeon, S.H.; Kim, S.S.; Kim, M.; Lee, C.S. Subfoveal choroidal thickness as a predictor of treatment response to anti-vascular endothelial growth factor therapy for polypoidal choroidal vasculopathy. *Graefe's Arch. Clin. Exp. Ophthalmol.* **2016**, *254*, 1497–1503.
64. Koh, A.; Lee, W.K.; Chen, L.J.; Chen, S.J.; Hashad, Y.; Kim, H.; Lai, T.Y.; Pilz, S.; Ruamviboonsuk, P.; Tokaji, E.; et al. EVEREST study: Efficacy and safety of verteporfin photodynamic therapy in combination with ranibizumab or alone versus ranibizumab monotherapy in patients with symptomatic macular polypoidal choroidal vasculopathy. *Retina* **2012**, *32*, 1453–1464. [CrossRef] [PubMed]
65. Oishi, A.; Miyamoto, N.; Mandai, M.; Honda, S.; Matsuoka, T.; Oh, H.; Kita, M.; Nagai, T.; Bessho, N.; Uenishi, M.; et al. LAPTOP study: A 24-month trial of verteporfin versus ranibizumab for polypoidal choroidal vasculopathy. *Ophthalmology* **2014**, *121*, 1151–1152. [CrossRef] [PubMed]
66. Won, K.L.; Yuichiro, O.; Tomohiro, I.; Shih-Jen, C.; Tien Yin, W.; Paul, M.; Tatsuro, I.; Eric, Z.; Sergio, L. Efficacy and Safety of Intravitreal Aflibercept in Polypoidal Choroidal Vasculopathy: 12-Month Results of the PLANET Study. *Investig. Ophthalmol. Vis. Sci.* **2017**, *58*, 1199.
67. Kokame, G.T.; Lai, J.C.; Wee, R.; Yanagihara, R.; Shantha, J.G.; Ayabe, J.; Hirai, K. Prospective clinical trial of Intravitreal aflibercept treatment for Polypoidal choroidal vasculopathy with hemorrhage or exudation (EPIC study): 6 month results. *BMC Ophthalmol.* **2016**, *16*, 127. [CrossRef] [PubMed]
68. Gulati, N.; Forooghian, F.; Lieberman, R.; Jabs, D.A. Vascular endothelial growth factor inhibition in uveitis: A systematic review. *Br. J. Ophthalmol.* **2011**, *95*, 162–165. [CrossRef] [PubMed]
69. Brown, D.M.; Kaiser, P.K.; Michels, M.; Soubrane, G.; Heier, J.S.; Kim, R.Y.; Sy, J.P.; Schneider, S. ANCHOR Study Group. Ranibizumab versus verteporfin for neovascular age-related macular degeneration. *N. Engl. J. Med.* **2006**, *355*, 1432–1444. [CrossRef]
70. Rosenfeld, P.J.; Brown, D.M.; Heier, J.S.; Boyer, D.S.; Kaiser, P.K.; Chung, C.Y.; Kim, R.Y. MARINA Study Group. Ranibizumab for neovascular age-related macular degeneration. *N. Engl. J. Med.* **2006**, *355*, 1419–1431. [CrossRef]
71. Busbee, B.G.; Ho, A.C.; Brown, D.M.; Heier, J.S.; Suñer, I.J.; Li, Z.; Rubio, R.G.; Lai, P.; HARBOR Study Group. Twelve-month efficacy and safety of 0.5 mg or 2.0 mg ranibizumab in patients with subfoveal neovascular age-related macular degeneration. *Ophthalmology* **2013**, *120*, 1046–1056. [CrossRef]
72. Forooghian, F.; Cukras, C.; Meyerle, C.B.; Chew, E.Y.; Wong, W.T. Tachyphylaxis after intravitreal bevacizumab for exudative age-related macular degeneration. *Retina* **2009**, *29*, 723–731. [CrossRef]
73. Ho, A.C.; Busbee, B.G.; Regillo, C.D.; Wieland, M.R.; Van Everen, S.A.; Li, Z.; Rubio, R.G.; Lai, P.; HARBOR Study Group. Twenty-four-month efficacy and safety of 0.5 mg or 2.0 mg ranibizumab in patients with subfoveal neovascular age-related macular degeneration. *Ophthalmology* **2014**, *121*, 2181–2192. [CrossRef]
74. Fung, A.T.; Kumar, N.; Vance, S.K.; Slakter, J.S.; Klancnik, J.M.; Spaide, R.S.; Freund, K.B. Pilot study to evaluate the role of high-dose ranibizumab 2.0 mg in the management of neovascular age-related macular degeneration in patients with persistent/recurrent macular fluid <30 days following treatment with intravitreal anti-VEGF therapy (the LAST Study). *Eye* **2012**, *26*, 1181–1187. [PubMed]

75. Brown, D.M.; Chen, E.; Mariani, A.; Major, J.C., Jr. The SAVE Study Group. Super-dose anti-VEGF (SAVE) trial: 2.0 mg intravitreal ranibizumab for recalcitrant neovascular macular degeneration-primary end point. *Ophthalmology* **2013**, *120*, 349–354. [CrossRef] [PubMed]
76. Stewart, M.W.; Rosenfeld, P.J.; Penha, F.M.; Wang, F.; Yehoshua, Z.; Bueno-Lopez, E.; Lopez, P.F. Pharmacokinetic rationale for dosing every 2 weeks versus 4 weeks with intravitreal ranibizumab, bevacizumab, and aflibercept (vascular endothelial growth factor Trap-eye). *Retina* **2012**, *32*, 434–457. [CrossRef] [PubMed]
77. Lumbroso, B.; Rispoli, M.; Savastano, M.C. Longitudinal optical coherence tomography–angiography study of type 2 naive choroidal neovascularization early response after treatment. *Retina* **2015**, *35*, 2242–2251. [CrossRef]
78. Hara, C.; Wakabayashi, T.; Fukushima, Y.; Sayanagi, K.; Kawasaki, R.; Sato, S.; Sakaguchi, H.; Nishida, K. Tachyphylaxis during treatment of exudative age-related macular degeneration with aflibercept. *Graefe's Arch. Clin. Exp. Ophthalmol.* **2019**, *257*, 2559–2569. [CrossRef]
79. Gasperini, J.L.; Fawzi, A.A.; Khondkaryan, A.; Lam, L.; Chong, L.P.; Eliott, D.; Walsh, A.C.; Hwang, J.; Sadda, S.R. Bevacizumab and ranibizumab tachyphylaxis in the treatment of choroidal neovascularisation. *Br. J. Ophthalmol.* **2012**, *96*, 14–20. [CrossRef]
80. Schaal, S.; Kaplan, H.J.; Tezel, T.H. Is there tachyphylaxis to intravitreal anti-vascular endothelial growth factor pharmacotherapy in age-related macular degeneration? *Ophthalmology* **2008**, *115*, 2199–2205. [CrossRef]
81. Lazzeri, S.; Ripandelli, G.; Sartini, M.S.; Parravano, M.; Varano, M.; Nardi, M.; Di Desidero, T.; Orlandi, P.; Bocci, G. Aflibercept administration in neovascular age-related macular degeneration refractory to previous anti-vascular endothelial growth factor drugs: A critical review and new possible approaches to move forward. *Angiogenesis* **2015**, *18*, 397–432. [CrossRef]
82. Yonekawa, Y.; Andreoli, C.; Miller, J.B.; Loewenstein, J.I.; Sobrin, L.; Eliott, D.; Vavvas, D.G.; Miller, J.W.; Kim, I.K. Conversion to aflibercept for chronic refractory or recurrent neovascular age-related macular degeneration. *Am. J. Ophthalmol.* **2013**, *156*, 29–35. [CrossRef]
83. Bakall, B.; Folk, J.C.; Boldt, H.C.; Sohn, E.H.; Stone, E.M.; Russell, S.R.; Mahajan, V.B. Aflibercept therapy for exudative age-related macular degeneration resistant to bevacizumab and ranibizumab. *Am. J. Ophthalmol.* **2013**, *156*, 15–22. [CrossRef]
84. Seguin-Greenstein, S.; Lightman, S.; Tomkins-Netzer, O. A Meta-Analysis of Studies Evaluating Visual and Anatomical Outcomes in Patients with Treatment Resistant Neovascular Age-Related Macular Degeneration following Switching to Treatment with Aflibercept. *J. Ophthalmol.* **2016**, *2016*, 4095852. [CrossRef] [PubMed]
85. Spooner, K.; Hong, T.; Wijeyakumar, W.; Chang, A.A. Switching to aflibercept among patients with treatment-resistant neovascular age-related macular degeneration: A systematic review with meta-analysis. *Clin. Ophthalmol.* **2017**, *11*, 161–177. [CrossRef] [PubMed]
86. Vazquez-Alfageme, C.; Nicholson, L.; Hamilton, R.D.; Patel, P.J. Incidence and long term visual acuit outcomes of retinal pigment eithelium tears after intravitreal anti vascular endothelial growth factor treatment of neovascular age related macular degeneration. *Retina* **2019**, *39*, 664–669. [CrossRef] [PubMed]
87. Mitchell, P.; Rodríguez, F.J.; Joussen, A.M.; Koh, A.; Eter, N.; Wong, D.T.; Korobelnik, J.F.; Okada, A.A. Management of retinal pigment epithelium tear during anti-vascular endothelial growth factor therapy. *Retina* **2021**, *41*, 671–678. [CrossRef]
88. Empeslidis, T.; Vardarinos, A.; Konidaris, V.; Ch'ng, S.W.; Kapoor, B.; Deane, J.; Tsaousis, K.T. Incidence of retinal pigment epithelial tears and associated risk factors after treatment of age-related macular degeneration with intravitreal anti-VEGF injections. *Open Ophthalmol. J.* **2014**, *8*, 101–104. [CrossRef]
89. Gutfleisch, M.; Heimes, B.; Schumacher, M.; Dietzel, M.; Lommatzsch, A.; Bird, A.; Pauleikhoff, D. Long-term visual outcome of pigment epithelial tears in association with anti-VEGF therapy of pigment epithelial detachment in AMD. *Eye* **2011**, *25*, 1181–1186. [CrossRef]
90. Levine, J.P.; Marcus, I.; Sorenson, J.A.; Spaide, R.F.; Cooney, M.J.; Freund, K.B. Macular hemorrhage in neovascular age-related macular degeneration after stabilization with antiangiogenic therapy. *Retina* **2009**, *29*, 1074–1079. [CrossRef]
91. Yang, S.; Zhao, J.; Sun, X. Resistance to anti-VEGF therapy in neovascular age-related macular degeneration: A comprehensive review. *Drug Des. Dev. Ther.* **2016**, *10*, 1857–1867.
92. Kuroda, Y.; Yamashiro, K.; Miyake, M.; Yoshikawa, M.; Nakanishi, H.; Oishi, A.; Tamura, H.; Ooto, S.; Tsujikawa, A.; Yoshimura, N. Factors associated with recurrence of age-related macular degeneration after anti-vascular endothelial growth factor treatment: A retrospective cohort study. *Ophthalmology* **2015**, *122*, 2303–2310. [CrossRef]
93. Grunwald, J.E.; Pistilli, M.; Daniel, E.; Ying, G.S.; Pan, W.; Jaffe, G.J.; Toth, C.A.; Hagstrom, S.A.; Maguire, M.G.; Martin, D.F.; et al. Incidence and growth of geographic atrophy during 5 years of comparison of age-related macular degeneration treatments trials. *Ophthalmology* **2017**, *124*, 97–104. [CrossRef]
94. Sadda, S.R.; Tuomi, L.L.; Ding, B.; Fung, A.E.; Hopkins, J.J. Macular atrophy in the HARBOR study for neovascular age-related macular degeneration. *Ophthalmology* **2018**, *125*, 878–886. [CrossRef] [PubMed]
95. Rofagha, S.; Bhisitkul, R.B.; Boyer, D.S.; Sadda, S.R.; Zhang, K.; SEVEN-UP Study Group. Seven-year outcomes in ranibizumab-treated patients in ANCHOR, MARINA, and HORIZON: A multicenter cohort study (SEVEN-UP). *Ophthalmology* **2013**, *120*, 2292–2299. [CrossRef] [PubMed]
96. Chakravarthy, U.; Harding, S.P.; Rogers, C.A.; Downes, S.M.; Lotery, A.J.; Culliford, L.A.; Reeves, B.C.; IVAN Study Investigators. Alternative treatments to inhibit VEGF in age-related choroidal neovascularisation: 2-year findings of the IVAN randomised controlled trial. *Lancet* **2013**, *382*, 1258–1267. [CrossRef]

97. Peters, S.; Heiduschka, P.; Julien, S.; Ziemssen, F.; Fietz, H.; Bartz-Schmidt, K.U.; Tübingen Bevacizumab Study Group; Schraermeyer, U. Ultrastructural findings in the primate eye after intravitreal injection of bevacizumab. *Am. J. Ophthalmol.* **2007**, *143*, 995–1002. [CrossRef] [PubMed]
98. Usui-Ouchi, A.; Friedlander, M. Anti-VEGF therapy: Higher potency and long-lasting antagonism are not necessarily better. *J. Clin. Investig.* **2019**, *129*, 3032–3034. [CrossRef] [PubMed]
99. Siedlecki, J.; Fischer, C.; Schworm, B.; Kreutzer, T.C.; Luft, N.; Kortuem, K.U.; Schumann, R.G.; Wolf, A.; Priglinger, S.G. Impact of Sub-Retinal Fluid on the Long-Term Incidence of Macular Atrophy in Neovascular Age-related Macular Degeneration under Treat & Extend Anti-Vascular Endothelial Growth Factor Inhibitors. *Sci. Rep.* **2020**, *10*, 8036.
100. Dhrami-Gavazi, E.; Balaratnasingam, C.; Lee, W.; Freund, K.B. Type 1 neovascularization may confer resistance to geographic atrophy amongst eyes treated for neovascular age-related macular degeneration. *Int. J. Retin. Vitr.* **2015**, *1*, 15. [CrossRef]
101. Mantel, I.; Dirani, A.; Zola, M.; Parvin, P.; De Massougnes, S.; Bergin, C. Macular atrophy incidence in anti-vascular endothelial growth factor- treated neovascular age—Related macular degeneration: Risk Factor Evaluation for Individualized Treatment Need of Ranibizumab or Aflibercept According to an Observe-and-Plan Regimen. *Retina* **2019**, *39*, 906–917. [CrossRef]
102. Bracha, P.; Moore, N.A.; Ciulla, T.A.; WuDunn, D.; Cantor, L.B. The acute and chronic effects of intravitreal anti-vascular endothelial growth factor injections on intraocular pressure: A review. *Surv. Ophthalmol.* **2018**, *63*, 281–295. [CrossRef]
103. Falavarjani, K.G.; Nguyen, Q.D. Adverse events and complications associated with intravitreal injection of anti-VEGF agents: A review of literature. *Eye* **2013**, *27*, 787–794. [CrossRef]
104. Bodaghi, B.; Souied, E.H.; Tadayoni, R.; Weber, M.; Ponthieux, A.; Kodjikian, L. Detection and Management of Intraocular Inflammation after Brolucizumab Treatment for Neovascular Age-Related Macular Degeneration. *Ophthalmol. Retin.* **2023**, *7*, 879–891. [CrossRef] [PubMed]
105. Witkin, A.J.; Hahn, P.; Murray, T.G.; Arevalo, J.F.; Blinder, K.J.; Choudhry, N.; Emerson, G.G.; Goldberg, R.A.; Kim, S.J.; Pearlman, J.; et al. Occlusive Retinal Vasculitis Following Intravitreal Brolucizumab. *J. Vitreoretin. Dis.* **2020**, *4*, 269–279. [CrossRef] [PubMed]
106. Kearns, J.D.; Wassmann, P.; Olgac, U.; Fichter, M.; Christen, B.; Rubic-Schneider, T.; Koepke, S.; Cochin de Billy, B.; Ledieu, D.; Andre, C.; et al. A root cause analysis to identify the mechanistic drivers of immunogenicity against the anti-VEGF biotherapeutic brolucizumab. *Sci. Transl. Med.* **2023**, *15*, eabq5068. [CrossRef] [PubMed]
107. Karle, A.C.; Wrobel, M.B.; Koepke, S.; Gutknecht, M.; Gottlieb, S.; Christen, B.; Rubic-Schneider, T.; Pruimboom-Brees, I.; Leber, X.C.; Scharenberg, M.; et al. Anti-brolucizumab immune response as one prerequisite for rare retinal vasculitis/retinal vascular occlusion adverse events. *Sci. Transl. Med.* **2023**, *15*, eabq5241. [CrossRef]
108. Matucci, A.; Nencini, F.; Vivarelli, E.; Bormioli, S.; Maggi, E.; Vultaggio, A. Immunogenicity-unwanted immune responses to biological drugs—Can we predict them? *Expert Rev. Clin. Pharmacol.* **2021**, *14*, 47–53. [CrossRef]
109. Adrean, S.D.; Chaili, S.; Grant, S.; Pirouz, A. Recurrence rate of choroidal neovascularization in neovascular age-related macular degeneration managed with a treat-extend-stop protocol. *Ophthalmol. Retin.* **2018**, *2*, 225–230. [CrossRef]
110. Arendt, P.; Yu, S.; Munk, M.R.; Ebneter, A.; Wolf, S.; Zinkernagel, M.S. Exit strategy in a treat-and-extend regimen for exudative age-related macular degeneration. *Retina* **2019**, *39*, 27–33. [CrossRef]
111. Lanzetta, P.; Loewenstein, A.; The Vision Academy Steering Committee. Fundamental principles of an anti-VEGF treatment regimen: Optimal application of intravitreal anti–vascular endothelial growth factor therapy of macular diseases. *Graefe's Arch. Clin. Exp. Ophthalmol.* **2017**, *255*, 1259–1273. [CrossRef]
112. Banerjee, I.; de Sisternes, L.; Hallak, J.A.; Leng, T.; Osborne, A.; Rosenfeld, P.J.; Gregori, G.; Durbin, M.; Rubin, D. Prediction of age-related macular degeneration disease using a sequential deep learning approach on longitudinal SD-OCT imaging biomarkers. *Sci. Rep.* **2020**, *10*, 15434. [CrossRef]
113. Chandra, R.S.; Ying, G.S. Evaluation of multiple machine learning models for Predicting Number of Anti-VEGF injections in the comparison of AMD Treatment Trials (CATT). *Transl. Vis. Sci. Technol.* **2023**, *12*, 18. [CrossRef]
114. Romo-Bucheli, D.; Erfurth, U.S.; Bogunovic, H. End-to-end Deep Learning Model for Predicting Treatment requirements in Neovascular AMD from longitudinal retinal OCT imaging. *IEEE J. Biomed. Health Inform.* **2020**, *24*, 3456–3465. [CrossRef] [PubMed]
115. Pfau, M.; Sahu, S.; Rupnow, R.A.; Romond, K.; Millet, D.; Holz, F.G.; Schmitz-Valckenberg, S.; Fleckenstein, M.; Lim, J.I.; de Sisternes, L.; et al. Probabilistic forecasting of Anti-VEGF treatment frequency in Neovascular Age-Related Macular Degeneration. *Transl. Vis. Sci. Technol.* **2021**, *10*, 30. [CrossRef] [PubMed]
116. Fu, D.J.; Faes, L.; Wagner, S.K.; Moraes, G.; Chopra, R.; Patel, P.J.; Balaskas, K.; Keenan, T.D.L.; Bachmann, L.M.; Keane, P.A. Predicting Incremental and Future Visual Change in Neovascular Age-Related Macular Degeneration using deep learning. *Ophthalmol. Retin.* **2021**, *5*, 1074–1084. [CrossRef] [PubMed]
117. Balaskas, K.; Glinton, S.; Keenan, T.D.L.; Faes, L.; Liefers, B.; Zhang, G.; Pontikos, N.; Struyven, R.; Wagner, S.K.; McKeown, A.; et al. Prediction of visual function from automatically quantified optical coherence tomography biomarkers in patients with geographic atrophy using machine learning. *Sci. Rep.* **2022**, *12*, 15565. [CrossRef]

life

MDPI

Review

The Co-Occurrence of 22q11.2 Deletion Syndrome and Epithelial Basement Membrane Dystrophy: A Case Report and Review of the Literature

Marta Armentano, Ludovico Alisi, Francesca Giovannetti, Valeria Iannucci, Luca Lucchino, Alice Bruscolini * and Alessandro Lambiase

Department of Sense Organs, Sapienza University of Rome, 00185 Rome, Italy;
marta.armentano@uniroma1.it (M.A.); ludovico.alisi@uniroma1.it (L.A.);
francesca.giovannetti@uniroma1.it (F.G.); valeria.iannucci@uniroma1.it (V.I.); luca.lucchino@uniroma1.it (L.L.);
alessandro.lambiase@uniroma1.it (A.L.)
* Correspondence: alice.bruscolini@uniroma1.it

Abstract: Background: 22q11.2 deletion syndrome (22q11.2DS) is a genetic disorder caused by the deletion of the q11.2 band of chromosome 22. It may affect various systems, including the cardiovascular, immunological, gastrointestinal, endocrine, and neurocognitive systems. Additionally, several ocular manifestations have been described. Results: We report a case of a 34-year-old female diagnosed with 22q11.2DS who presented with visual discomfort and foreign body sensation in both eyes. She had no history of recurrent ocular pain. A comprehensive ophthalmological examination was performed, including anterior segment optical coherence tomography and in vivo confocal microscopy. Overall, the exams revealed bilateral corneal map-like lines, dots, and fingerprint patterns, consistent with a diagnosis of epithelial basement membrane dystrophy (EBMD). In addition to presenting with this novel corneal manifestation for 22q11.2 DS, we review the ocular clinical features of 22q11.2DS in the context of our case. Conclusions: The EBMD may represent a new corneal manifestation associated with 22q11.2 syndrome, although the link between these conditions is unknown. Further research is warranted to investigate potentially shared genetic or molecular pathways to the understanding of the phenotypic variety observed among this rare syndrome.

Keywords: confocal microscopy; DiGeorge syndrome; 22q11.2 deletion syndrome; map-dot-fingerprint dystrophy; ocular rare diseases

1. Introduction

22q11.2 deletion syndrome (22q11.2DS) is the most common microdeletion human disorder, caused by meiotic chromosome rearrangements. This condition affects approximately 1 in 4000 live births, regardless of sex and ethnic background [1,2]. Although 22q11.2DS is an autosomal dominant condition, more than 90% of patients have unaffected parents, resulting from sporadic microdeletions in the q11.2 region of chromosome 22 [1,3]. It is well known that the disease is caused by microdeletions ranging from 0.7 to 3 million base pairs in size, most of the time included between the low copy number repeats (LCRs) A-D. Within this region, over 90 genes are found, with T-box 1 (TBX1) being the most studied [4]. TBX1 is involved in a myriad of developmental pathways, is expressed in all three germ layers, and is responsible for the communications between the three germ layers and the neural crest [5,6]. Many of the physical abnormalities commonly seen in individuals with 22q11.2DS result from issues in the development and functioning of structures originating from the pharyngeal arch system. This includes craniofacial features, the thymus, parathyroid glands, aortic arch, and cardiac outflow tract. These structures are formed from a combination of cells from the three primary germ layers of the embryo (endoderm, mesoderm, and ectoderm) as well as neural crest cells originating from the closing neural tube [4]. Currently, despite the relatively common occurrence of ocular manifestations in 22q11.2DS, there is a significant lack of information about the genetic determinants of such alterations [7].

Clinically, it manifests with extremely varied symptoms, grouped into different phenotypes defined as DiGeorge syndrome, velocardiofacial (Shprintzen) syndrome, and conotruncal anomaly face (Takao) syndrome [8,9]. These disorders present a variable expressivity and heterogeneous presentation. The most common manifestations are congenital cardiovascular disease (74%), predominantly conotruncal heart malformations; facial dysmorphia and palatal dysfunction (69%); immune deficiency, especially thymic hypoplasia (77%); and endocrinopathies (50%), including thyroid dysfunction, hypoparathyroidism with resultant hypocalcemia, and growth hormone deficiency [2,10,11]. Moreover, affected individuals typically exhibit neurodevelopmental and behavioral disorders such as cognitive delay, learning difficulties (70–90%), attention-deficit hyperactivity disorder (ADHD), and schizophrenia [12–15]. The diagnostic suspicion is based on clinical evaluation. In particular, the finding of specific cardiac anomalies, such as Fallot tetralogy; truncus arteriosus; ventricular abnormalities; right aortic arch or interrupted aortic arch, detected by echographic examinations in association with facial; palatal; and vertebral bone dysmorphisms, is very suggestive. The definitive diagnosis is established by genomic analysis to confirm the chromosomal deletion performing fluorescence in situ hybridization (FISH) or Multiplex Ligation-dependent Probe Amplification (MLPA) [16].

2. Case Description

A 34-year-old female diagnosed with 22q11.2DS was referred to our department for an ophthalmologic evaluation in May 2023. She complained of blurred vision and foreign body sensation at the presentation in both eyes. The patient denied any history of eye pain and ocular trauma. The family history was negative for genetic or ophthalmic diseases. The patient was diagnosed with 22q11.2DS following the recognition of ventricular septal defect, for which she underwent surgical repair shortly after birth. The diagnosis was confirmed by FISH. Her medical therapy consisted of bisoprolol for cardiac support. The patient applied no topical eye treatments.

The best corrected visual acuity was 20/40 in the right eye (RE) and 20/20 in the left eye (LE), with a refraction of sph-4 cyl-1 ax 50° and sph-3.5 cyl-1 ax 150°, respectively. Slit lamp biomicroscopy showed the presence of bilateral inferior paracentral corneal lesions, suggestive of map-dot-fingerprint dystrophy (Figure 1). There was no corneal fluorescein staining. Posterior embryotoxon was also observed in both eyes. Additional exams were conducted to better characterize the corneal lesions, including Placido disk-based corneal topography, corneal pachymetry, specular microscopy, anterior segment optical coherence tomography, and in vivo confocal microscopy. Corneal topography was performed using the Sirius Scheimpflug–Placido disk topographer (Sirius, CSO, Firenze, Italy). The analysis of topographic maps showed no pathological alterations compatible with corneal ectasia. Specifically, the Kmax and Kmean values were 49.01 D (RE) and 48.73 D (LE), and 46.66 D (RE) and 46.74 D (LE), respectively. Additionally, no displacement of the thinnest point (490 μm RE and 498 μm LE) was observed, nor was there any correspondence with areas of posterior elevation. The anterior tangential map reveals irregularities in corneal curvature, likely attributable to changes in the epithelial basement membrane complex, leading to tear film instability. Overall, the exam showed no significant alterations, highlighting mild astigmatism in both eyes (Kast RE: −1.52 D; LE: −1.69 D). Central corneal thickness was 494 μm in the right eye and 499 μm in the left eye. The inferior peripheral corneal thickness at 8 mm on the pachymetry map was at the upper limits of normal in the right eye (710 μm RE; 658 μm LE). This finding may partially be attributable to the presence of a thickened basement membrane with an irregular overlying epithelial layer. In addition, specular microscopy (Perseus, CSO, Firenze, Italy) was performed, showing no alterations in the endothelial mosaic and no pathological changes in the endothelial cell density (RE: 2436 cells/mm^2; LE: 2679 cells/mm^2). Anterior segment optical coherence tomography

(RTVue, Optovue Inc., Fremont, CA, USA) revealed small epithelial and subepithelial hyperreflective areas, with a thickening of the epithelial basement membrane and absence of stromal opacities (Figure 1). Both results support the suspicion of EBMD.

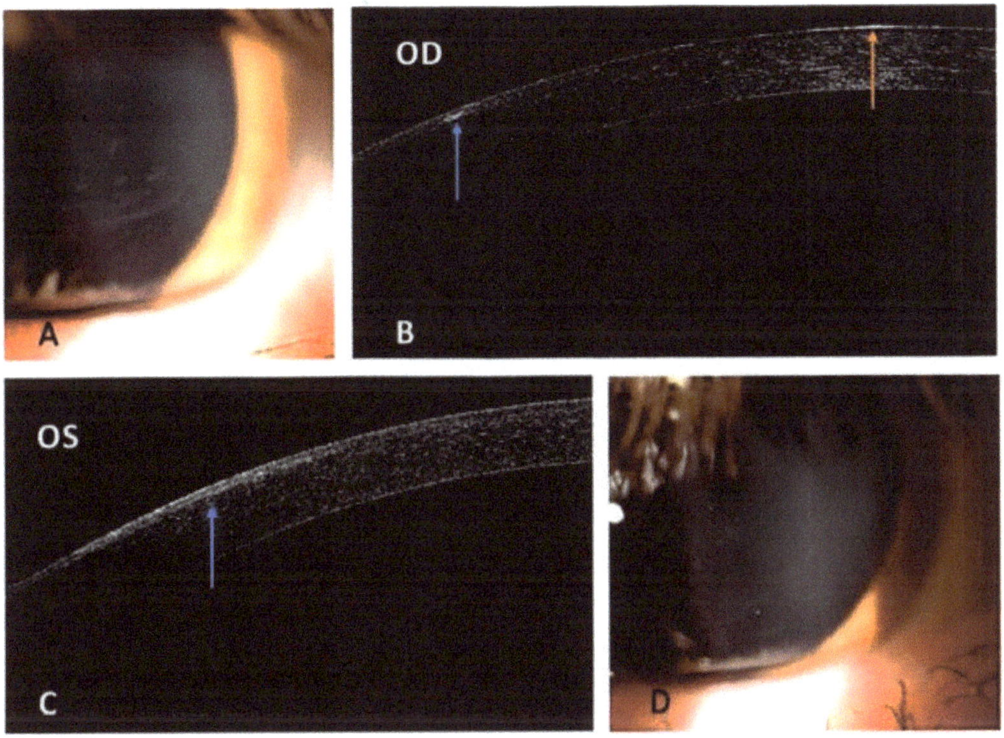

Figure 1. Patient's slit-lamp and anterior segment optical coherence tomography images. (**A**) Slit-lamp photograph of the right eye showing elongated irregular opacities of the corneal epithelium. (**B**,**C**) Anterior segment optical coherence tomography scans of both eyes. The corneal stroma and the underlying layers have a normal aspect. (**B**) Presence of an abnormal spot of the epithelial basement membrane (blue arrow) and an irregular hyperreflective region of the corneal epithelium (orange arrow) in RE. (**C**) Evidence of diffuse thickening of the epithelial basement membrane, resulting in a large highly reflective area (blue arrow) involving the overlying epithelium in LE. (**D**) Slit-lamp photograph of the left eye demonstrating geographic map-like lines surrounding epithelial dots. RE: right eye; LE: left eye.

Moreover, the patient underwent in vivo confocal microscopy (Heidelberg Engineering, Heidelberg, Germany) (Figure 2). Corneal map lines appeared as hyperreflective extracellular material located in the basal epithelium and Bowman's membrane layer. The deposits were variously arranged in linear, rounded, geographic, and multilaminar patterns. Conversely, the fingerprints microscopically correspond to multiple hypo-reflective lines in the epithelium and Bowman's membrane. In the same layers and the anterior stroma, microdots were detected as highly reflective spots. There were no abnormalities in the posterior stroma and the underlying layers.

Finally, a dilated funduscopic examination showed significant bilateral retinal vascular tortuosity and a tilted optic disk (Figure 3). The rest of the fundus oculi was within normal limits.

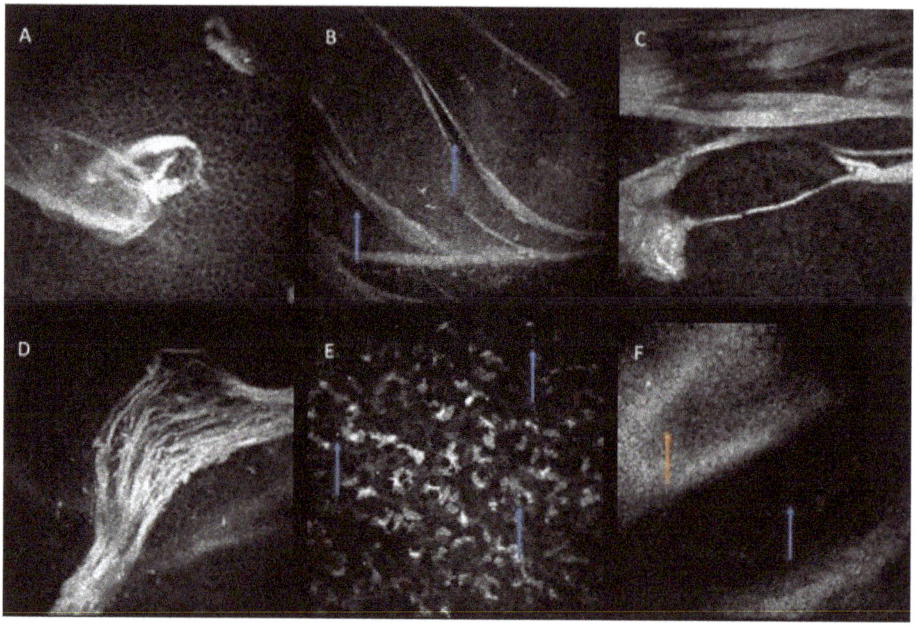

Figure 2. In vivo confocal microscopy images of EBMD-affected corneal layers. (**A**) Irregularly shaped extracellular hyperreflective deposits in the basal epithelium (depth 44 μm). (**B**) Hyporeflective lines (blue arrows) interspersed between highly reflective curvilinear changes in the basal epithelium (depth 46 μm). (**C**) Linear and ring-shaped highly reflective material in the epithelial basement membrane (depth 55 μm). (**D**) Sheetlike deposits in epithelial basement membrane (depth 63 μm). (**E**) Highly reflective microdots (blue arrows) spread in the anterior stroma (depth 82 μm). (**F**) Descemet membrane folds (orange arrow) and hyporeflective striae (blue arrow) in the posterior stroma (depth 465 μm). These findings may represent pressure-induced artifacts and should be distinguished from pathological changes.

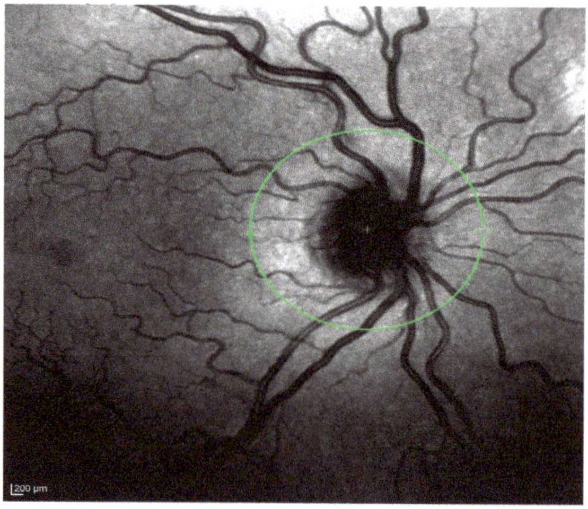

Figure 3. Near-infrared OCT of the posterior pole highlighting marked vascular tortuosity and tilted optic disk.

3. Focus on EBMD

EBMD is the most frequent anterior corneal dystrophy, occurring in about 2–43% of individuals [17]. It is often referred to as map-dot-fingerprint dystrophy, as it typically presents with various combinations of geographic map-like lines, epithelial dots, and subepithelial fingerprints on slit-lamp examination. The map-like lines are represented by irregular, slightly grayish areas flanked by clearer zones, typically arranged around the epithelial dots or Cogan's microcysts. Occasionally, fingerprint patterns are also observed in the same patient [18–20]. The basis of these alterations lies in an abnormal thickening of the Bowman's membrane, which protrudes towards the corneal epithelium, determining the onset of opacities of variable shape and altering the normal desquamation of the epithelial cells, which remain trapped in the corneal layers, forming microcysts [18,21].

EBMD pathophysiology is still unclear. Since its prevalence increases with age, the latest IC3D classification of corneal dystrophies reported that the disease typically results from age-dependent corneal degeneration [22]. Nevertheless, in a minority of cases, a genetic role has been assessed, and some authors suggest a hereditary nature of the condition [23,24]. Recently, *TGFBI* (transforming growth factor b-induced) pathogenic variants have been identified as the cause of several corneal dystrophies, including EBMD. According to Boutboul et al. work, 10% of EBMD patients had *TGFBI* variants [23]. These data were subsequently validated by Evans et al., in which the incidence was 9%, although the mutations were different from those previously known [25]. The multiple TGFBI variants causative of EBMD highlight a genetic heterogeneity of the dystrophy and suggest the need for future research in this field. While the deletion of the 22q11.2 region is probably not causative for EBMD, our patient showed the presence of this genetic entity in both eyes, a first in the literature. The patient's young age strongly indicates genetic etiology, since the epithelial basal membrane linked to degenerative causes is associated with old age. EBMD is associated with the mutation of TGFBI in chromosome 5, but not all the affected patients show the mutation. We can hypothesize that other genetic alterations can be causative for this clinical condition. 22q11.2DS is known to compromise many loci involved in systemic and ocular developmental pathways, and we can hypothesize that some of them can be responsible for EBDM. However, other causative genes for this corneal manifestation need to be identified.

The disease is usually asymptomatic; however, central lesions may lead to corneal astigmatism, resulting in blurred vision and photophobia [26]. Moreover, as the clinical case reported in the present study, up to 30% of patients experience recurrent episodes of ocular pain, foreign body sensation, and tearing, following spontaneous erosions of the corneal epithelium [27,28]. The symptoms are usually exacerbated on awakening due to nocturnal corneal dehydration. For this reason, hypertonic nighttime lubricants, tear substitutes, and/or therapeutic contact lenses may help prevent epithelial damage and reduce daytime symptoms. In addition, Labetoulle et al. proposed the use of topical heparan sulfate mimetic polymer to reduce ocular discomfort in patients with EBMD resistant to conventional symptomatic treatments, with a high success rate [29]. In cases of severe recurrent corneal erosions, epithelial debridement, anterior stromal puncture, and phototherapeutic keratectomy (PTK) is indicated [30–34].

The diagnosis is achieved by a careful slit-lamp examination. Recently, anterior segment optical coherence tomography and in vivo confocal microscopy have shown great usefulness in elucidating the morphologic alterations of EBMD and facilitated its diagnosis, especially in doubtful cases on slit lamp examination [35–37]. In particular, confocal microscopy allows for in vivo visualization of EBMD signs at the cellular level, enabling their differentiation from other similar basement membrane disorders. Except for the microcysts, all the distinguishing EBMD features have been documented in our patient extending the set of corneal manifestations already described in association with this syndrome [36,38,39]. As the genetic mechanisms underlying the dystrophy are still largely unexplained, further research is warranted to investigate a potential molecular basis between the two conditions.

4. Review of the Main Ocular Manifestations in 22q11.2 DS

Different studies and case reports highlighted the association between the 22q11.2DS and ocular pathologies over time even though the knowledge and frequency of eye involvement are still not well established.

4.1. Adnexa, External Eye Structures and Globe Involvement

A wide range of manifestations involving the ocular adnexa are reported in the recent literature on patients affected by 22q11.2DS.

Chandramohan et al. described a case of unilateral inferior orbital mass, responsible for motility abnormalities and eyelid alterations. Magnetic resonance imaging (MRI) was used to better characterize the lesion, which was defined as a congenital colobomatous intraorbital cyst involving the optic nerve and displacing the eyeball. The cystic lesion determined microphthalmia, restricted eye movement, and mechanical ectropion [40].

A single case report described a complete and bilateral lack of the inferior lacrimal ducts in association with the absence of the membranous nasolacrimal ducts in a 5-year-old child presenting 22q11.2DS. The patient underwent a bilateral endoscopic dacryocystorhinostomy. The authors concluded that due to the potential occurrence of the dysgenesis of the nasolacrimal duct in patients with systemic syndromes, symptoms such as mucous discharge or epiphora should be investigated thoroughly [41].

Moreover, cases of eyelid hooding and congenital ptosis have been identified. In 2005 a large study involving 240 patients affected by congenital heart diseases was conducted. The study aimed to collect ocular characteristics in association with cardiac anomalies. Among the cohort, 24 patients with 22q11.2DS were enrolled. The authors detected one case of Duane retraction syndrome and three cases of palpebral ptosis [42]. In another study conducted by Forbes et al. on 90 patients, eyelid hooding and ptosis were the most common findings involving the ocular adnexa. The authors suggested that eyelid hooding contributes to the facial feature of 22q11.2DS despite being present in 20% of the enrolled patients. Another relevant feature reported was a relatively high frequency of strabismus and motility disorders (18% compared to 4% of the general population). The most commonly reported feature was exotropia [43].

Eyelid hooding, narrow palpebral fissures, and floppy eyelids are also described by Gokturk et al. and Mansour AM et al. [42,44,45].

Microphthalmia is frequently described in the literature in association with this genetic condition, with bilateral or unilateral presentation. The reported cases include association with bilateral sclerocornea (one patient-one eye) [46], intraorbital cyst with a large chorioretinal coloboma, and complete chorioretinal coloboma, with visible retrolental persistent fetal vasculature (one patient-bilateral presentation) [40] and contralateral mild sclerocornea, corneal staphyloma, and congenital aphakia (one patient, one eye) [47]. These findings suggest that the genes responsible for anterior segment dysgenesis such as *CRYBB1*, *CRYBB2*, and *CRYBB3*, which are located in 22q11.2, may also influence the development of the whole globe [48].

4.2. Corneal Involvement

Corneal involvement in 22q11.2 DS is quite characteristic and presents multiple expressions. Keratoconus is a corneal ectasia characterized by a progressive thinning and steepening of the corneal stroma, which is commonly localized in the inferotemporal sector, but it can compromise the central region as well [49]. Different authors who described ophthalmological manifestation in 22q11.2 DS identified some cases of keratoconus [50–52].

Sclerocornea is a rare congenital condition presenting with different degrees of corneal opacification proceeding from the limbus to the central cornea. The cause of sclerocornea is attributable to a defective migration of neural crest cells determining a failure in the limbus development [53]. Sclerocornea has been described in patients affected by 22q11.2DS mostly in combination with other dysgenic features involving the anterior segment such as descemetocele, microphthalmia, corneal staphyloma, congenital aphakia, and iridocorneal adhesions [46,47].

Descemetocele is the protrusion of the Descemet membrane through a deep corneal stromal defect [54] and has been described as a single case series by Binenbaum and colleagues in five eyes of 5 patients with 22q11.2DS [46].

Corneal staphyloma is an extremely rare congenital condition encountered among the causes of congenital corneal opacification. This condition manifests with severe anterior corneal protrusion and opacification, often requiring penetrating keratoplasty [55]. Tarlan et al. reported a unilateral case of corneal staphyloma in a 2-year-old child affected by 22q11.2 DS. Fluorescence in situ hybridization analysis showed a heterozygous 250 kb region deletion in the 22q11.2DS critical region 2 [47]. Corneal manifestations are reported in Table 1.

Table 1. Corneal manifestations and relative frequency. The sclerocornea frequency appears higher than expected as Binenbaum et al. only recruited patients affected by sclerocornea [46].

Manifestation	Number of Patients	Author
Keratoconus	1 (case report)	Saffra et al., 2015 [50]
	1 out of 10	Bassett et al., 1998 [51]
	1 out of 128	Midbari et al., 2016 [52]
Sclerocornea	7 (100%)	Binenbaum et al., 2008 [46]
	1 (case report)	Tarlan et al., 2014 [47]
Corneal staphyloma	1 (case report)	Tarlan et al., 2014 [47]
Descemetocele	3 (42.8%)	Binenbaum et al., 2008 [46]

4.3. Anterior Segment Involvement

The most commonly described dysgenetic feature in 22q11.2DS patients is posterior embryotoxon. It manifests with an anterior displacement of the Schwalbe's line and the terminal portion of the Descemet membrane. Glaucoma represents one of the main complications affecting 50% of patients with embryotoxon due to concomitant iridogoniodysgenesis [56,57]. Many clinicians described the presence of posterior embryotoxon in consistent percentages of patients affected by 22q11.2DS. Among them, Mansour et al. identified posterior embryotoxon in 23% of their sample (five patients out of twenty-two) [45]. Casteels and coworkers evaluated 36 children affected by 22q11.2DS, and they identified posterior embryotoxon in 32 eyes [58]. Forbes et al. evaluated 90 patients with confirmed 22q11.2DS and described posterior embryotoxon in 44 cases (49% of the sample) [43]. Gokturk et al. identified posterior embryotoxon in 50% of their sample (eight patients), becoming one of the most diffuse alterations among their group of patients [44].

Aniridia is a congenital dysembryogenic disorder causing various grades of iris hypoplasia. It is usually related to autosomal dominant mutations involving the *PAX6* gene. This pathology can be associated with other ocular findings such as corneal opacification, glaucoma, or cataract [59]. In association with 22q11.2DS, researchers have described isolated cases of aniridia or iris hypoplasia. Moreover, bilateral iridocorneal adhesions or other severe anterior segment dysgenic anomalies such as crystalline lens congenital absence or lens subluxation have been reported [40,44,46,47].

Peters anomaly is a congenital malformation of the eye's anterior segment, resulting from inherited or sporadic mutations in key developmental genes such as PAX6 [60]. Reis et al. described an 8-year-old female with 22q11.2DS who developed glaucoma at birth, alongside the Peters anomaly. Genetic testing revealed a heterozygous variant in the CYP1B1 gene, a common mutation associated with congenital and juvenile glaucoma [61]. Other reports also link Peters anomaly with 22q11.2DS. Erdogan et al. documented a 4-month-old with facial dysmorphism and right eye leukocoria. Slit lamp examination confirmed Peters anomaly and subsequent fluorescent in situ hybridization identified

22q11.2DS [62]. In a study by Casteels et al., one out of thirty-six young patients with 22q11.2DS had Peters anomaly [58]. Another case involved a 3-year-old with unilateral corneal opacity, where Peters anomaly was accompanied by peripheral corneal scleralization. The development of Peters anomaly in these patients is likely due to defective neural crest cell maturation [63]. Other particular features involving the iris within the framework of this pathology are iris coloboma, prominent iris processes, prominent iris crypts, iris remnants, and iris nodules [43–45,58]. Isolated congenital cataracts or lens opacities have also been described in a few papers [45,64]. Table 2 describes the alterations of the anterior segment most frequently associated with 22q11.2DS.

Table 2. Anterior segment manifestations and relative frequency. * The number expresses eyes, not patients.

Manifestation	Number of Patients	Author
Posterior embryotoxon	44 (49%)	Forbes et al., 2007 [43]
	8 (50%)	Gokturk et al., 2016 [44]
	5 (23%)	Mansour et al., 1987 [45]
	32 (44%) *	Casteels et al., 2008 [58]
Peters anomaly	1 (out of 36)	Casteels et al., 2008 [58]
	3 (case reports)	Reis et al., 2015 [61]; Erdogan et al., 2008 [62]; Casteels et al., 2005 [63]
Aniridia	1 (case report)	Chandramohan et al., 2021 [40]
Lens subluxation	1 (case report)	Chandramohan et al., 2021 [40]
Congenital aphakia	1 (case report)	Tarlan et al., 2014 [47]
Cataract	1 out of 22	Mansour et al., 1987 [45]
	1 (case report)	Allegrini et al., 2017 [64]
	1 out of 36	Casteels et al., 2008 [58]
Iridocorneal adhesions	1 out of 7	Binenbaum et al., 2008 [46]
Severe anterior segment dysgenesis	1 out of 7	Binenbaum et al., 2008 [46]
	2 (case reports)	Erdogan et al., 2008 [62]; Tarlan et al., 2014 [47]

4.4. Posterior Segment Involvement

One of the most frequently reported features involving the posterior segment in this genetic condition is vascular retinal tortuosity also observed in our clinical case. Mansour et al. identified eight cases of retinal tortuosity in a cohort of twenty-two DiGeorge patients, and years later, eleven cases in a sample of twenty-four patients [42,45]. Casteels and coworkers evaluated 36 children affected by 22q11.2DS, and the posterior segment evaluation demonstrated retinal vessel tortuosity in 56 eyes (28 patients) [58]. Saffra et al. presented the case of a 23-year-old male patient affected by 22q11.2DS, and keratoconus, and additionally, the posterior segment examination revealed the presence of a tortuous retinal vascular tree [50]. A large group of 128 patients with 22q11.2DS were enrolled in 2016 by Kufert et al. The patients underwent a full-body clinical evaluation and a psychiatric assessment. The study had the purpose of collecting information about the variety of medical conditions and disorders affecting these patients. The clinicians identified ophthalmological involvement in 30.5% of the sample. They described tortuous retinal vessels in 3.9% of the sample (five patients) [52]. Forbes et al. in their study involving 90 patients with confirmed 22q11.2DS identified tortuous retinal vasculature in 31 subjects (34% of the sample) [43]. Several other works described this vascular anomaly in patients with this genetic condition [44,65,66]. Different optic disk anomalies have been recognized in this genetic condition, particularly optic disk atrophy, optic nerve drusen, and small or tilted optic disk as noted in the patients described above [42–45,60,66].

Chorioretinal coloboma is an ocular malformation occurring during embryogenesis, due to a failure in the closure of the embryonic fissure. This anomaly can develop as a sporadic manifestation with an autosomal dominant inheritance, or it can be familiar with autosomal recessive inheritance more commonly. Chorioretinal colobomas are also described in the context of systemic genetic diseases [67,68].

Many researchers described chorioretinal colobomas in patients with 22q11.2DS syndrome. Chandramohan et al., during the examination of a 4-month patient, identified an extensive chorioretinal coloboma compromising the posterior pole structures in the RE. The left eye (LE) was affected by a complete coloboma involving the retina and choroid. Moreover, the persistence of fetal retrolental vasculature was observed in the LE [40]. Midbari Kufert et al., in a large cohort of one hundred twenty-eight patients, described one case of chorioretinal coloboma [52]. The literature has also described the case report of a child affected by 22q11.2DS, presenting familial exudative vitreoretinopathy (FEVR), in the absence of the pathognomonic mutations *LRP5* and *FZD4* [69]. Many other sporadic alterations of the posterior segment in patients with 22q11.2DS are reported in the literature and summarized in Table 3.

Table 3. Posterior segment manifestations and relative frequency.

Manifestation	Number of Patients	Author
Retinal vascular tortuosity	11 (61%)	Mansour et al., 2005 [42]
	31 (34%)	Forbes et al., 2007 [43]
	9 (56.2%)	Gokturk et al., 2016 [44]
	8 (36.3%)	Mansour et al., 1987 [45]
	4 (case reports)	Saffra et al., 2015 [50]; Kozak et al., 2022 [69]; Allegrini et al., 2017 [64]; De Niro et al., 2013 [65]
	5 (3.9%)	Midbari et al., 2016 [52]
	28 (77.7%)	Casteels et al., 2008 [58]
	8 (80%)	Crewther et al., 1998 [66]
Disk drusen	1 out of 24	Mansour et al., 2005 [42]
	1 (case report)	Allegrini et al., 2017 [64]
Chorioretinal colobomas	1 (case report)	Chandramohan et al., 2021 [40]
	1 out of 128	Midbari et al., 2016 [52]
Retrolental persistent fetal vasculature	1 (case report)	Chandramohan et al., 2021 [40]
Familial exudative vitreoretinopathy	1 (case report)	Gilmour et al., 2009 [69]
Diffuse retinal, vitreous, and papillar hemorrhages with vascular dysplasia	1 (case report)	Kozak et al., 2022 [70]
Retinopathy of prematurity	1 (case report)	Paulus et al., 2013 [71]
Optic disk hypoplasia	6 (33%)	Mansour et al., 2005 [42]
	1 out of 16	Gokturk et al., 2016 [44]
	4 (18%)	Mansour et al., 1987 [45]
	3 (30%)	Crewther et al., 1998 [66]
Tilted optic nerve	1 out of 90	Forbes et al., 2007 [43]
Optic disk swelling	1 (case report)	Girgis et al., 2004 [72]

5. Conclusions

In conclusion, we report the first case of coincident EBMD and 22q11.2DS in a young adult patient. Several papers reported extensive case series of systemic manifestations including ocular features in childhood. However, there is poor evidence of potential new manifestations that may develop in the adult population. It seemed interesting to report this association, which has never been described before in the literature, even though it is not possible to determine if there is a connection between the two conditions. Given that EBMD typically develops between the third and sixth decades of life, it would be suggested that patients with 22q11.2DS undergo regular ocular examinations until adulthood to promptly identify and manage corneal and ocular changes.

Author Contributions: A.B. conceptualization, V.I. methodology, M.A. acquisition of data, M.A., L.A., L.L. and F.G. writing—review and editing, A.L. supervision. All authors have read and agreed to the published version of the manuscript.

Funding: This research received no external funding.

Institutional Review Board Statement: Not applicable.

Informed Consent Statement: Written informed consent was obtained from the patients for publication of these case reports and any accompanying images.

Data Availability Statement: Not applicable.

Conflicts of Interest: The authors declare no conflicts of interest.

References

1. Oskarsdóttir, S.; Vujic, M.; Fasth, A. Incidence and prevalence of the 22q11 deletion syndrome: A population-based study in Western Sweden. *Arch. Dis. Child.* **2004**, *89*, 148–151. [CrossRef] [PubMed]
2. Shprintzen, R.J. Velo-cardio-facial syndrome: 30 Years of study. *Dev. Disabil. Res. Rev.* **2008**, *14*, 3–10. [CrossRef] [PubMed]
3. Driscoll, D.A.; Salvin, J.; Sellinger, B.; Budarf, M.L.; McDonald-McGinn, D.M.; Zackai, E.H.; Emanuel, B.S. Prevalence of 22q11 microdeletions in DiGeorge and velocardiofacial syndromes: Implications for genetic counselling and prenatal diagnosis. *J. Med. Genet.* **1993**, *30*, 813–817. [CrossRef] [PubMed]
4. McDonald-McGinn, D.M.; Sullivan, K.E. Chromosome 22q11.2 deletion syndrome (DiGeorge syndrome/velocardiofacial syndrome). *Medicine* **2011**, *90*, 1–18. [CrossRef] [PubMed]
5. Morrow, B.E.; McDonald-McGinn, D.M.; Emanuel, B.S.; Vermeesch, J.R.; Scambler, P.J. Molecular genetics of 22q11.2 deletion syndrome. *Am. J. Med. Genet. A* **2018**, *176*, 2070–2081. [CrossRef] [PubMed]
6. Papangeli, I.; Scambler, P. The 22q11 deletion: DiGeorge and velocardiofacial syndromes and the role of TBX1. *Wiley Interdiscip. Rev. Dev. Biol.* **2013**, *2*, 393–403. [CrossRef] [PubMed]
7. Funato, N. Craniofacial Phenotypes and Genetics of DiGeorge Syndrome. *J. Dev. Biol.* **2022**, *10*, 18. [CrossRef]
8. Shprintzen, R.J.; Goldberg, R.B.; Lewin, M.L.; Sidoti, E.J.; Berkman, M.D.; Argamaso, R.V.; Young, D. A new syndrome involving cleft palate, cardiac anomalies, typical facies, and learning disabilities: Velo-cardio-facial syndrome. *Cleft. Palate J.* **1978**, *15*, 56–62.
9. Wulfsberg, E.A.; Leana-Cox, J.; Neri, G. What's in a name? Chromosome 22q abnormalities and the DiGeorge, velocardiofacial, and conotruncal anomalies face syndromes. *Am. J. Med. Genet.* **1996**, *65*, 317–319. [CrossRef]
10. McDonald-McGinn, D.M.; Sullivan, K.E.; Marino, B.; Philip, N.; Swillen, A.; Vorstman, J.A.S.; Zackai, E.H.; Emanuel, B.S.; Vermeesch, J.R.; Morrow, B.E.; et al. 22q11.2 deletion syndrome. *Nat. Rev. Dis. Primers* **2015**, *1*, 15071. [CrossRef]
11. Bassett, A.S.; Chow, E.W.C.; Husted, J.; Weksberg, R.; Caluseriu, O.; Webb, G.D.; Gatzoulis, M.A. Clinical features of 78 adults with 22q11 Deletion Syndrome. *Am. J. Med. Genet. A* **2005**, *138*, 307–313. [CrossRef]
12. Murphy, K.C.; Jones, L.A.; Owen, M.J. High rates of schizophrenia in adults with velo-cardio-facial syndrome. *Arch. Gen. Psychiatry* **1999**, *56*, 940–945. [CrossRef] [PubMed]
13. Gothelf, D.; Schaer, M.; Eliez, S. Genes, brain development and psychiatric phenotypes in velo-cardio-facial syndrome. *Dev. Disabil. Res. Rev.* **2008**, *14*, 59–68. [CrossRef] [PubMed]
14. Rizvi, S.; Khan, A.M.; Saeed, H.; Aribara, A.M.; Carrington, A.; Griffiths, A.; Mohit, A. Schizophrenia in DiGeorge Syndrome: A Unique Case Report. *Cureus* **2018**, *10*, e3142. [CrossRef] [PubMed]
15. Schneider, M.; Debbané, M.; Bassett, A.S.; Chow, E.W.C.; Fung, W.L.A.; Bree, M.B.M.v.D.; Owen, M.; Murphy, K.C.; Niarchou, M.; Kates, W.R.; et al. Psychiatric disorders from childhood to adulthood in 22q11.2 deletion syndrome: Results from the International Consortium on Brain and Behavior in 22q11.2 Deletion Syndrome. *Am. J. Psychiatry* **2014**, *171*, 627–639. [CrossRef] [PubMed]
16. Cortés-Martín, J.; Peñuela, N.L.; Sánchez-García, J.C.; Montiel-Troya, M.; Díaz-Rodríguez, L.; Rodríguez-Blanque, R. Deletion Syndrome 22q11.2: A Systematic Review. *Children* **2022**, *9*, 1168. [CrossRef] [PubMed]
17. Werblin, T.P.; Hirst, L.W.; Stark, W.J.; Maumenee, I.H. Prevalence of map-dot-fingerprint changes in the cornea. *Br. J. Ophthalmol.* **1981**, *65*, 401–409. [CrossRef]
18. Cogan, D.G.; Donaldson, D.D.; Kuwabara, T.; Marshall, D. Microcystic Dystrophy of the Corneal Epithelium. *Trans. Am. Ophthalmol. Soc.* **1964**, *62*, 213–225. [PubMed]
19. Guerry, D. Observations on Cogan's microcystic dystrophy of the corneal epithelium. *Trans. Am. Ophthalmol. Soc.* **1965**, *63*, 320–334.

20. Trobe, J.D.; Laibson, P.R. Dystrophic changes in the anterior cornea. *Arch. Ophthalmol.* **1972**, *87*, 378–382. [CrossRef]
21. Rodrigues, M.M.; Fine, B.S.; Laibson, P.R.; Zimmerman, L.E. Disorders of the corneal epithelium. A clinicopathologic study of dot, geographic, and fingerprint patterns. *Arch. Ophthalmol.* **1974**, *92*, 475–482. [CrossRef] [PubMed]
22. Møller, H.U.; Weiss, J.S. IC3D classification of corneal dystrophies. *Dev. Ophthalmol.* **2011**, *48*, 1–8. [CrossRef] [PubMed]
23. Boutboul, S.; Black, G.C.M.; Moore, J.E.; Sinton, J.; Menasche, M.; Munier, F.L.; Laroche, L.; Abitbol, M.; Schorderet, D.F. A subset of patients with epithelial basement membrane corneal dystrophy have mutations in TGFBI/BIGH3. *Hum. Mutat.* **2006**, *27*, 553–557. [CrossRef] [PubMed]
24. Laibson, P.R.; Krachmer, J.H. Familial occurrence of dot (microcystic), map, fingerprint dystrophy of the cornea. *Investig. Ophthalmol.* **1975**, *14*, 397–399.
25. Evans, C.J.; Davidson, A.E.; Carnt, N.; López, K.E.R.; Veli, N.; Thaung, C.M.; Tuft, S.J.; Hardcastle, A.J. Genotype-Phenotype Correlation for TGFBI Corneal Dystrophies Identifies p.(G623D) as a Novel Cause of Epithelial Basement Membrane Dystrophy. *Investig. Ophthalmol. Vis. Sci.* **2016**, *57*, 5407–5414. [CrossRef] [PubMed]
26. Ehlers, N.; Møller, H.U. Dot-map-fingerprint dystrophy--Cogan's microcystic dystrophy--normal reactions of the corneal epithelium? *Acta Ophthalmol.* **1987**, *182*, 62–66. [CrossRef] [PubMed]
27. Laibson, P.R. Recurrent corneal erosions and epithelial basement membrane dystrophy. *Eye Contact Lens* **2010**, *36*, 315–317. [CrossRef]
28. Hykin, P.G.; Foss, A.E.; Pavesio, C.; Dart, J.K. The natural history and management of recurrent corneal erosion: A prospective randomised trial. *Eye* **1994**, *8 Pt 1*, 35–40. [CrossRef] [PubMed]
29. Labetoulle, M.; Rousseau, A.; M'Garrech, M.; Kaswin, G.; Dupas, B.; Baudouin, C.; Barreau, E.; Bourcier, T.; Chiambaretta, F. Efficacy of a Topical Heparan Sulfate Mimetic Polymer on Ocular Surface Discomfort in Patients with Cogan's Epithelial Basement Membrane Dystrophy. *J. Ocul. Pharmacol. Ther.* **2019**, *35*, 359–365. [CrossRef]
30. Orndahl, M.J.; Fagerholm, P.P. Phototherapeutic keratectomy for map-dot-fingerprint corneal dystrophy. *Cornea* **1998**, *17*, 595–599. [CrossRef]
31. Lee, W.S.; Lam, C.K.; Manche, E.E. Phototherapeutic keratectomy for epithelial basement membrane dystrophy. *Clin. Ophthalmol.* **2017**, *11*, 15–22. [CrossRef]
32. McLean, E.N.; MacRae, S.M.; Rich, L.F. Recurrent erosion. Treatment by anterior stromal puncture. *Ophthalmology* **1986**, *93*, 784–788. [CrossRef]
33. Pogorelov, P.; Langenbucher, A.; Kruse, F.; Seitz, B. Long-term results of phototherapeutic keratectomy for corneal map-dot-fingerprint dystrophy (Cogan-Guerry). *Cornea* **2006**, *25*, 774–777. [CrossRef]
34. Vo, R.C.; Chen, J.L.; Sanchez, P.J.; Yu, F.; Aldave, A.J. Long-Term Outcomes of Epithelial Debridement and Diamond Burr Polishing for Corneal Epithelial Irregularity and Recurrent Corneal Erosion. *Cornea* **2015**, *34*, 1259–1265. [CrossRef]
35. Ramos, J.L.B.; Li, Y.; Huang, D. Clinical and research applications of anterior segment optical coherence tomography—A review. *Clin Exp. Ophthalmol.* **2009**, *37*, 81–89. [CrossRef]
36. Hernández-Quintela, E.; Mayer, F.; Dighiero, P.; Briat, B.; Savoldelli, M.; Legeais, J.-M.; Renard, G. Confocal microscopy of cystic disorders of the corneal epithelium. *Ophthalmology* **1998**, *105*, 631–636. [CrossRef]
37. El Sanharawi, M.; Sandali, O.; Basli, E.; Bouheraoua, N.; Ameline, B.; Goemaere, I.; Georgeon, C.; Hamiche, T.; Borderie, V.; Laroche, L. Fourier-domain optical coherence tomography imaging in corneal epithelial basement membrane dystrophy: A structural analysis. *Am. J. Ophthalmol.* **2015**, *159*, 755–763. [CrossRef]
38. Rosenberg, M.E.; Tervo, T.M.; Petroll, W.M.; Vesaluoma, M.H. In vivo confocal microscopy of patients with corneal recurrent erosion syndrome or epithelial basement membrane dystrophy. *Ophthalmology* **2000**, *107*, 565–573. [CrossRef] [PubMed]
39. Kobayashi, A.; Yokogawa, H.; Sugiyama, K. In vivo laser confocal microscopy findings in patients with map-dot-fingerprint (epithelial basement membrane) dystrophy. *Clin. Ophthalmol.* **2012**, *6*, 1187–1190. [CrossRef] [PubMed]
40. Chandramohan, A.; Sears, C.M.; Huang, L.C.; Beres, S.; Fredrick, D.; Kossler, A.L. Microphthalmia and orbital cysts in DiGeorge syndrome. *J. AAPOS* **2021**, *25*, 358–360. [CrossRef] [PubMed]
41. Prabhakaran, V.C.; Davis, G.; Wormald, P.J.; Selva, D. Congenital absence of the nasolacrimal duct in velocardiofacial syndrome. *J. AAPOS* **2008**, *12*, 85–86. [CrossRef] [PubMed]
42. Mansour, A.M.; Bitar, F.F.; Traboulsi, E.I.; Kassak, K.M.; Obeid, M.Y.; Megarbane, A.; I Salti, H. Ocular pathology in congenital heart disease. *Eye* **2005**, *19*, 29–34. [CrossRef] [PubMed]
43. Forbes, B.J.; Binenbaum, G.; Edmond, J.C.; DeLarato, N.; McDonald-McGinn, D.M.; Zackai, E.H. Ocular findings in the chromosome 22q11.2 deletion syndrome. *J. AAPOS* **2007**, *11*, 179–182. [CrossRef]
44. Gokturk, B.; Topcu-Yilmaz, P.; Bozkurt, B.; Yildirim, M.S.; Guner, S.N.; Sayar, E.H.; Reisli, I. Ocular Findings in Children With 22q11.2 Deletion Syndrome. *J. Pediatr. Ophthalmol. Strabismus* **2016**, *53*, 218–222. [CrossRef] [PubMed]
45. Mansour, A.M.; Goldberg, R.B.; Wang, F.M.; Shprintzen, R.J. Ocular findings in the velo-cardio-facial syndrome. *J. Pediatr. Ophthalmol. Strabismus* **1987**, *24*, 263–266. [CrossRef]
46. Binenbaum, G.; McDonald-McGinn, D.M.; Zackai, E.H.; Walker, B.M.; Coleman, K.; Mach, A.M.; Adam, M.; Manning, M.; Alcorn, D.M.; Zabel, C.; et al. Sclerocornea associated with the chromosome 22q11.2 deletion syndrome. *Am. J. Med. Genet. A* **2008**, *146A*, 904–909. [CrossRef]
47. Tarlan, B.; Kiratli, H.; Kılıç, E.; Utine, E.; Boduroğlu, K. A case of 22q11.2 deletion syndrome with right microphthalmia and left corneal staphyloma. *Ophthalmic Genet.* **2014**, *35*, 248–251. [CrossRef]

48. Mataftsi, A.; Islam, L.; Kelberman, D.; Sowden, J.C.; Nischal, K.K. Chromosome abnormalities and the genetics of congenital corneal opacification. *Mol. Vis.* **2011**, *17*, 1624–1640.
49. Santodomingo-Rubido, J.; Carracedo, G.; Suzaki, A.; Villa-Collar, C.; Vincent, S.J.; Wolffsohn, J.S. Keratoconus: An updated review. *Cont. Lens Anterior. Eye* **2022**, *45*, 101559. [CrossRef]
50. Saffra, N.; Reinherz, B. Keratoconus in an adult with 22q11.2 deletion syndrome. *BMJ Case Rep.* **2015**, *2015*, bcr2014203737. [CrossRef]
51. Bassett, A.S.; Hodgkinson, K.; Chow, E.W.; Correia, S.; Scutt, L.E.; Weksberg, R. 22q11 deletion syndrome in adults with schizophrenia. *Am. J. Med. Genet.* **1998**, *81*, 328–337. [CrossRef]
52. Midbari Kufert, Y.; Nachmani, A.; Nativ, E.; Weizman, A.; Gothelf, D. Association between prematurity and the evolution of psychotic disorders in 22q11.2 deletion syndrome. *J. Neural Transm.* **2016**, *123*, 1491–1497. [CrossRef]
53. Quiroz-Casian, N.; Chacon-Camacho, O.F.; Barragan-Arevalo, T.; Nava-Valdez, J.; Lieberman, E.; Salgado-Medina, A.; Navas, A.; Graue-Hernandez, E.O.; Zenteno, J.C. Sclerocornea-Microphthalmia-Aphakia Complex: Description of Two Additional Cases Associated With Novel FOXE3 Mutations and Review of the Literature. *Cornea* **2018**, *37*, 1178–1181. [CrossRef]
54. Agarwal, R.; Nagpal, R.; Todi, V.; Sharma, N. Descemetocele. *Surv. Ophthalmol.* **2021**, *66*, 2–19. [CrossRef]
55. Wan, Y.; Xiao, G.; Yu, T.; Zhang, P.; Hong, J. Histopathological examination of congenital corneal staphyloma and prognosis after penetrating keratoplasty. *Medicine* **2020**, *99*, e21892. [CrossRef]
56. Rennie, C.A.; Chowdhury, S.; Khan, J.; Rajan, F.; Jordan, K.; Lamb, R.J.; Vivian, A.J. The prevalence and associated features of posterior embryotoxon in the general ophthalmic clinic. *Eye* **2005**, *19*, 396–399. [CrossRef]
57. Michels, K.; Bohnsack, B.L. Ophthalmological Manifestations of Axenfeld-Rieger Syndrome: Current Perspectives. *Clin. Ophthalmol.* **2023**, *17*, 819–828. [CrossRef]
58. Casteels, I.; Casaer, P.; Gewillig, M.; Swillen, A.; Devriendt, K. Ocular findings in children with a microdeletion in chromosome 22q11.2. *Eur. J. Pediatr.* **2008**, *167*, 751–755. [CrossRef]
59. Landsend, E.C.S.; Lagali, N.; Utheim, T.P. Congenital aniridia—A comprehensive review of clinical features and therapeutic approaches. *Surv. Ophthalmol.* **2021**, *66*, 1031–1050. [CrossRef]
60. Bhandari, R.; Ferri, S.; Whittaker, B.; Liu, M.; Lazzaro, D.R. Peters anomaly: Review of the literature. *Cornea* **2011**, *30*, 939–944. [CrossRef]
61. Reis, L.M.; Tyler, R.C.; Zori, R.; Burgess, J.; Mueller, J.; Semina, E.V. A case of 22q11.2 deletion syndrome with Peters anomaly, congenital glaucoma, and heterozygous mutation in CYP1B1. *Ophthalmic Genet.* **2015**, *36*, 92–94. [CrossRef] [PubMed]
62. Erdoğan, M.K.; Utine, G.E.; Alanay, Y.; Aktaş, D. Unilateral Peters' anomaly in an infant with 22q11.2 deletion syndrome. *Clin. Dysmorphol.* **2008**, *17*, 289–290. [CrossRef] [PubMed]
63. Casteels, I.; Devriendt, K. Unilateral Peters' anomaly in a patient with DiGeorge syndrome. *J. Pediatr. Ophthalmol. Strabismus* **2005**, *42*, 311–313. [CrossRef] [PubMed]
64. Allegrini, D.; Penco, S.; Pece, A.; Autelitano, A.; Montesano, G.; Paci, S.; Montanari, C.; Maver, A.; Peterlin, B.; Damante, G. Cataract and optic disk drusen in a patient with glycogenosis and di George syndrome: Clinical and molecular report. *BMC Ophthalmol.* **2017**, *17*, 107. [CrossRef] [PubMed]
65. De Niro, J.E.; Randhawa, S.; McDonald, H.R. Retinal vascular tortuosity in DiGeorge syndrome complicated by solar retinopathy. *Retin Cases Brief Rep.* **2013**, *7*, 343–346. [CrossRef] [PubMed]
66. Crewther, S.G.; Kiely, P.M.; Kok, L.L.; Crewther, D.P. Anomalies of genetic development as predictors of oculo-visual abnormalities in velo-cardio-facial syndrome. *Optom. Vis. Sci.* **1998**, *75*, 748–757. [CrossRef] [PubMed]
67. Uhumwangho, O.M.; Jalali, S. Chorioretinal coloboma in a paediatric population. *Eye* **2014**, *28*, 728–733. [CrossRef] [PubMed]
68. Pagon, R.A. Ocular coloboma. *Surv. Ophthalmol.* **1981**, *25*, 223–236. [CrossRef]
69. Gilmour, D.F.; Downey, L.M.; Sheridan, E.; Long, V.; Bradbury, J.; Inglehearn, C.F.; Toomes, C. Familial exudative vitreoretinopathy and DiGeorge syndrome: A new locus for familial exudative vitreoretinopathy on chromosome 22q11.2? *Ophthalmology* **2009**, *116*, 1522–1524. [CrossRef]
70. Kozak, I.; Ali, S.A.; Wu, W.C. Novel retinal observations in a child with DiGeorge (22q11.2 deletion) syndrome. *Am. J. Ophthalmol. Case Rep.* **2022**, *27*, 101608. [CrossRef]
71. Paulus, Y.M.; Moshfeghi, D.M. Persistent plus disease after laser in retinopathy of prematurity with tetralogy of Fallot. *Eur. J. Ophthalmol.* **2013**, *23*, 764–766. [CrossRef]
72. Girgis, R.a.M.; McKee, H.D.R.; Innes, J.R. Swollen optic discs in a patient with the chromosome 22q11.2 deletion syndrome. *Br. J. Ophthalmol.* **2004**, *88*, 591–592. [CrossRef] [PubMed]

life

MDPI

Review

Vernal Keratoconjunctivitis: Immunopathological Insights and Therapeutic Applications of Immunomodulators

Navpreet K. Hehar * and DeGaulle I. Chigbu

Pennsylvania College of Optometry, Salus University, Elkins Park, PA 19027, USA; dchigbu@salus.edu
* Correspondence: nhehar@salus.edu

Abstract: Vernal keratoconjunctivitis (VKC) is a complex and multifactorial disease process that employs Th2 cell-mediated immunologic processes, which involves the overexpression of interleukin 4 (IL-4), IL-5, IL-9, IL-13, and IL-31, and the activation of mast cells that release IL-5 and CCL-11, recruiting eosinophils to the site of inflammation. The disease primarily affects young males and is more common in regions with warm climates. VKC is characterized by persistent and recurrent conjunctival inflammation that can adversely affect the patient's quality of life, and, when inadequately treated, may lead to a host of ocular complications, such as corneal shield ulcers and scarring. The major distinct forms of VKC include limbal or palpebral, which may occur in combination. The clinicopathological features of VKC include the presence of pseudogerontoxon, limbal gelatinous hyperplasia, and perilimbal hyperpigmentation. Topical immunomodulators are effective anti-steroidal options for controlling severe and chronic cases of VKC. This review will provide a brief overview of topical immunomodulators, including cyclosporin and tacrolimus, and will highlight the clinical manifestations, pathological mechanisms, and fibroproliferative changes in the conjunctiva that can result from recurrent disease.

Keywords: Th2 cells; IL-4; IL-5; IL-13; vernal keratoconjunctivitis; immunomodulators; cyclosporine A (CsA); tacrolimus

1. Introduction

Vernal keratoconjunctivitis (VKC) is a chronic, and potentially severe, allergic inflammatory disease that affects the ocular surface [1–3]. Although the name "vernal" implies a seasonal pattern, with repeated bouts of inflammation occurring during warm seasons, VKC becomes perennial in approximately 25% of patients who experience symptoms throughout the year [1]. VKC is classified into three distinct categories based on the ocular area that is predominantly affected: namely, either limbal, palpebral, or a mixed form of VKC [1,4,5]. The palpebral form of VKC is characterized by the presence of giant papillae on the upper tarsal lid, while the limbal form is characterized by the presence of gelatinous limbal infiltrates, and Trantas dots [6]. Transient yellow-white deposits with an opaque appearance may be present in limbal VKC and are termed Horner–Trantas dots [1,7]. Histological examination reveals epithelial cell debris with dense infiltration of eosinophils [1,8,9]. In the mixed form, both the upper tarsal lid and limbus are involved. The etiology of this condition is considered to be a combination of type I and type IV hypersensitivity reactions that are characterized by an overexpression of mast cells, eosinophils, Th2 cells, cytokines, and chemokines, which play a significant inflammatory role [1,4,5]. This inflammatory cascade contributes to the characteristic symptoms and ocular surface changes seen in VKC, which include intense pruritis, redness, photophobia, ropy mucus discharge, and foreign-body sensations [1]. Pathognomonic signs of VKC include the presence of yellow-white limbal deposits, known as Horner–Trantas dots, cobblestone giant papillae of the upper tarsal lids, and shield ulcers [1,6]. Additional ocular signs observed in patients with VKC include perilimbal conjunctival pigmentation, punctate epithelial keratitis, and pseudogerontoxon [1,6].

Management of VKC involves a combination of topical therapy including mast cell stabilizers, antihistamines, NSAIDs, corticosteroids, or immunomodulators [4,5,9]. Immunomodulators have been used in clinical practice since 1959 [10]. The utilization of these agents is prevalent in ophthalmic care for addressing a spectrum of ocular conditions including dry eye disease [11,12], allergic conjunctivitis [13], non-infectious uveitis [14,15], and other recalcitrant ocular surface diseases [16]. Immunomodulator therapy offers new therapeutic options in the management of chronic inflammatory conditions as they are steroid-sparing agents. Topical immunomodulators are well tolerated, have a better safety profile, and play a crucial role in the management of moderate to severe allergic eye disease.

This paper will review the disease process of VKC, including the clinicopathological features of VKC, and discuss the anti-inflammatory and immunomodulatory agents that can be used to treat moderate, severe, or recurrent forms of the disease. While VKC is typically not sight-threatening, its impact on the patient's quality of life can be substantial. Understanding its clinical features, underlying mechanisms, and appropriate treatment strategies is crucial in order to provide symptomatic relief and prevent serious ocular sequelae.

2. Epidemiology of VKC

VKC is characterized by persistent allergic inflammation that affects the conjunctiva and culminates in acute symptoms, including intense pruritis and ropy mucus discharge. Patients may also complain of ocular irritation, photophobia, foreign-body sensations, and excessive tearing. The epidemiology of VKC reveals certain patterns regarding its demographic distribution and its prevalence. VKC has an extreme geographical distribution but is more prevalent in regions with warm and dry climates, such as Central and South America, West Africa, the Indian and Mediterranean subcontinent, the Middle East, and parts of Asia [1–3]. This particular ocular disorder primarily affects pre-pubescent individuals, wherein the majority of cases have been reported to occur in the first decade of life [1,2]. While most cases of VKC resolve after puberty, some cases may persist into adulthood [17]. Interestingly, the great majority of patients that develop VKC are male, with the male-to-female ratio reported to be from 2:1 to 4:1 [1,2]. This male preponderance dissipates after puberty, where both genders are affected almost equally [1]. VKC is commonly a bilateral condition (98%) and can occur alone or be associated with atopic diseases such as asthma, allergic rhinitis, and eczema [1,3]. Sex-related hormonal influences have been postulated in the pathogenesis of VKC due to the observation of a predilection for males, with spontaneous recovery after puberty [18,19]. Estrogen and progesterone receptors are found to be overexpressed in the epithelium of the tarsal and bulbar conjunctiva in VKC patients and are reported to modulate the activity of eosinophils, specifically resulting in degranulation of eosinophils [18,20]. The role of the endocrine system may explain the recurrent nature of this disease in the adult population. Recurrent VKC in adulthood is different from adult VKC-like disease, which is described as a new onset after puberty with signs and symptoms similar to those in the pediatric form of the disease, but with a lower male-to-female ratio, lower incidence, and less corneal involvement [18,19]. VKC in adults is not common and is reported to account for 12% of VKC cases [21]. Adult patients with recurrent VKC tend to have more severe inflammatory reactions compared to childhood VKC patients, which has been confirmed by the increased level of acute inflammatory markers present in this adult form [22,23]. As such, these patients are at a higher risk of developing severe chronic complications of VKC, including scarring, corneal ectasia, and limbal stem cell deficiency; therefore, this dictates the increased need for topical corticosteroids and immunosuppressive therapy to adequately manage the inflammation [22,23].

3. Immunopathophysiology of VKC

The immunopathogenesis of VKC involves a complex interplay of the immune system that leads to the activation of an exaggerated immune response to specific allergens. Exposure of susceptible individuals to dust, pollen, and other wind-borne allergens is thought to contribute to conjunctival hyper-reactivity and lead to an inflammatory cascade [5]. VKC is classically considered a type IV hypersensitivity reaction, in which Th2 lymphocytes produce pro-inflammatory mediators including IL-3, IL-4, IL-5, IL-9, IL-13, and IL-31. These Th2 cell-derived cytokines are responsible for the clinicopathological expression in the conjunctivae and corneas of patients with vernal keratoconjunctivitis. Additionally, IL-9 is produced by Th9 cells and mast cells [24]. As such, Th2 and Th9 cells have a role to play in the immunopathophysiology of VKC.

There is an overexpression of IgE that primes the conjunctival mast cells as well as the activation and recruitment of eosinophils [1,5,9,25]. Histopathological analysis reveals conjunctival infiltration with immune cells, including eosinophils, lymphocytes, and basophils, which produce inflammatory mediators that promote tissue damage and post-inflammatory tissue remodeling [5,25]. Epithelial cells, mast cells, and fibroblasts are present in the conjunctiva, and these cells play a role in the immunopathophysiology of vernal keratoconjunctivitis. Epithelial cells express receptors for IL-9 [26,27], IL-33 [28], and histamine [29,30], and as such, epithelial cells can participate in mediating the immune and pathological changes that occur in the conjunctivae and corneas of individuals with vernal keratoconjunctivitis [4].

In a murine model of allergic experimental conjunctivitis, it was shown that IL-9 bound to IL-9R expressed on conjunctival and corneal epithelial cells induced a breach of the barrier function of the epithelium of the ocular surface [31]. This can manifest as punctate epithelial erosions due to the breakdown of the tight and adherent junctions that link the individual epithelial cells of the ocular surface. Furthermore, the breach of the epithelium can facilitate the access of allergens to antigen-presenting cells resident in the subepithelial layer of the conjunctiva to promote type 2 allergic immune responses in the conjunctiva. Additionally, allergens can induce the crosslinking of IgE-attached receptors on sensitized conjunctival mast cells, leading to activation and degranulation of the mast cells and resulting in a type 2-mediated immune response during allergic inflammation of the conjunctiva [29,32–34].

A dysfunctional epithelial barrier of the cornea can provide a portal for immune mediators in the tear film to gain access to the corneal stroma. Cytokines such as IL-4 and TNF-alpha can activate the corneal fibroblasts to produce matrix metalloproteinase (MMP) that breaks down the corneal stroma. Additionally, MMP released from degranulated eosinophils and activated ocular surface epithelial cells can degrade the collagen matrix of the corneal stroma, leading to the development of a sterile corneal ulcer [4,9]. Conjunctival epithelial cells can act as a mediator of type 2 immune responses during allergen-induced conjunctival inflammation since activated epithelial cells of the conjunctiva can produce cytokines such as IL-25, TSLP, and IL-33 [35]. IL-33 produced by epithelial cells and fibroblasts of the ocular surface cells promotes the chronic inflammatory process that is characteristic of vernal keratoconjunctivitis, because it can activate mast cells and eosinophils during type 2 immune responses in allergic diseases [36–39]. Furthermore, IL-33 has been demonstrated to induce barrier dysfunction of ocular surface epithelium [31]. TSLP is a cytokine derived from conjunctival epithelial cells. It activates dendritic cells to promote the generation of Th2 cells that mediate type 2 allergic immune responses [40], as well as activating mast cells to secrete IL-4, IL-5, TNF-alpha, and IL-13 [41]. As such, conjunctival epithelial cells, along with IL-25, TSLP, and IL-33, have a role to play in the immunopathophysiology of chronic allergic disorders of the ocular surface, such as vernal keratoconjunctivitis.

Connective tissue mast cells contain tryptase and chymase, and they are usually located in the subepithelial layer of the conjunctiva and skin [42]. Histamine, proteases, and heparin are preformed mediators released by mast cells [43]. Histamine interacts with its receptors to induce various clinical expressions observed in individuals with VKC. Mast cell-derived tryptase can activate C3 and C5 to generate C3a and C5a, respectively [44]. C3a and C5a generated by the mast cell-derived tryptase can also mediate the recruitment of eosinophils to the site of allergic inflammation [45]. Fukuoka et al. [46] demonstrated that the complement components C3 and C5 are produced by human connective mast cells located in the skin. TNF-alpha and IL-4, or TNF-alpha and IL-13, can induce fibroblasts to secrete C3 [47]. The results of these studies have shown that connective tissue mast cells and fibroblasts can secrete C3. Protease secreted by domestic dust allergens can generate C3a from C3, and the generated C3a can interact with C3aR on mast cells to induce the activation and degranulation of mast cells with the consequential release of histamine, lipid mediators, chemokines, and cytokines [48–50]. This demonstrates that C3a generated via immune and non-immune mechanisms during the activation of the complement system can play a role in the immunopathophysiology of vernal keratoconjunctivitis [51].

Leukotriene B4 (LTB4), leukotriene C4 (LTC4), platelet-activating factor (PAF), prostaglandin D2 (PGD2), and prostaglandin E2 (PGE2) are lipid mediators released by mast cells [43]. Lipid mediators such as leukotrienes (LTB4 and LTC4) and prostaglandins (PGD2 and PGE2) induce changes in the diameter (vasodilation) and permeability (increased vasopermeability) of conjunctival blood vessels during allergic inflammation of the conjunctiva [52–54]. Lipid mediators play a role in promoting the influx of immune cells such as eosinophils to the conjunctiva during allergic inflammation [54]. PAF [55,56], PGD2 [57], and LTB4 [58,59] mediate the recruitment of eosinophils to the conjunctiva. The pro-inflammatory mediators released by eosinophils cause inflammation, damage, and remodeling of the ocular surface in VKC [7,53,60].

Cytokines (IL-4, IL-5, IL-9, IL-13, IL-25, IL-31, and IL-33) and chemokines (CCL5, CCL11, CCL17) are released by degranulated mast cells [4,43]. Conjunctival fibroblasts express receptors for IL-4 and IL-13. The binding of IL-4 or IL-13 to their receptors expressed on fibroblasts in the conjunctiva results in the proliferation and excess production of extracellular matrix by these activated conjunctival fibroblasts [61]. The overgrowth of fibroblasts in the conjunctiva during allergic inflammation results in the development of papillae [4,61]. Because IL-4- or IL-13-activated conjunctival fibroblasts do not undergo apoptosis by virtue of their activation of the phosphatidylinositol-3-kinase (PI3K)/AKT signaling pathway, these cytokines contribute to the development of papillae in vernal keratoconjunctivitis [61]. Similar to IL-4 and IL-13 [62,63], IL-9 can promote the production of IgE-secreting plasma cells [64,65]. IL-9 induces the upregulation of the IL-5R alpha chain on eosinophils [66]. IL-5 induces the proliferation, maturation, differentiation, and chemotaxis of eosinophils to the site of allergen-induced inflammation in the conjunctiva [4,29,67]. IL-25 can exacerbate the inflammatory process because of its ability to recruit eosinophils to the site of allergic inflammation [68]. CCL5 and CCL11 recruit eosinophils [69] and recruit Th2 cells [70] to the conjunctiva during the allergic inflammatory process to mediate the immunopathology of VKC [4]. As such, lipid mediators, cytokines, and chemokines play a role in the immunopathophysiology of VKC.

4. Differential Diagnosis

The clinical features of VKC overlap with a similar condition known as atopic keratoconjunctivitis (AKC), where both represent a severe ocular allergic reaction. AKC affects all ages but has a peak incidence in the fourth and fifth decades of life and is characterized by chronic inflammation that involves the conjunctiva and cornea, where patients typically have concurrent systemic atopic diseases [71]; in fact, more than 95% of AKC patients have eczema, and 87% have a history of asthma [72]. AKC differs from VKC in that there is significant eyelid/dermal involvement that presents as thickened and fissured eyelids with an eczematous, erythematous appearance [71,73]. Corneal complications are common in AKC, ranging from punctate keratitis to the development of persistent epithelial defects and plaque formation [73].

5. Ocular Involvement: Signs and Symptoms

Patients with VKC present with complaints of intense ocular pruritis, which could be attributed to the interaction between histamine and histamine receptor 1 expressed on the conjunctival sensory nerve fibers [74,75]. The interaction between IL-31, a cytokine released by traumatized ocular surface epithelial cells, degranulated mast cells, eosinophils, and Th2 cells and their receptors expressed on sensory nerve fibers in the conjunctiva are also responsible for this intense itch sensation [76,77]. Additionally, the chronic itch sensation experienced by individuals with VKC could also be attributed to IL-4 and IL-13 [78]. Frequent eye rubbing secondary to chronic itching is a risk factor for the development of corneal ectasia, which is a well-reported complication of chronic VKC [9,77,79]. The incidence of ectasia development has been reported to be as high as 26.8%, with higher rates of incidence being associated with chronic disease and those of male gender [80]. Patients with the limbal form of the disease are reported to have an increased incidence of keratoconus compared to the other forms of the disease [81]. The bulbar conjunctival hyperemia and perilimbal chemosis observed during clinical evaluation of the ocular surface are clinical signs attributed to the action of mediators derived from mast cells and Th2 cells. Mast cell-derived histamine interacts with histamine receptor 1 (H1R) expressed on blood vessels in the conjunctiva to induce vasodilation and capillary leakage, which manifests as conjunctival hyperemia and chemosis, respectively [82,83]. Similar to the effect of histamine on conjunctival blood vessels, leukotrienes mediate the dilation and permeability of conjunctival blood vessels, which presents as conjunctival hyperemia and chemosis in individuals with VKC, respectively [4]. Furthermore, the conjunctival chemosis and hyperemia in individuals with VKC could be attributed to the action of PGE2 on vascular smooth muscle cells, which leads to increased vascular leakage and vasodilation [29,84,85]. PGD2 induces the dilation and increased permeability of blood vessels in the conjunctiva [84,86] and intensifies the ocular itch sensation [29,87]. Additionally, the binding of IL-4 to its receptors expressed on conjunctival vascular endothelial cells can induce the upregulation of vascular cell adhesion molecule 1 (VCAM-1), which culminates in vasodilation and vasopermeability, observed as conjunctival hyperemia and conjunctiva chemosis, respectively [88,89]. The complaint of mucus discharge could be attributed to the action of IL-13 and histamine. IL-13 is a pleiotropic cytokine secreted by Th2 cells and degranulated mast cells. It can induce the hyperplasia of goblet cells located in the conjunctival epithelium, as well as induce the hypersecretion of mucin from these activated conjunctival goblet cells [4,74,90]. Furthermore, IL-9 also induces the hyperplasia of goblet cells [91]. Additionally, mucoid discharge has been shown to occur when histamine binds to histamine receptors expressed on goblet cells [74,92]. Thus, Th2- and Th9-derived cytokines are contributors to the complaint of mucoid discharge.

Ocular involvement in VKC primarily includes changes in the conjunctiva and limbus. The hallmark sign of VKC is papillary hyperplasia of varying degrees and severity, which can affect the upper tarsal conjunctiva and the limbal bulbar conjunctiva [8,93]. Conjunctival fibroblasts express receptors for histamine, IL-4, and IL-13. These mediators act on their cognate receptors expressed on conjunctival fibroblasts to induce hyperproliferation of conjunctival fibroblasts, as well as to promote excess production of extracellular matrix proteins from these fibroblasts [3,4,94]. Additionally, IL-9 secreted by Th2 cells, Th9 cells, eosinophils, and mast cells can synergize with IL-4 in promoting the remodeling of the conjunctival tissue [95,96]. Therefore, activated conjunctival fibroblasts in VKC patients promote fibroproliferative changes and tissue remodeling in the conjunctiva, which is observed as papillae on the palpebral conjunctiva [4,8,93]. Histological examination of papillae in VKC reveals hyperplastic epithelium with a fibrovascular core and the presence of a massive influx of inflammatory cells in the subepithelial layer of the conjunctival tissue [5,8,93]. These inflammatory cells present in a characteristic distribution where lymphocytes localize to the center of the papillae and eosinophils localize to the periphery of the papillae [93]. This massive cell infiltration and hypervascularization, along with hyperproliferation of the conjunctival fibroblasts, results in the appearance of the giant papillae that are seen in VKC. The papillae can vary in size from 0.1 to 5.0 mm, where those larger than 1.0 mm are classified as giant papillae, and, when confluent, give the classic "cobblestone" appearance [5]. This papillary hypertrophy typically manifests in the superior palpebral conjunctiva in VKC, and inferior palpebral conjunctiva in AKC [71,73]. Limbal VKC is characterized by the presence of confluent, gelatinous papillae located mainly on the limbal region of the bulbar conjunctiva (Figure 1). Increased pigmentation of the perilimbal intrapalpebral conjunctiva can occur in non-Caucasian patients with VKC (Figure 2) [5,97–99]. The color of the pigment can vary from light golden-brown to dark brownish-black and can be seen in active or quiescent disease forms [98,99]. There is an abundance of melanocytes and mast cells within the limbal region of the bulbar conjunctiva [99]. It is postulated that immune molecules such as histamine and stem cell factors can activate histamine receptor 2 and CD117 expressed on melanocytes located within the limbal region of the bulbar conjunctiva, respectively. This interaction induces the melanocytes to produce excess melanin, which causes pigmentary changes within the intrapalpebral bulbar conjunctiva [99]. The presence of perilimbal hyperpigmentation can help confirm the diagnosis of VKC, especially when signs and symptoms are subtle, since it appears to be a consistent finding in certain populations with VKC [99,100].

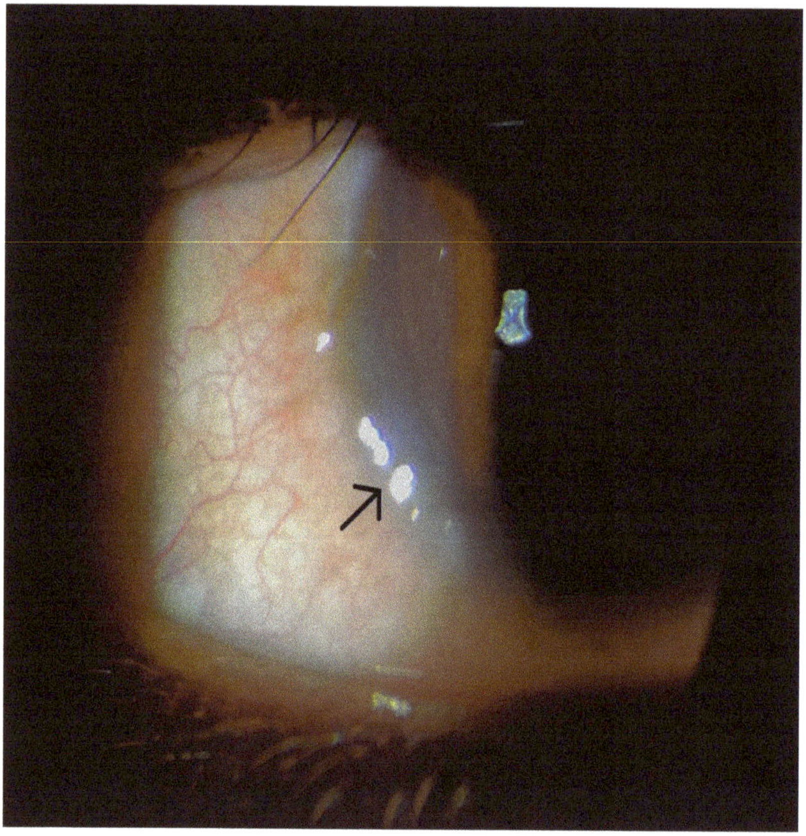

Figure 1. Slit-lamp examination of a right eye that reveals limbal VKC with the presence of perilimbal chemosis and gelatinous limbal papillae (black arrow). Note the hyper-reflectivity in the area of the gelatinous limbal papillae. This patient had previously been treated with 1.0% prednisolone acetate.

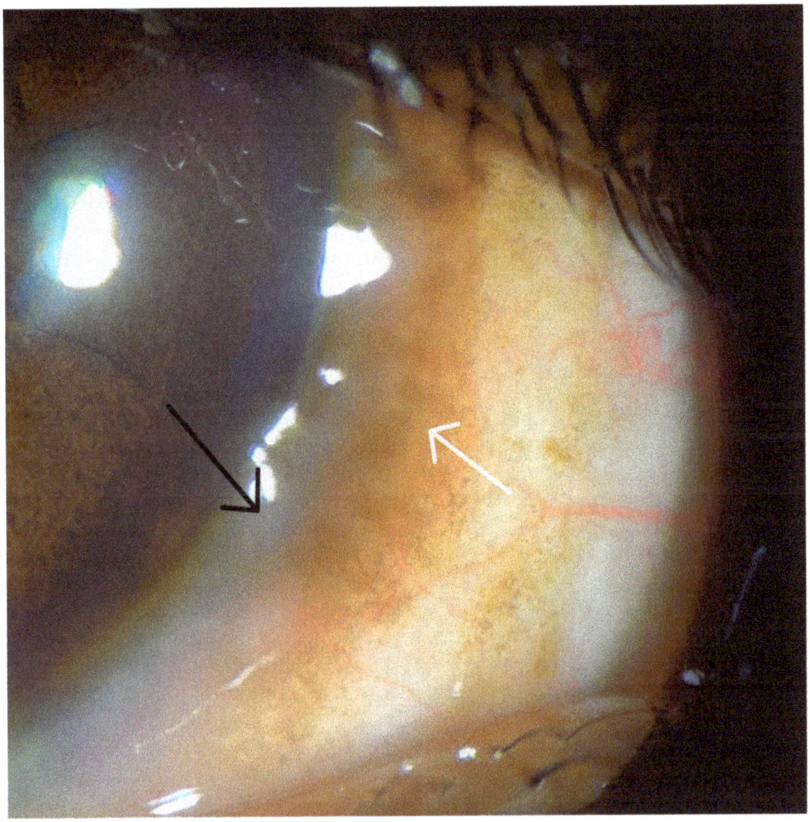

Figure 2. Slit-lamp examination of a left eye that reveals corneal involvement in the form of pseudogerontoxon (black arrow) and perilimbal bulbar conjunctival hyperpigmentation (white arrow).

While the conjunctiva is the primary site of ocular involvement in VKC, the corneal tissue may become compromised in response to the chronic and exaggerated immune response, leading to permanent vision loss in some cases. Corneal involvement occurs in around 50% of patients and is common in the tarsal, mixed, and perennial forms of the disease [9,101]. Corneal changes include punctate epithelial keratitis, macroerosions, neovascularization, microbial keratitis, shield ulcers, scarring, and plaque formation [1,101,102]. IL-5 derived from degranulating mast cells and Th2 cells recruits and activates eosinophil, a granulocyte that participates in the inflammation-associated damage and remodeling of the ocular surface observed in chronic forms of ocular allergy such as vernal keratoconjunctivitis [103–105]. The pathogenesis of corneal involvement is secondary to the toxic effects from mediators released during the degranulation of eosinophils in the conjunctiva, including the eosinophilic cationic protein (ECP), major basic protein (MBP), and matrix metalloproteinase-9 (MMP-9) [3,9]. These mediators induce degradation of the extracellular matrix proteins present in the corneal epithelial basement membrane. This results in the persistent epithelial keratopathy that is seen in VKC [102,106]. Additionally, IL-9 can interact with epithelial cells of the ocular surface to cause a breach of the barrier function of the epithelium, which culminates in the development of punctate epithelial erosions due to the compromised ocular surface epithelium [31]. Persistent corneal epithelial compromise extending into the Bowman's layer, along with degradation of the collagen type 1 present in the corneal stroma, can lead to an oval-shaped defect with elevated margins and can present as a shield ulcer, a vision-threatening complication of VKC [9,107]. Patients may also present with pseudogerontoxon, which appears as a gelatinous grey-white segment in the peripheral corneal stroma and is the result of lipid deposition from chronic increased limbal vasopermeability (Figure 2) [1,101]. It is of note that vascular endothelial cells express receptors for IL-4 and histamine. As such, the persistent IL-4 activation of these endothelial cells on limbal blood vessels results in the upregulation of VCAM-1 on these vascular endothelial cells, which culminates in a breach of the endothelial barrier function [88,89].

6. Management of VKC

The main goals of VKC treatment include controlling acute symptoms and preventing recurrent disease. Currently, there are no well-established treatment guidelines for VKC, and options are individualized based on disease stage, severity, and duration [108]. Because the immunopathogenesis of VKC is multifactorial, the use of a combination of agents with more direct effects on the inflammatory processes is ideal to control acute symptoms and prevent recurrent disease [4]. Non-pharmacological disease management includes the identification and avoidance of specific allergens, and pharmacological therapy includes antihistamines, mast cell stabilizers, and non-steroidal anti-inflammatory drugs (NSAIDs) [4,108,109]. Mild disease is typically managed with topical mast cell stabilizers, antihistamines, or dual-acting agents [5,110,111]. Mast cell stabilizers work by inhibiting mast cell degranulation, which thereby prohibits the release of pro-inflammatory mediators [4,6]. Mast cell stabilizers have also been shown to act on additional cells involved in ocular allergy, including neutrophils, macrophages, eosinophils, and monocytes [112]. Antihistamines block histamine from interacting with their receptors on immune and non-immune cells [4,6]. Most antihistamines target the H1 receptor to provide acute symptomatic relief, whereas mast cell stabilizers exhibit a slow onset of action and aid in chronic management [110]. Dual-acting agents, which contain both mast cell stabilizers and antihistamines, offer the advantage of providing rapid symptomatic relief, coupled with long-term mast cell stabilization [4,6,110]. These agents are well tolerated, and dual-therapy agents are generally preferred over monotherapy with mast cell stabilizers or antihistamines alone [112]. Topical non-steroidal anti-inflammatory drugs (NSAIDs) work by inhibiting cyclooxygenase (COX)-1 and COX-2 enzymes, which thereby prohibits the release of prostaglandin E2 and I2 [4,110]. Prostaglandins are reported to have pruritogenic properties; therefore, the inhibition of these prostaglandins allows for the mitigation of ocular itching [1,113]. While NSAIDs provide symptomatic relief, they do not have any effect on the papillary hyperplasia or limbal changes seen in VKC [113,114]. Additionally, due to the side effects of corneal toxicity from these agents, prolonged use is ill-advised, especially if patients present with corneal involvement. While these agents provide symptomatic relief, they do not fully target the complex immune processes involved in VKC.

Moderate to severe forms of the disease require effective therapy to target the specific immune responses involved in VKC. Anti-inflammatory agents that are more effective include corticosteroids; however, these agents are associated with potentially serious adverse effects, including cataract formation, increased intraocular pressure, delayed wound healing, and increased susceptibility to infection [29]. In severe VKC, topical steroids are administered for a greater duration due to the intensity of the inflammation in these patients [22]. While long-term and indiscriminate use of topical corticosteroids is ill-advised, a "pulse" regimen of four drops per day for 5 days is preferred to manage acute episodes of VKC, and limiting longer treatment regimens to between one and three weeks with a slow taper is preferred for chronic episodes of VKC [109]. Low-potency steroids are initially used and include agents such as loteprednol and fluorometholone. In cases where low-potency steroids fail, higher-potency steroids can be administered, including agents such as prednisolone, dexamethasone, and diflurprednate. While corticosteroids are efficacious in controlling signs and symptoms of VKC, steroid-resistant forms of VKC exist and may necessitate alternative therapeutic management [115,116]. Additionally, VKC is associated with frequent recurrences of inflammation and often requires steroid-sparing agents to manage the condition [115,116].

Topical immunomodulators play a crucial role in the management of VKC as they are effective and have a better safety profile in the treatment of severe and recalcitrant disease [4]. These immunomodulators, such as calcineurin inhibitors, work by modulating the immune response and have achieved breakthrough results in the treatment of severe disease. Immunomodulators exert their therapeutic effects by binding to immunophilins (cyclophilin and FK506-binding protein) to form an immunomodulator–immunophilin complex that binds to calcineurin [117,118]. The binding of this complex to calcineurin interferes with the signaling pathway that is responsible for the proliferation of T cells. Cyclosporin binds to cyclophilin to form the cyclosporin–cyclophilin complex, which binds to calcineurin, thereby preventing calcineurin from the dephosphorylating nuclear factor of activated T cells (NFAT). This action blocks the migration of the cytoplasmic NFAT into the nucleus [118–120]. It is important to note that calcineurin is required for the activation of NFAT, and this is followed by the migration of the activated NFAT into the nucleus, where it binds to the regulatory region of T cell-derived cytokines to mediate transcription of genes that encode for IL-2 and other T cell-derived cytokines [118,119]. While corticosteroids are often used for short-term relief of acute episodes, calcineurin inhibitors are employed for long-term immunosuppression of chronic episodes. Specifically, calcineurin inhibitors, such as cyclosporine and tacrolimus, modulate the immune response by inhibiting the IL-2-mediated clonal expansion of Th2 cells, thereby inhibiting the release of Th2 cell-derived cytokines [4,109] such as IL-3 and IL-9, which have been shown to promote the growth and development of mast cells in ocular allergies [121]. Topical cyclosporine A (CsA) is effective in controlling inflammation of the ocular surface as it has been found to reduce the number of neutrophils, eosinophils, and lymphocytes infiltrating the conjunctiva, and is efficacious even at low concentrations such as 0.05% [4,111,122]. CsA has been shown to inhibit mast cell-mediated cytokine production by inhibiting Th2 lymphocyte proliferation, IL-2 production, and TNF-alpha production, thereby leading to an inhibitory effect on the development of ocular allergies [122]. Additional effects of CsA include inhibiting IL-5 production, which thereby prevents the recruitment of eosinophils, and ultimately inhibits the release of eosinophil-derived mediators such as eosinophil major basic protein to the site of ocular allergies [1,4,111]. CsA has been shown to significantly reduce tear levels of IL-4, IL-5, IL-17, TNF-alpha, IFN-gamma, and eotaxin, which have been shown to be increased in the tear films of patients with VKC [122,123]. Different concentrations of CsA range from 0.05% to 2.0% and are available in select countries [112]. Commercially available forms include 0.05%, which is authorized for dry eye disease, and 0.1%, which is authorized for severe VKC. Both the low- and high-dose ends of the spectrum, 0.1% and 2.0%, respectively, have been shown to have comparable efficacy and safety profiles in treating severe VKC, where both dosages were found to enable a substantial reduction in the use of topical corticosteroids [124]. In a study evaluating the efficacy of 0.1% CsA in a cationic emulsion versus a hospital preparation of 2.0% CsA via dilution of an intravenous preparation, both dosages were found to induce comparable improvements in clinical signs and patient symptoms [124]. Interestingly, the 0.1% CsA group was able to control their symptoms with a lower number of daily instillations (two drops per day on inclusion, then one drop per day) compared to the 2.0% CsA group (three drops per day on inclusion, then two drops per day). This is likely due to the fact that CsA is a lipophilic substance, making it insoluble in water [125]. Because the 0.1% CsA formulation was delivered in a lipid-based system, there was increased retention on the ocular surface, allowing for a lower dose to provide similar therapeutic effects [124]. In a study [123] evaluating the efficacy of 0.05% CsA in VKC, patients were treated with a loading dose of four times a day for two weeks, followed by gradual tapering to three times a day for a week, then twice a day for the next week, once a day for a week, and finally a maintenance dose of one drop per day until the final follow up. The results of this study revealed a beneficial effect of 0.05% CsA in reducing signs and symptoms as early as two weeks, which was maintained after three months [123]. CsA has been shown to be efficacious in treating signs and symptoms of VKC: specifically, 91% of patients treated with 2% CsA four times daily showed decreased symptoms, and 66% showed improvement in clinical signs of VKC [126]. It has also been observed through the VEKTIS trial that one month of treatment with 0.1% CsA four times daily improved symptoms and quality of life, and was well tolerated in children and adults with severe VKC [127,128]. This finding was additionally supported by the NOVATIVE trial, which evaluated the efficacy of both 0.05% and 0.1% CsA [129]. This trial found that improvement was most notable with the 0.1% CsA, where patients had improved signs and symptoms as early as 1 week, which continued throughout the first month of treatment [130]. A pooled analysis of the data from both studies demonstrated that both high and low dosages of CsA were safely tolerated, where the most frequent adverse events were mild to moderate pain at the instillation site (high dose, 9.4%; low dose, 7.5%), and pruritus (high dose, 5.2%; low dose, 7.5%) [129]. Recommendations from the Expert Working Group in Asia (MOVIA) suggest considering the initiation of topical 0.1% CsA for patients with moderate to severe or persistent VKC [112]. This finding is also supported by the European Expert Consensus (Eur-VKC Group), who recommend topical CsA in order to provide a corticosteroid-sparing effect [114]. The MOVIA group recommend initiating CsA as a first line of treatment for patients presenting with moderate to severe VKC, and only prescribing corticosteroids as a short-pulse treatment if there is an inadequate response to the CsA, or if there are corneal complications. In contrast, the EUR-VKC Group recommend starting with short-pulse corticosteroids before CsA in the treatment sequence. While there is no consensus on the specific concentration or dosage of CsA, both groups suggest the use of CsA for long-term control [112,114]. This long-term control was demonstrated in a case report of a 12-year-old male with a recurrent vernal shield ulcer after discontinuing CsA [131]. Once 0.1% CsA was reinitiated, there was complete resolution of his shield ulcer with no reported recurrence. This benefit was additionally observed in a case report of multiple patients, where initiation of topical CsA was found to cause marked improvements in corneal shield ulcers [132]. All patients in this case were treated with 0.1% CsA, dosed eight times per day, and were concurrently treated with a corticosteroid. Gradual tapering of the treatment was initiated once improvement was noted, and topical CsA was maintained at twice or four times daily to prevent recurrent disease. CsA has been shown to be safe and effective and is used in varying concentrations, on-label and off-label, for the treatment of VKC [109,127,129].

Tacrolimus is another calcineurin inhibitor that works to modulate the inflammatory response by binding to FK506-binding protein (FKBP) to form a tacrolimus–FKBP complex that binds to calcineurin. This interferes with the ability of calcineurin to dephosphorylate NFAT [120]. Thus, tacrolimus suppresses the production of cytokines such as IL-2, IL-4, and IL-5 [133] and also suppresses histamine release by mast cells [134]. This agent has a long history of being used as an immunosuppressant after organ transplantation [109] and is significantly more potent than cyclosporine [134,135]. This increased potency of tacrolimus is beneficial in treating cases refractory to cyclosporine [136]. Tacrolimus drops and ointments come in varying concentrations, ranging from 0.005% to 0.1% [13,109,137], with 0.1% being the most common [133]. Tacrolimus 0.1% eye drops are not FDA-approved and are currently used off-label for the treatment of VKC. In a study evaluating the safety and efficacy of 0.1% tacrolimus in pediatric patients who responded poorly to CsA, significant improvements were noted in clinical signs including marked improvements in giant papillae in all forms of the disease [138]. This finding was additionally supported by a study evaluating the effect of 0.03% tacrolimus in patients who were unsuccessfully treated with CsA and corticosteroids [139]. In this study, the patients experienced significant reductions in their signs and symptoms after 4 weeks of treatment with the following dosing schedule: topical tacrolimus ointment 0.03% twice daily for 8 weeks, and then once daily for 2 months, followed by three times daily for 8 weeks. Resolution of giant papillae and corneal lesions was noted within 8 weeks of treatment. In a study evaluating the efficacy of 0.03% versus 0.1% tacrolimus in recalcitrant VKC, both strengths were effective in treating VKC, where 88% of patients receiving 0.03% and 94% of patients receiving 0.1% experienced significant improvements in their clinical signs and symptoms [137]. Resolution of the papillary component of VKC depends on the strength of treatment, where a higher strength (0.1%) provides increased efficacy in controlling papillary hyperplasia [137]. This effect was also observed in another study evaluating the efficacy of 0.03% tacrolimus in VKC [134], which reported a significant reduction in papillae in the tacrolimus-treated group compared to the control group (fluorometholone 0.1%). In another study evaluating the efficacy of 0.1% tacrolimus, patients previously treated with 2 months of 0.1% cyclosporine only experienced significant resolution of their papillae with administration of 0.1% tacrolimus for 1 month [140]. Patients treated with tacrolimus can exhibit improvements in their clinical signs and symptoms as early as three days [141], where the most common adverse events reported are transient burning [137,140,142,143] and ocular stinging [134,137]. Both cyclosporin and tacrolimus reduce the transcription of cytokine genes required for encoding T cell-derived cytokines [119,120] and are effective immunomodulators for controlling the inflammatory reaction seen in VKC. In a study evaluating the efficacy of 0.03% tacrolimus versus 2% CsA, tacrolimus was reported to be more effective in treating signs and symptoms of VKC compared to 2% CsA [144]. Interestingly, another study comparing 0.1% tacrolimus with 2% CsA revealed that both were equally effective in the treatment of VKC [145]. Currently, there are no established protocols for VKC treatment using immunomodulators. A treatment protocol that has been proposed includes initiating 0.03% tacrolimus as a first line of therapy for severe VKC, increasing the dose to 0.1% if no improvement is noted, or for cases that do not show improvement with corticosteroid therapy [146]. Patients who received tacrolimus as first-line treatment were shown to have shorter treatment periods and follow-up durations compared to patients who received tacrolimus as second-line treatment. Monitoring these patients closely every 2–4 weeks initially is advised, as tacrolimus can take up to one month to take effect. Gradual tapering of the treatment is initiated once improvement in clinical signs and symptoms is noted [146]. In a study evaluating the efficacy and safety of prolonged treatment of severe VKC with topical 0.1% tacrolimus, it was demonstrated that 2 years of treatment was effective in improving clinical scores and remission rates, with limited adverse effects compared to a group treated for 6 months [133]. In fact, no adverse events occurred from the 12th to the 24th month of treatment use. Another study evaluating the safety of 0.1% tacrolimus in the treatment of refractory AKC for 48 months demonstrated similar findings, with complete clinical resolution and remission of disease in the absence of other medications, and with mild adverse effects that were limited to a mild burning sensation [147]. These findings suggest that patients with severe forms of VKC likely require therapy for longer periods of time in order to prevent recurrences, and they highlight the safety of long-term application.

Both CsA and tacrolimus have been used off-label for the treatment of severe or steroid-intolerant disease. The use of a combination of immunomodulators was first evaluated in the treatment of patients with steroid-dependent AKC [148]. The results from this study demonstrated a reduction in the number of recurrences, while limiting the use of corticosteroids. In a study evaluating the role of combined immunomodulator therapy in severe steroid-intolerant VKC, the use of CsA and tacrolimus had a synergistic effect and provided rapid resolution of signs and symptoms once the tacrolimus was introduced into the treatment regimen [115]. The patients in this study were initially treated with 0.1% CsA four times daily, which showed significant improvement within 2 weeks of therapy; however, the response was considered suboptimal, which prompted the inclusion of a 0.03% tacrolimus ointment twice daily to the treatment regimen. The addition of tacrolimus resulted in significant improvement and resolution of clinical signs and symptoms including itching, photophobia, discharge, tarsal papillae, and punctate keratopathy. The improved response is likely due to the higher potency of tacrolimus. It is also worth noting that while both drugs inhibit the calcineurin receptor, they do so by binding to different sites (CsA binds to cyclophilin A, and tacrolimus binds to

FKBP12). Combined immunomodulator therapy allows for the rapid control of symptoms and should be considered in cases of severe inflammation [115,148]. While there have been no head-to-head randomized controlled studies of 0.1% tacrolimus and cyclosporine, varying concentrations of both agents, used both on-label and off-label, are safe and effective in the treatment of VKC. However, although these topical immunomodulators are effective in treating and controlling VKC, it is suggested to reserve cyclosporine and tacrolimus for severe or refractory forms of VKC, or for cases where corticosteroids are contraindicated [111,137,149]. Patients that do not respond to corticosteroids (Figure 1) can access therapeutic benefits with the use of immunomodulators (Figure 3).

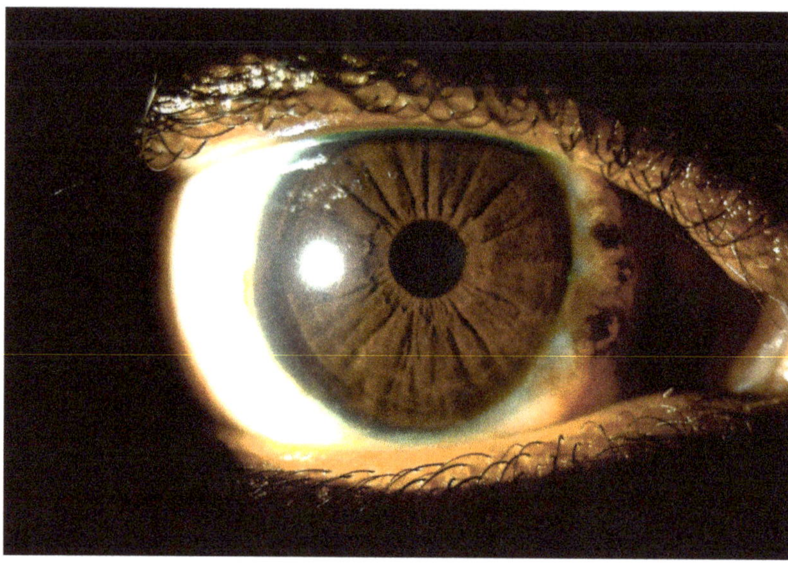

Figure 3. Slit-lamp examination of a right eye that reveals resolution of the limbal papillae with no active signs of vernal keratoconjunctivitis after initiation of 0.1% CsA for 6 weeks.

7. Future Directions

In recent years, therapy employing biologics and monoclonal antibodies has been developed to treat allergic diseases [150]. Such therapies are currently not approved for allergic eye disease; however, it has been reported that the off-label use of these agents provides promising results in the treatment of ocular allergic disease. Specifically, omalizumab, a humanized monoclonal anti-IgE antibody, appears to offer therapeutic relief in patients with severe VKC by targeting the IgE-mediated pathophysiology of the condition [108,151]. Larger controlled clinical trials are needed to establish the role of biologics and monoclonal antibodies, and to determine the appropriate dosage and administration of these agents in the treatment of VKC. Additional efforts in research are needed to identify the specific pathogenesis of VKC to allow the formulation of new molecules that target the diverse pathogenic mechanisms of this condition. Additionally, practitioners would benefit from established diagnostic criteria and treatment guidelines, especially for moderate, severe, and refractory cases of VKC.

8. Conclusions

VKC is a sight-threatening chronic inflammatory condition that primarily affects pre-pubescent males in warm climates. The conjunctiva and cornea are the major ocular sites affected, where prolonged and chronic inflammation can result in impaired visual function and quality of life. This review highlighted the importance of understanding the fibroproliferative changes that occur in VKC and selecting appropriate therapy to control the inflammatory cascade. The VKC treatment armamentarium includes both on- and off-label therapeutic options, including the use of immunomodulators in severe and refractory cases of VKC. Correct management is imperative to prevent adverse effects and ocular complications associated with this challenging condition of the ocular surface.

Funding: This research received no external funding.

Institutional Review Board Statement: Not applicable.

Informed Consent Statement: Not applicable.

Data Availability Statement: No new data were created or analyzed in this study. Data sharing is not applicable to this article.

Conflicts of Interest: The authors declare no conflicts of interest.

References

1. Kumar, S. Vernal keratoconjunctivitis: A major review. *Acta Ophthalmol.* **2009**, *87*, 133–147. [CrossRef]
2. Leonardi, A.; Busca, F.; Motterle, L.; Cavarzeran, F.; Fregona, I.; Plebani, M.; Secchi, A. Case series of 406 vernal keratoconjunctivitis patients: A demographic and epidemiological study. *Acta Ophthalmol. Scand.* **2006**, *84*, 406–410. [CrossRef]
3. Chigbu, D.I.; Sandrasekaramudaly-Brown, S. Ocular surface disease: A case of vernal keratoconjunctivitis. *Contact Lens Anterior Eye* **2011**, *34*, 39–44. [CrossRef]
4. Chigbu, D.I.; Labib, B.A. Immunopharmacology in Vernal Keratoconjunctivitis: Current and Future Perspectives. *Pharmaceuticals* **2021**, *14*, 658. [CrossRef]
5. Singhal, D.; Sahay, P.; Maharana, P.K.; Raj, N.; Sharma, N.; Titiyal, J.S. Vernal Keratoconjunctivitis. *Surv. Ophthalmol.* **2019**, *64*, 289–311. [CrossRef]
6. Bruschi, G.; Ghiglioni, D.G.; Cozzi, L.; Osnaghi, S.; Viola, F.; Marchisio, P. Vernal Keratoconjunctivitis: A Systematic Review. *Clin. Rev. Allergy Immunol.* **2023**, *65*, 277–329. [CrossRef] [PubMed]
7. Chigbu, D.I.; Jain, P.; Khan, Z.K. Immune Mechanisms, Pathology, and Management of Allergic Ocular Diseases. In *Advanced Concepts in Human Immunology: Prospects for Disease Control*; Jain, P., Ndhlovu, L.C., Eds.; Springer Nature: Cham, Switzerland, 2020; pp. 229–277.
8. Kumagai, N.; Fukuda, K.; Fujitsu, Y.; Yamamoto, K.; Nishida, T. Role of structural cells of the cornea and conjunctiva in the pathogenesis of vernal keratoconjunctivitis. *Prog. Retin. Eye Res.* **2006**, *25*, 165–187. [CrossRef] [PubMed]
9. Feizi, S.; Javadi, M.A.; Alemzadeh-Ansari, M.; Arabi, A.; Shahraki, T.; Kheirkhah, A. Management of corneal complications in vernal keratoconjunctivitis: A review. *Ocul. Surf.* **2021**, *19*, 282–289. [CrossRef] [PubMed]
10. Allison, A.C. Immunosuppressive drugs: The first 50 years and a glance forward. *Immunopharmacology* **2000**, *47*, 63–83. [CrossRef]
11. McMonnies, C.W. Dry eye disease immune responses and topical therapy. *Eye Vis.* **2019**, *6*, 12. [CrossRef]
12. Periman, L.M.; Perez, V.L.; Saban, D.R.; Lin, M.C.; Neri, P. The Immunological Basis of Dry Eye Disease and Current Topical Treatment Options. *J. Ocul. Pharmacol. Ther.* **2020**, *36*, 137–146. [CrossRef]
13. Erdinest, N.; Ben-Eli, H.; Solomon, A. Topical tacrolimus for allergic eye diseases. *Curr. Opin. Allergy Clin. Immunol.* **2019**, *19*, 535–543. [CrossRef] [PubMed]
14. Chan, N.S.; Choi, J.; Cheung, C.M.G. Pediatric Uveitis. *Asia Pac. J. Ophthalmol.* **2018**, *7*, 192–199.
15. Abdel-Aty, A.; Gupta, A.; Del Priore, L.; Kombo, N. Management of noninfectious scleritis. *Ther. Adv. Ophthalmol.* **2022**, *14*, 25158414211070879. [CrossRef]
16. Katz, E.A.; Sunshine, S.; Mun, C.; Sarwar, M.; Surenkhuu, B.; Pradeep, A.; Jain, S. Combinatorial therapy with immunosuppressive, immunomodulatory and tear substitute eyedrops ("Triple Play") in Recalcitrant Immunological Ocular Surface Diseases. *Ocul. Surf.* **2022**, *23*, 1–11. [CrossRef]
17. Di Zazzo, A.; Bonini, S.; Fernandes, M. Adult vernal keratoconjunctivitis. *Curr. Opin. Allergy Clin. Immunol.* **2020**, *20*, 501–506. [CrossRef]
18. Bonini, S.; Coassin, M.; Aronni, S.; Lambiase, A. Vernal keratoconjunctivitis. *Eye* **2004**, *18*, 345–351. [CrossRef] [PubMed]
19. Leonardi, A.; Lazzarini, D.; Motterle, L.; Bortolotti, M.; Deligianni, V.; Curnow, S.J.; Bonini, S.; Fregona, I.A. Vernal keratoconjunctivitis-like disease in adults. *Am. J. Ophthalmol.* **2013**, *155*, 796–803. [CrossRef]
20. Chigbu, D.I. The pathophysiology of ocular allergy: A review. *Contact Lens Anterior Eye* **2009**, *32*, 3–15, quiz 43-4. [CrossRef]
21. Saboo, U.S.; Jain, M.; Reddy, J.C.; Sangwan, V.S. Demographic and clinical profile of vernal keratoconjunctivitis at a tertiary eye care center in India. *Indian J. Ophthalmol.* **2013**, *61*, 486–489. [CrossRef]
22. Di Zazzo, A.; Micera, A.; De Piano, M.; Coassin, M.; Sharma, S.; Bonini, S.; Fernandes, M. Adult Vernal Keratoconjunctivitis: Clinical and biochemical profile of a rare disease. *Ocul. Surf.* **2019**, *17*, 737–742. [CrossRef] [PubMed]
23. Micera, A.; Di Zazzo, A.; De Piano, M.; Sharma, S.; Mori, T.; De Gregorio, C.; Coassin, M.; Fernandes, M. Tissue remodeling in adult vernal keratoconjunctivitis. *Exp. Eye Res.* **2022**, *225*, 109301. [CrossRef] [PubMed]
24. Eskandarpour, M.; Zhang, X.; Micera, A.; Zaher, S.; Larkin, F.D.P.; Nunn, M.; Bonini, S.; Weston-Davies, W.; Calder, V.L. Allergic eye disease: Blocking LTB4/C5 in vivo suppressed disease and Th2 & Th9 cells. *Allergy* **2022**, *77*, 660–664.

25. Leonardi, A. Vernal keratoconjunctivitis: Pathogenesis and treatment. *Prog. Retin. Eye Res.* **2002**, *21*, 319–339. [CrossRef]
26. Goswami, R.; Kaplan, M.H. A brief history of IL-9. *J. Immunol.* **2011**, *186*, 3283–3288. [CrossRef]
27. Pajulas, A.; Fu, Y.; Cheung, C.C.L.; Chu, M.; Cannon, A.; Alakhras, N.; Zhang, J.; Ulrich, B.J.; Nelson, A.S.; Zhou, B.; et al. Interleukin-9 promotes mast cell progenitor proliferation and CCR2-dependent mast cell migration in allergic airway inflammation. *Mucosal Immunol.* **2023**, *16*, 432–445. [CrossRef] [PubMed]
28. Drake, L.Y.; Kita, H. IL-33: Biological properties, functions, and roles in airway disease. *Immunol. Rev.* **2017**, *278*, 173–184. [CrossRef]
29. Labib, B.A.; Chigbu, D.I. Therapeutic Targets in Allergic Conjunctivitis. *Pharmaceuticals* **2022**, *15*, 547. [CrossRef]
30. Thangam, E.B.; Jemima, E.A.; Singh, H.; Baig, M.S.; Khan, M.; Mathias, C.B.; Church, M.K.; Saluja, R. The Role of Histamine and Histamine Receptors in Mast Cell-Mediated Allergy and Inflammation: The Hunt for New Therapeutic Targets. *Front. Immunol.* **2018**, *9*, 1873. [CrossRef]
31. Hu, J.; Gao, N.; Zhang, Y.; Chen, X.; Li, J.; Bian, F.; Chi, W.; Liu, Z.; de Paiva, C.S.; Pflugfelder, S.C.; et al. IL-33/ST2/IL-9/IL-9R signaling disrupts ocular surface barrier in allergic inflammation. *Mucosal Immunol.* **2020**, *13*, 919–930. [CrossRef]
32. Singh, N.; Diebold, Y.; Sahu, S.K.; Leonardi, A. Epithelial barrier dysfunction in ocular allergy. *Allergy* **2022**, *77*, 1360–1372. [CrossRef]
33. Enriquez-de-Salamanca, A.; Calder, V.; Gao, J.; Galatowicz, G.; Garcia-Vazquez, C.; Fernandez, I.; Stern, M.E.; Diebold, Y.; Calonge, M. Cytokine responses by conjunctival epithelial cells: An in vitro model of ocular inflammation. *Cytokine* **2008**, *44*, 160–167. [CrossRef]
34. Leonardi, A.; De Dominicis, C.; Motterle, L. Immunopathogenesis of ocular allergy: A schematic approach to different clinical entities. *Curr. Opin. Allergy Clin. Immunol.* **2007**, *7*, 429–435. [CrossRef]
35. Divekar, R.; Kita, H. Recent advances in epithelium-derived cytokines (IL-33, IL-25, and thymic stromal lymphopoietin) and allergic inflammation. *Curr. Opin. Allergy Clin. Immunol.* **2015**, *15*, 98–103. [CrossRef]
36. Cherry, W.B.; Yoon, J.; Bartemes, K.R.; Iijima, K.; Kita, H. A novel IL-1 family cytokine, IL-33, potently activates human eosinophils. *J. Allergy Clin. Immunol.* **2008**, *121*, 1484–1490. [CrossRef]
37. Williams, C.M.; Rahman, S.; Hubeau, C.; Ma, H.L. Cytokine pathways in allergic disease. *Toxicol. Pathol.* **2012**, *40*, 205–215. [CrossRef]
38. Ninomiya, I.; Yamatoya, K.; Mashimo, K.; Matsuda, A.; Usui-Ouchi, A.; Araki, Y.; Ebihara, N. Role of Oncostatin M in the Pathogenesis of Vernal Keratoconjunctivitis: Focus on the Barrier Function of the Epithelium and Interleukin-33 Production by Fibroblasts. *Investig. Ophthalmol. Vis. Sci.* **2022**, *63*, 26. [CrossRef] [PubMed]
39. Matsuda, A.; Okayama, Y.; Terai, N.; Yokoi, N.; Ebihara, N.; Tanioka, H.; Kawasaki, S.; Inatomi, T.; Katoh, N.; Ueda, E.; et al. The Role of Interleukin-33 in Chronic Allergic Conjunctivitis. *Investig. Ophthalmol. Vis. Sci.* **2009**, *63*, 26. [CrossRef] [PubMed]
40. Matsuda, A.; Ebihara, N.; Yokoi, N.; Kawasaki, S.; Tanioka, H.; Inatomi, T.; de Waal Malefyt, R.; Hamuro, J.; Kinoshita, S.; Murakami, A. Functional role of thymic stromal lymphopoietin in chronic allergic keratoconjunctivitis. *Investig. Ophthalmol. Vis. Sci.* **2010**, *51*, 151–155. [CrossRef] [PubMed]
41. Comeau, M.R.; Ziegler, S.F. The influence of TSLP on the allergic response. *Mucosal Immunol.* **2010**, *3*, 138–147. [CrossRef]
42. Katelaris, C. Ocular allergy: Implications for the clinical immunologist. *Ann. Allergy Asthma Immunol.* **2003**, *90* (Suppl. S3), 23–27. [CrossRef]
43. Solimando, A.G.; Desantis, V.; Ribatti, D. Mast Cells and Interleukins. *Int. J. Mol. Sci.* **2022**, *23*, 14004. [CrossRef]
44. Fukuoka, Y.; Xia, H.Z.; Sanchez-Munoz, L.B.; Dellinger, A.L.; Escribano, L.; Schwartz, L.B. Generation of anaphylatoxins by human beta-tryptase from C3, C4, and C5. *J. Immunol.* **2008**, *180*, 6307–6316. [CrossRef]
45. DiScipio, R.G.; Schraufstatter, I.U. The role of the complement anaphylatoxins in the recruitment of eosinophils. *Int. Immunopharmacol.* **2007**, *7*, 1909–1923. [CrossRef] [PubMed]
46. Fukuoka, Y.; Hite, M.R.; Dellinger, A.L.; Schwartz, L.B. Human skin mast cells express complement factors C3 and C5. *J. Immunol.* **2013**, *191*, 1827–1834. [CrossRef]
47. Katz, Y.; Stav, D.; Barr, J.; Passwell, J.H. IL-13 results in differential regulation of the complement proteins C3 and factor B in tumour necrosis factor (TNF)-stimulated fibroblasts. *Clin. Exp. Immunol.* **1995**, *101*, 150–156. [CrossRef]
48. Zhang, X.; Kohl, J. A complex role for complement in allergic asthma. *Expert Rev. Clin. Immunol.* **2010**, *6*, 269–277. [CrossRef]
49. Wills-Karp, M.; Koehl, J. New insights into the role of the complement pathway in allergy and asthma. *Curr. Allergy Asthma Rep.* **2005**, *5*, 362–369. [CrossRef] [PubMed]
50. Maruo, K.; Akaike, T.; Ono, T.; Okamoto, T.; Maeda, H. Generation of anaphylatoxins through proteolytic processing of C3 and C5 by house dust mite protease. *J. Allergy Clin. Immunol.* **1997**, *100*, 253–260. [CrossRef] [PubMed]
51. Ballow, M.; Donshik, P.C.; Mendelson, L. Complement proteins and C3 anaphylatoxin in the tears of patients with conjunctivitis. *J. Allergy Clin. Immunol.* **1985**, *76*, 473–476. [CrossRef]
52. Galli, S.J.; Tsai, M.; Piliponsky, A.M. The development of allergic inflammation. *Nature* **2008**, *454*, 445–454. [CrossRef]
53. Hirakata, T.; Lee, H.C.; Ohba, M.; Saeki, K.; Okuno, T.; Murakami, A.; Matsuda, A.; Yokomizo, T. Dietary omega-3 fatty acids alter the lipid mediator profile and alleviate allergic conjunctivitis without modulating T(h)2 immune responses. *FASEB J.* **2019**, *33*, 3392–3403. [CrossRef]
54. Luna-Gomes, T.; Bozza, P.T.; Bandeira-Melo, C. Eosinophil recruitment and activation: The role of lipid mediators. *Front. Pharmacol.* **2013**, *4*, 27. [CrossRef] [PubMed]

55. Kimani, G.; Tonnesen, M.G.; Henson, P.M. Stimulation of eosinophil adherence to human vascular endothelial cells in vitro by platelet-activating factor. *J. Immunol.* **1988**, *140*, 3161–3166. [CrossRef] [PubMed]
56. Little, M.M.; Casale, T.B. Comparison of platelet-activating factor-induced chemotaxis of normodense and hypodense eosinophils. *J. Allergy Clin. Immunol.* **1991**, *88*, 187–192. [CrossRef] [PubMed]
57. Monneret, G.; Cossette, C.; Gravel, S.; Rokach, J.; Powell, W.S. 15R-methyl-prostaglandin D2 is a potent and selective CRTH2/DP2 receptor agonist in human eosinophils. *J. Pharmacol. Exp. Ther.* **2003**, *304*, 349–355. [CrossRef]
58. Tager, A.M.; Dufour, J.H.; Goodarzi, K.; Bercury, S.D.; von Andrian, U.H.; Luster, A.D. BLTR mediates leukotriene B(4)-induced chemotaxis and adhesion and plays a dominant role in eosinophil accumulation in a murine model of peritonitis. *J. Exp. Med.* **2000**, *192*, 439–446. [CrossRef] [PubMed]
59. Patnode, M.L.; Bando, J.K.; Krummel, M.F.; Locksley, R.M.; Rosen, S.D. Leukotriene B4 amplifies eosinophil accumulation in response to nematodes. *J. Exp. Med.* **2014**, *211*, 1281–1288. [CrossRef]
60. Leonardi, A.; Secchi, A.G. Vernal keratoconjunctivitis. *Int. Ophthalmol. Clin.* **2003**, *43*, 41–58. [CrossRef]
61. Fujitsu, Y.; Fukuda, K.; Kimura, K.; Seki, K.; Kumagai, N.; Nishida, T. Protection of human conjunctival fibroblasts from NO-induced apoptosis by interleukin-4 or interleukin-13. *Investig. Ophthalmol. Vis. Sci.* **2005**, *46*, 797–802. [CrossRef]
62. McKenzie, G.J.; Fallon, P.G.; Emson, C.L.; Grencis, R.K.; McKenzie, A.N. Simultaneous disruption of interleukin (IL)-4 and IL-13 defines individual roles in T helper cell type 2-mediated responses. *J. Exp. Med.* **1999**, *189*, 1565–1572. [CrossRef] [PubMed]
63. Huang, H.; Li, Y.; Liu, B. Transcriptional regulation of mast cell and basophil lineage commitment. *Semin. Immunopathol.* **2016**, *38*, 539–548. [CrossRef]
64. Demoulin, J.B.; Renauld, J.C. Interleukin 9 and its receptor: An overview of structure and function. *Int. Rev. Immunol.* **1998**, *16*, 345–364. [CrossRef]
65. Temann, U.A.; Geba, G.P.; Rankin, J.A.; Flavell, R.A. Expression of interleukin 9 in the lungs of transgenic mice causes airway inflammation, mast cell hyperplasia, and bronchial hyperresponsiveness. *J. Exp. Med.* **1998**, *188*, 1307–1320. [CrossRef] [PubMed]
66. Gounni, A.S.; Gregory, B.; Nutku, E.; Aris, F.; Latifa, K.; Minshall, E.; North, J.; Tavernier, J.; Levit, R.; Nicolaides, N.; et al. Interleukin-9 enhances interleukin-5 receptor expression, differentiation, and survival of human eosinophils. *Blood* **2000**, *96*, 2163–2171. [CrossRef]
67. Solomon, A.; Shmilowich, R.; Shasha, D.; Frucht-Pery, J.; Pe'er, J.; Bonini, S.; Levi-Schaffer, F. Conjunctival fibroblasts enhance the survival and functional activity of peripheral blood eosinophils in vitro. *Investig. Ophthalmol. Vis. Sci.* **2000**, *41*, 1038–1044.
68. Peng, B.; Sun, L.; Zhang, M.; Yan, H.; Shi, G.; Xia, Z.; Dai, R.; Tang, W. Role of IL-25 on Eosinophils in the Initiation of Th2 Responses in Allergic Asthma. *Front. Immunol.* **2022**, *13*, 842500. [CrossRef]
69. Isgro, M.; Bianchetti, L.; Marini, M.A.; Bellini, A.; Schmidt, M.; Mattoli, S. The C-C motif chemokine ligands CCL5, CCL11, and CCL24 induce the migration of circulating fibrocytes from patients with severe asthma. *Mucosal Immunol.* **2013**, *6*, 718–727. [CrossRef]
70. Zhang, Y.; Guan, X.Y.; Jiang, P. Cytokine and Chemokine Signals of T-Cell Exclusion in Tumors. *Front. Immunol.* **2020**, *11*, 594609. [CrossRef]
71. Leonardi, A. Allergy and allergic mediators in tears. *Exp. Eye Res.* **2013**, *117*, 106–117. [CrossRef]
72. Bielory, L. Allergic and immunologic disorders of the eye. Part II: Ocular allergy. *J. Allergy Clin. Immunol.* **2000**, *106*, 1019–1032. [CrossRef] [PubMed]
73. Zhan, H.; Smith, L.; Calder, V.; Buckley, R.; Lightman, S. Clinical and immunological features of atopic keratoconjunctivitis. *Int. Ophthalmol. Clin.* **2003**, *43*, 59–71. [CrossRef] [PubMed]
74. Chigbu, D.I. Minhas, B.K. Immunopathology of allergic conjunctivitis. *Eur. Med. J.* **2018**, *3*, 76–83. [CrossRef]
75. Ohbayashi, M.; Manzouri, B.; Morohoshi, K.; Fukuda, K.; Ono, S.J. The Role of Histamine in Ocular Allergy. *Adv. Exp. Med. Biol.* **2010**, *709*, 43–52. [PubMed]
76. Nemmer, J.M.; Kuchner, M.; Datsi, A.; Olah, P.; Julia, V.; Raap, U.; Homey, B. Interleukin-31 Signaling Bridges the Gap between Immune Cells, the Nervous System and Epithelial Tissues. *Front. Med.* **2021**, *8*, 639097. [CrossRef] [PubMed]
77. Zhang, Q.; Putheti, P.; Zhou, Q.; Liu, Q.; Gao, W. Structures and biological functions of IL-31 and IL-31 receptors. *Cytokine Growth Factor Rev.* **2008**, *19*, 347–356. [CrossRef]
78. Oetjen, L.K.; Mack, M.R.; Feng, J.; Whelan, T.M.; Niu, H.; Guo, C.J.; Chen, S.; Trier, A.M.; Xu, A.Z.; Tripathi, S.V.; et al. Sensory Neurons Co-opt Classical Immune Signaling Pathways to Mediate Chronic Itch. *Cell* **2017**, *171*, 217–228.e13. [CrossRef]
79. Dantas, P.; Alves, M.; Nishiwaki-Dantas, M. Topographic corneal changes in patients with vernal keratoconjunctivitis. *Arq. Bras. Oftalmol.* **2005**, *68*, 593–598. [CrossRef]
80. Totan, Y.; Hepşen, I.; Cekiç, O.; Gündüz, A.; Aydin, E. Incidence of keratoconus in subjects with vernal keratoconjunctivitis: A videokeratographic study. *Ophthalmology* **2001**, *108*, 824–827. [CrossRef]
81. Zhang, X.; Huang, F.; Qiu, J.; Yang, Y.; Zhang, C. Corneal biomechanical properties in vernal keratoconjunctivitis and its subtypes: A preliminary study. *Int. Ophthalmol.* **2023**, *43*, 2083–2090. [CrossRef]
82. Ashina, K.; Tsubosaka, Y.; Nakamura, T.; Omori, K.; Kobayashi, K.; Hori, M.; Ozaki, H.; Murata, T. Histamine Induces Vascular Hyperpermeability by Increasing Blood Flow and Endothelial Barrier Disruption In Vivo. *PLoS ONE* **2015**, *10*, e0132367. [CrossRef]
83. Kugelmann, D.; Rotkopf, L.T.; Radeva, M.Y.; Garcia-Ponce, A.; Walter, E.; Waschke, J. Histamine causes endothelial barrier disruption via Ca^{2+}-mediated RhoA activation and tension at adherens junctions. *Sci. Rep.* **2018**, *8*, 13229. [CrossRef]

84. Smyth, E.M.; Grosser, T.; Wang, M.; Yu, Y.; FitzGerald, G.A. Prostanoids in health and disease. *J. Lipid Res.* **2009**, *50*, S423–S428. [CrossRef] [PubMed]
85. Gomez, I.; Foudi, N.; Longrois, D.; Norel, X. The role of prostaglandin E2 in human vascular inflammation. *Prostaglandins Leukot. Essent. Fat. Acids* **2013**, *89*, 55–63. [CrossRef]
86. Domingo, C.; Palomares, O.; Sandham, D.A.; Erpenbeck, V.J.; Altman, P. The prostaglandin D(2) receptor 2 pathway in asthma: A key player in airway inflammation. *Respir. Res.* **2018**, *19*, 189. [CrossRef] [PubMed]
87. Lee, K.; Lee, S.H.; Kim, T.H. The Biology of Prostaglandins and Their Role as a Target for Allergic Airway Disease Therapy. *Int. J. Mol. Sci.* **2020**, *21*, 1851. [CrossRef]
88. Kotowicz, K.; Callard, R.E.; Friedrich, K.; Matthews, D.J.; Klein, N. Biological activity of IL-4 and IL-13 on human endothelial cells: Functional evidence that both cytokines act through the same receptor. *Int. Immunol.* **1996**, *8*, 1915–1925. [CrossRef]
89. Skaria, T.; Burgener, J.; Bachli, E.; Schoedon, G. IL-4 Causes Hyperpermeability of Vascular Endothelial Cells through Wnt5A Signaling. *PLoS ONE* **2016**, *11*, e0156002. [CrossRef] [PubMed]
90. Tukler Henriksson, J.; Coursey, T.G.; Corry, D.B.; De Paiva, C.S.; Pflugfelder, S.C. IL-13 Stimulates Proliferation and Expression of Mucin and Immunomodulatory Genes in Cultured Conjunctival Goblet Cells. *Investig. Ophthalmol. Vis. Sci.* **2015**, *56*, 4186–4197. [CrossRef]
91. Pajulas, A.; Zhang, J.; Kaplan, M.H. The World according to IL-9. *J. Immunol.* **2023**, *211*, 7–14. [CrossRef]
92. Galicia-Carreon, J.; Santacruz, C.; Hong, E.; Jimenez-Martinez, M.C. The ocular surface: From physiology to the ocular allergic diseases. *Rev. Alerg. Mex.* **2013**, *60*, 172–183.
93. Kato, N.; Fukagawa, K.; Dogru, M.; Fujishima, H.; Tsubota, K. Mechanisms of giant papillary formation in vernal keratoconjunctivitis. *Cornea* **2006**, *25* (Suppl. S1), S47–S52. [CrossRef] [PubMed]
94. Fujitsu, Y.; Fukuda, K.; Kumagai, N.; Nishida, T. IL-4-induced cell proliferation and production of extracellular matrix proteins in human conjunctival fibroblasts. *Exp. Eye Res.* **2003**, *76*, 107–114. [CrossRef] [PubMed]
95. Stassen, M.; Schmitt, E.; Bopp, T. From interleukin-9 to T helper 9 cells. *Ann. N. Y. Acad. Sci.* **2012**, *1247*, 56–68. [CrossRef]
96. Soroosh, P.; Doherty, T.A. Th9 and allergic disease. *Immunology* **2009**, *127*, 450–458. [CrossRef] [PubMed]
97. Rao, S.; Padmanabhan, P. Perilimbal conjunctival pigmentation in vernal keratoconjunctivitis: A new sign. *Cornea* **2002**, *21*, 432. [CrossRef] [PubMed]
98. Rao, S.; Meenakshi, S.; Srinivasan, B.; Baluswamy, S. Perilimbal bulbar conjunctival pigmentation in vernal conjunctivitis: Prospective evaluation of a new clinical sign in an Indian population. *Cornea* **2004**, *23*, 356–359. [CrossRef] [PubMed]
99. Luk, F.; Wong, V.; Rao, S.; Lam, D. Perilimbal conjunctival pigmentation in Chinese patients with vernal keratoconjunctivitis. *Eye* **2008**, *22*, 1011–1014. [CrossRef] [PubMed]
100. Dubbaka, S.; Agrawal, M.; Sati, A.; Vats, S.; Mahajan, S. An observational study on the presence of perilimbal conjunctival pigmentation in vernal keratoconjunctivitis. *Indian J. Ophthalmol.* **2023**, *71*, 1816–1821. [CrossRef]
101. Leonardi, A.; Righetti, G.; Giovannini, G.; De Marchi, V.; Occhiuto, M. Diagnostic criteria of chronic conjunctivitis: Atopic keratoconjunctivitis and vernal keratoconjunctivitis. *Curr. Opin. Allergy Clin. Immunol.* **2023**, *23*, 390–396. [CrossRef]
102. Solomon, A. Corneal complications of vernal keratoconjunctivitis. *Curr. Opin. Allergy Clin. Immunol.* **2015**, *15*, 489–494. [CrossRef]
103. Wong, A.H.; Barg, S.S.; Leung, A.K. Seasonal and perennial allergic conjunctivitis. *Recent Pat. Inflamm. Allergy Drug Discov.* **2014**, *8*, 139–153. [CrossRef]
104. Chigbu, D.I. The management of allergic eye diseases in primary eye care. *Contact Lens Anterior Eye* **2009**, *32*, 260–272. [CrossRef]
105. Abbas, A.; Lichtman, A.; Pillai, S. Allergy. In *Cellular and Molecular Immunology*; Elsevier Saunders: Philadelphia, PA, USA, 2015; pp. 239–264.
106. Trocme, S.D.; Hallberg, C.K.; Gill, K.S.; Gleich, G.J.; Tyring, S.K.; Brysk, M.M. Effects of eosinophil granule proteins on human corneal epithelial cell viability and morphology. *Investig. Ophthalmol. Vis. Sci.* **1997**, *38*, 593–599.
107. Reddy, J.C.; Basu, S.; Saboo, U.S.; Murthy, S.I.; Vaddavalli, P.K.; Sangwan, V.S. Management, clinical outcomes, and complications of shield ulcers in vernal keratoconjunctivitis. *Am. J. Ophthalmol.* **2013**, *155*, 550–559.e1. [CrossRef] [PubMed]
108. Doan, S.; Papadopoulos, N.G.; Lee, J.K.; Leonardi, S.; Manti, S.; Lau, S.; Rondon, C.; Sharma, V.; Pleyer, U.; Jaumont, X.; et al. Vernal keratoconjunctivitis: Current immunological and clinical evidence and the potential role of omalizumab. *World Allergy Organ. J.* **2023**, *16*, 100788. [CrossRef]
109. Ali, A.; Bielory, L.; Dotchin, S.; Hamel, P.; Strube, Y.N.J.; Koo, E.B. Management of vernal keratoconjunctivitis: Navigating a changing treatment landscape. *Surv. Ophthalmol.* 2023, *in press*.
110. Leonardi, A. Management of vernal keratoconjunctivitis. *Ophthalmol. Ther.* **2013**, *2*, 73–88. [CrossRef]
111. Gokhale, N.S. Systematic approach to managing vernal keratoconjunctivitis in clinical practice: Severity grading system and a treatment algorithm. *Indian J. Ophthalmol.* **2016**, *64*, 145–148. [CrossRef] [PubMed]
112. Mehta, J.S.; Chen, W.L.; Cheng, A.C.K.; Cung, L.X.; Dualan, I.J.; Kekunnaya, R.; Khaliddin, N.; Kim, T.I.; Lam, D.K.; Leo, S.W.; et al. Diagnosis, Management, and Treatment of Vernal Keratoconjunctivitis in Asia: Recommendations from the Management of Vernal Keratoconjunctivitis in Asia Expert Working Group. *Front. Med.* **2022**, *9*, 882240. [CrossRef]
113. Andoh, T.; Kuraishi, Y. Lipid Mediators and Itch. In *Itch: Mechanisms and Treatment*; Carstens, E., Akiyama, T., Eds.; CRC Press: Boca Raton, FL, USA, 2014.

114. Dahlmann-Noor, A.; Bonini, S.; Bremond-Gignac, D.; Heegaard, S.; Leonardi, A.; Montero, J.; Silva, E.D.; Group, E.-V. Novel Insights in the Management of Vernal Keratoconjunctivitis (VKC): European Expert Consensus Using a Modified Nominal Group Technique. *Ophthalmol. Ther.* **2023**, *12*, 1207–1222. [CrossRef]
115. Maharana, P.K.; Singhal, D.; Raj, N.; Sharma, N.; Titiyal, J.S. Role of combined immunomodulator therapy in severe steroid intolerant vernal keratoconjunctivitis. *Eye* **2021**, *35*, 979–987. [CrossRef] [PubMed]
116. Chatterjee, A.; Bandyopadhyay, S.; Kumar Bandyopadhyay, S. Efficacy, Safety and Steroid-sparing Effect of Topical Cyclosporine A 0.05% for Vernal Keratoconjunctivitis in Indian Children. *J. Ophthalmic Vis. Res.* **2019**, *14*, 412–418. [CrossRef]
117. Roy, J.; Cyert, M.S. Identifying New Substrates and Functions for an Old Enzyme: Calcineurin. *Cold Spring Harb. Perspect. Biol.* **2020**, *12*, a035436. [CrossRef] [PubMed]
118. Abbas, A.K.; Licthman, A.H.; Pillai, S. Immune Receptors and Signal Transduction. In *Cellular and Molecular Immunology*; Elsevier Saunders: Philadelphia, PA, USA, 2017; pp. 145–178.
119. Murphy, K.; Weaver, C. Manipulation of the Immune Response. In *Janeway's Immunobiology*; Garland Science: New York, NY, USA, 2017; pp. 701–748.
120. Gutfreund, K.; Bienias, W.; Szewczyk, A.; Kaszuba, A. Topical calcineurin inhibitors in dermatology. Part I: Properties, method and effectiveness of drug use. *Postepy Dermatol. Alergol.* **2013**, *30*, 165–169. [CrossRef]
121. Murphy, K.P.; Weaver, C. Allergy and Allergic Diseases. In *Janeway's Immunobiology*; Garland Science: New York, NY, USA, 2017; pp. 601–641.
122. Oray, M.; Toker, E. Tear cytokine levels in vernal keratoconjunctivitis: The effect of topical 0.05% cyclosporine a therapy. *Cornea* **2013**, *32*, 1149–1154. [CrossRef]
123. Subedi, K.; Sharma, B.; Shrestha, S. Efficacy of Topical Cyclosporine 0.05% the Treatment of Vernal Keratoconjunctivitis. *Nepal. J. Ophthalmol.* **2020**, *12*, 39–47. [CrossRef]
124. Bourcier, T.; Dory, A.; Dormegny, L.; Alcazar, J.; Gaucher, D.; Sauer, A. Efficacy and Safety of 0.1% Cyclosporine versus 2% Cyclosporine in the Treatment of Severe Vernal Keratoconjunctivitis in Children. *Clin. Ophthalmol.* **2022**, *16*, 3589–3596. [CrossRef] [PubMed]
125. Giannaccare, G.; Rossi, C.; Borselli, M.; Bonzano, C.; Carnovale Scalzo, G.; Nicolo, M.; Scorcia, V.; Traverso, C.E.; Vagge, A. Clinical Outcomes of Topical 0.1% Ciclosporin Cationic Emulsion Used on Label in Children with Vernal Keratoconjunctivitis. *Ophthalmol. Ther.* **2023**, *12*, 1787–1793. [CrossRef]
126. Gupta, V.; Sahu, P. Topical cyclosporin A in the management of vernal keratoconjunctivitis. *Eye* **2001**, *15 Pt 1*, 39–41. [CrossRef]
127. Leonardi, A.; Doan, S.; Amrane, M.; Ismail, D.; Montero, J.; Nemeth, J.; Aragona, P.; Bremond-Gignac, D.; Group, V.S. A Randomized, Controlled Trial of Cyclosporine A Cationic Emulsion in Pediatric Vernal Keratoconjunctivitis: The VEKTIS Study. *Ophthalmology* **2019**, *126*, 671–681. [CrossRef]
128. Bremond-Gignac, D.; Doan, S.; Amrane, M.; Ismail, D.; Montero, J.; Nemeth, J.; Aragona, P.; Leonardi, A.; Group, V.S. Twelve-Month Results of Cyclosporine A Cationic Emulsion in a Randomized Study in Patients With Pediatric Vernal Keratoconjunctivitis. *Am. J. Ophthalmol.* **2020**, *212*, 116–126. [CrossRef]
129. Leonardi, A.; Doan, S.; Aragona, P.; Amrane, M.; Ismail, D.; Montero, J.; Nemeth, J.; Bremond-Gignac, D. Topical cyclosporine A cationic ophthalmic emulsion in paediatric vernal keratoconjunctivitis: Pooled analysis of randomised NOVATIVE and VEKTIS trials. *Eye* **2023**, *37*, 2320–2326. [CrossRef]
130. Leonardi, A.; Pisella, P.J.; Benitez-Del-Castillo, J.M.; Amrane, M.; Ismail, D.; Doan, S.; Bremond-Gignac, D. NOVATIVE: A Phase II/III, Multicenter, Double-masked, Randomized Study of Cyclosporine A 0.05% and 0.1% Ophthalmic Cationic Emulsion Versus Vehicle in Patients with Vernal Keratoconjunctivitis. *Clin. Ther.* **2023**, *45*, 1284–1288. [CrossRef]
131. Ozkaya, D.; Usta, G.; Karaca, U. A Case of Shield Ulcer Due to Vernal Keratoconjunctivitis. *Iran. J. Allergy Asthma Immunol.* **2021**, *20*, 505–508.
132. Westland, T.; Patryn, E.K.; Nieuwendaal, C.P.; van der Meulen, I.J.E.; Mourits, M.P.; Lapid-Gortzak, R. Vernal shield ulcers treated with frequently installed topical cyclosporine 0.05% eyedrops. *Int. Ophthalmol.* **2018**, *38*, 363–368. [CrossRef]
133. Hirota, A.; Shoji, J.; Inada, N.; Shiraki, Y.; Yamagami, S. Evaluation of Clinical Efficacy and Safety of Prolonged Treatment of Vernal and Atopic Keratoconjunctivitis Using Topical Tacrolimus. *Cornea* **2022**, *41*, 23–30. [CrossRef]
134. Eltagoury, M.; Abou Samra, W.; Ghoneim, E. Safety and efficacy of topical tacrolimus 0.03% in the management of vernal keratoconjunctivitis: A non-randomized controlled clinical trial. *Med. Hypothesis Discov. Innov. Ophthalmol.* **2022**, *11*, 52–63. [CrossRef]
135. Armstrong, V.W.; Oellerich, M. New developments in the immunosuppressive drug monitoring of cyclosporine, tacrolimus, and azathioprine. *Clin. Biochem.* **2001**, *34*, 9–16. [CrossRef] [PubMed]
136. Pucci, N.; Caputo, R.; di Grande, L.; de Libero, C.; Mori, F.; Barni, S.; di Simone, L.; Calvani, A.; Rusconi, F.; Novembre, E. Tacrolimus vs. cyclosporine eyedrops in severe cyclosporine-resistant vernal keratoconjunctivitis: A randomized, comparative, double-blind, crossover study. *Pediatr. Allergy Immunol.* **2015**, *26*, 256–261. [CrossRef] [PubMed]
137. Saha, B.C.; Kumari, R.; Ambasta, A. Comparision of efficacy and safety of 0.03% and 0.1% tacrolimus ointment in children with vernal keratoconjunctivitis. *Ther. Adv. Ophthalmol.* **2023**, *15*, 25158414231173532. [CrossRef] [PubMed]
138. Caputo, R.; Marziali, E.; de Libero, C.; Di Grande, L.; Danti, G.; Virgili, G.; Villani, E.; Mori, F.; Bacci, G.M.; Lucenteforte, E.; et al. Long-Term Safety and Efficacy of Tacrolimus 0.1% in Severe Pediatric Vernal Keratoconjunctivitis. *Cornea* **2021**, *40*, 1395–1401. [CrossRef]

139. Fiorentini, S.F.; Khurram, D. Therapeutic effects of topical 0.03% Tacrolimus ointment in children with refractory vernal keratoconjunctivitis in Middle East. *Saudi J. Ophthalmol.* **2019**, *33*, 117–120. [CrossRef]
140. Barot, R.K.; Shitole, S.C.; Bhagat, N.; Patil, D.; Sawant, P.; Patil, K. Therapeutic effect of 0.1% Tacrolimus Eye Ointment in Allergic Ocular Diseases. *J. Clin. Diagn Res.* **2016**, *10*, NC05-9. [CrossRef]
141. Kheirkhah, A.; Zavareh, M.K.; Farzbod, F.; Mahbod, M.; Behrouz, M.J. Topical 0.005% tacrolimus eye drop for refractory vernal keratoconjunctivitis. *Eye* **2011**, *25*, 872–880. [CrossRef]
142. Fukushima, A.; Ohashi, Y.; Ebihara, N.; Uchio, E.; Okamoto, S.; Kumagai, N.; Shoji, J.; Takamura, E.; Nakagawa, Y.; Namba, K.; et al. Therapeutic effects of 0.1% tacrolimus eye drops for refractory allergic ocular diseases with proliferative lesion or corneal involvement. *Br. J. Ophthalmol.* **2014**, *98*, 1023–1027. [CrossRef]
143. Bardoloi, P.; Vanathi, M.; Velpandian, T.; Laxmi, M.; Gupta, N.; Lomi, N.; Tandon, R. Tear Tacrolimus Levels and Clinical Response after Adjunct Therapy with Cutaneous Application of Tacrolimus 0.1% over Upper Eyelid Skin in Chronic Vernal Keratoconjunctivitis. *Cornea* 2023; *in press*.
144. Heikal, M.A.; Soliman, T.T.; Abousaif, W.S.; Shebl, A.A. A comparative study between ciclosporine A eye drop (2%) and tacrolimus eye ointment (0.03%) in management of children with refractory vernal keratoconjunctivitis. *Graefes Arch. Clin. Exp. Ophthalmol.* **2022**, *260*, 353–361. [CrossRef]
145. Labcharoenwongs, P.; Jirapongsananuruk, O.; Visitsunthorn, N.; Kosrirukvongs, P.; Saengin, P.; Vichyanond, P. A double-masked comparison of 0.1% tacrolimus ointment and 2% cyclosporine eye drops in the treatment of vernal keratoconjunctivitis in children. *Asian Pac. J. Allergy Immunol.* **2012**, *30*, 177–184. [PubMed]
146. Arnon, R.; Rozen-Knisbacher, I.; Yahalomi, T.; Stanescu, N.; Niazov, Y.; Goldberg, D.; Sharabi-Nov, A.; Mostovoy, D. When to start tacrolimus ointment for vernal keratoconjunctivitis? A proposed treatment protocol. *Int. Ophthalmol.* **2022**, *42*, 1771–1780. [CrossRef]
147. Al-Amri, A.M. Long-term follow-up of tacrolimus ointment for treatment of atopic keratoconjunctivitis. *Am. J. Ophthalmol.* **2014**, *157*, 280–286. [CrossRef] [PubMed]
148. Tzu, J.H.; Utine, C.A.; Stern, M.E.; Akpek, E.K. Topical calcineurin inhibitors in the treatment of steroid-dependent atopic keratoconjunctivitis. *Cornea* **2012**, *31*, 649–654. [CrossRef] [PubMed]
149. Takamura, E.; Uchio, E.; Ebihara, N.; Ohno, S.; Ohashi, Y.; Okamoto, S.; Kumagai, N.; Satake, Y.; Shoji, J.; Nakagawa, Y.; et al. Japanese guidelines for allergic conjunctival diseases 2017. *Allergol. Int.* **2017**, *66*, 220–229. [CrossRef] [PubMed]
150. Cox, L. Biologics and Allergy Immunotherapy in the Treatment of Allergic Diseases. *Immunol. Allergy Clin. N. Am.* **2020**, *40*, 687–700. [CrossRef] [PubMed]
151. Fukuda, K.; Kishimoto, T.; Sumi, T.; Yamashiro, K.; Ebihara, N. Biologics for allergy: Therapeutic potential for ocular allergic diseases and adverse effects on the eye. *Allergol. Int.* **2023**, *72*, 234–244. [CrossRef] [PubMed]

MDPI AG
Grosspeteranlage 5
4052 Basel
Switzerland
Tel.: +41 61 683 77 34

Life Editorial Office
E-mail: life@mdpi.com
www.mdpi.com/journal/life

www.ingramcontent.com/pod-product-compliance
Lightning Source LLC
LaVergne TN
LVHW070448061126
851858LV00011B/184
9783725884070